# Pituitary Surgery

*Editors*

JEAN ANDERSON ELOY
CHRISTINA H. FANG
VIJAY AGARWAL

# OTOLARYNGOLOGIC CLINICS OF NORTH AMERICA

www.oto.theclinics.com

*Consulting Editor*
SUJANA S. CHANDRASEKHAR

April 2022 • Volume 55 • Number 2

**ELSEVIER**

1600 John F. Kennedy Boulevard • Suite 1800 • Philadelphia, Pennsylvania, 19103-2899

http://www.oto.theclinics.com

**OTOLARYNGOLOGIC CLINICS OF NORTH AMERICA Volume 55, Number 2**
**April 2022 ISSN 0030-6665, ISBN-13: 978-0-323-91977-7**

Editor: Stacy Eastman
Developmental Editor: Diana Grace Ang

*Otolaryngologic Clinics of North America* (ISSN 0030-6665) is published bimonthly by Elsevier, Inc., 360 Park Avenue South, New York, NY 10010-1710. Months of issue are February, April, June, August, October, and December. Business and Editorial Offices: 1600 John F. Kennedy Blvd., Suite 1800, Philadelphia, PA 19103-2899. Customer Service Office: 6277 Sea Harbor Drive, Orlando, FL 32887-4800. Periodicals postage paid at New York, NY and additional mailing offices. Subscription prices are $450.00 per year (US individuals), $1336.00 per year (US institutions), $100.00 per year (US & Canadian student/resident), $576.00 per year (Canadian individuals), $1396.00 per year (Canadian institutions), $628.00 per year (international individuals), $1396.00 per year (international institutions), $270.00 per year (international student/resident). Foreign air speed delivery is included in all *Clinics'* subscription prices. All prices are subject to change without notice. **POSTMASTER:** Send address changes to *Otolaryngologic Clinics of North America,* Elsevier Health Sciences Division, Subscription Customer Service, 3251 Riverport Lane, Maryland Heights, MO 63043. **Telephone: 1-800-654-2452 (U.S. and Canada); 314-447-8871 (outside U.S. and Canada). Fax: 314-447-8029. E-mail: journalscustomerservice-usa@elsevier.com (for print support); journalsonlinesupport-usa@elsevier.com (for online support).**

*Reprints.* For copies of 100 or more of articles in this publication, please contact the Commercial Reprints Department, Elsevier Inc., 360 Park Avenue South, New York, NY 10010-1710. Tel.: 212-633-3874; Fax: 212-633-3820; E-mail: reprints@elsevier.com.

*Otolaryngologic Clinics of North America* is also published in Spanish by McGraw-Hill Interamericana Editores S.A., P.O. Box 5-237, 06500 Mexico D.F., Mexico.

*Otolaryngologic Clinics of North America* is covered in *MEDLINE/PubMed (Index Medicus), Current Contents/Clinical Medicine, Excerpta Medica, BIOSIS, Science Citation Index,* and *ISI/BIOMED.*

# Contributors

## CONSULTING EDITOR

**SUJANA S. CHANDRASEKHAR, MD, FACS, FAAOHNS**
Past President, American Academy of Otolaryngology–Head and Neck Surgery,
Secretary-Treasurer, American Otological Society, Partner, ENT & Allergy Associates,
LLP, Clinical Professor, Department of Otolaryngology–Head and Neck Surgery,
Donald and Barbara Zucker School of Medicine at Hofstra-Northwell, Hempstead,
New York; Clinical Associate Professor, Department of Otolaryngology–Head and
Neck Surgery, Icahn School of Medicine at Mount Sinai, New York,
New York

## EDITORS

**JEAN ANDERSON ELOY, MD, FARS, FACS**
Department of Otolaryngology–Head and Neck Surgery, Department of Neurological
Surgery, Center for Skull Base and Pituitary Surgery, Professor and Vice Chairman,
Director, Rhinology and Sinus Surgery, Director, Otolaryngology Research, Co-Director,
Endoscopic Skull Base Surgery Program, Professor of Neurological Surgery, Professor of
Ophthalmology and Visual Science, Neurological Institute of New Jersey, Department of
Ophthalmology and Visual Science, Rutgers New Jersey Medical School, Newark,
New Jersey; Chairman and Chief of Service, Department of Otolaryngology and Facial
Plastic Surgery, Saint Barnabas Medical Center - RWJBarnabas Health, Livingston,
New Jersey

**CHRISTINA H. FANG, MD**
Assistant Professor, Department of Otorhinolaryngology–Head and Neck Surgery,
Montefiore Medical Center, The University Hospital for the Albert Einstein College of
Medicine, Bronx, New York

**VIJAY AGARWAL, MD**
Department of Neurological Surgery, Chief, Division of Skull Base and Minimally
Invasive Neurosurgery, Assistant Director, Residency Training Program, Associate
Professor, Leo M. Davidoff Department of Neurological Surgery, Associate Professor,
Department of Otorhinolaryngology–Head and Neck Surgery, Montefiore Medical
Center, The University Hospital for the Albert Einstein College of Medicine, Bronx,
New York

## AUTHORS

**NITHIN D. ADAPPA, MD**
Division of Neurosurgery, Children's Hospital of Philadelphia, Department of
Otorhinolaryngology and Head and Neck Surgery, Perelman School of Medicine at the
University of Pennsylvania, Philadelphia, Pennsylvania

**VIJAY AGARWAL, MD**
Department of Neurological Surgery, Chief, Division of Skull Base and Minimally Invasive Neurosurgery, Assistant Director, Residency Training Program, Associate Professor, Leo M. Davidoff Department of Neurological Surgery, Associate Professor, Department of Otorhinolaryngology–Head and Neck Surgery, Montefiore Medical Center, The University Hospital for the Albert Einstein College of Medicine, Bronx, New York

**PANKAJ K. AGARWALLA, MD**
Department of Neurosurgery, Rutgers New Jersey Medical School, Assistant Professor of Neurosurgery, Newark, New Jersey

**NADEEM AKBAR, MD**
Department of Otolaryngology, Albert Einstein College of Medicine, Bronx, New York

**CASSIDY ANDERSON, BS**
Albert Einstein College of Medicine, Bronx, New York

**MARK A. ARNOLD, MD**
Department of Otolaryngology–Head and Neck Surgery, Emory University School of Medicine, Atlanta, Georgia

**ADA BAISRE De LEÓN, MD**
Associate Professor, Department of Pathology, Immunology and Laboratory Medicine, Rutgers New Jersey Medical School, Newark, New Jersey

**ANDREW B. BOUCHER, MD**
Department of Neurosurgery, Emory University School of Medicine, Atlanta, Georgia

**DAVID P. BRAY, MD**
Department of Neurosurgery, Emory University School of Medicine, Atlanta, Georgia

**BENJAMIN P. BROWNLEE, MD**
Department of Otolaryngology–Head and Neck Surgery, University of Oklahoma Health Sciences Center, Oklahoma City, Oklahoma

**RICARDO CARRAU, MD**
Department of Neurological Surgery, Department of Otolaryngology–Head and Neck Surgery, The Ohio State University Wexner Medical Center, Columbus, Ohio

**PATRICK COLLEY, MD**
Department of Otolaryngology, Albert Einstein College of Medicine, Bronx, New York

**WILLIAM T. COULDWELL, MD, PhD**
Professor and Chair, Department of Neurosurgery, University of Utah, Salt Lake City, Utah

**JOHN R. CRAIG, MD**
Department of Otolaryngology–Head and Neck Surgery, Henry Ford Hospital, Detroit, Michigan

**REEM A. DAWOUD, BS**
Emory University School of Medicine, Atlanta, Georgia

**JEAN ANDERSON ELOY, MD, FARS, FACS**
Department of Otolaryngology–Head and Neck Surgery, Department of Neurological Surgery, Center for Skull Base and Pituitary Surgery, Professor and Vice Chairman, Director, Rhinology and Sinus Surgery, Director, Otolaryngology Research, Co-Director, Endoscopic Skull Base Surgery Program, Professor of Neurological Surgery, Professor of

Ophthalmology and Visual Science, Neurological Institute of New Jersey, Department of Ophthalmology and Visual Science, Rutgers New Jersey Medical School, Newark, New Jersey; Chairman and Chief of Service, Department of Otolaryngology and Facial Plastic Surgery, Saint Barnabas Medical Center - RWJBarnabas Health, Livingston, New Jersey

**CHIKEZIE I. ESEONU, MD, FAANS**
Neurosurgeon, Neurosurgery and Neuroscience Institute, University of Pittsburgh Medical Center, Central Pennsylvania, Harrisburg, Pennsylvania

**TIMOTHY FAN, BS**
Department of Otolaryngology–Head and Neck Surgery, Harvard Medical School, Department of Otolaryngology–Head and Neck Surgery, Massachusetts Eye and Ear Infirmary, Boston, Massachusetts

**CHRISTINA H. FANG, MD**
Assistant Professor, Department of Otorhinolaryngology–Head and Neck Surgery, Montefiore Medical Center, The University Hospital for the Albert Einstein College of Medicine, Bronx, New York

**JUAN C. FERNÁNDEZ-MIRANDA, MD**
Departments of Neurosurgery and Otolaryngology–Head and Neck Surgery, Stanford University School of Medicine, Palo Alto, California

**VANCE L. FREDRICKSON, MD**
Fellow, Department of Neurosurgery, University of Utah, Salt Lake City, Utah

**PAUL A. GARDNER, MD**
Department of Neurological Surgery, University of Pittsburgh School of Medicine, Pittsburgh, Pennsylvania

**ALEXANDRA M. GIANTINI-LARSEN, MD**
Department of Neurological Surgery, Weill Cornell Medical College, Resident, Department of Neurosurgery, NewYork-Presbyterian Hospital, New York, New York

**CHAD GLENN, MD**
Assistant Professor, Department of Neurological Surgery, University of Oklahoma Health Sciences Center, Oklahoma City, Oklahoma

**SANIYA GODIL, MD**
Department of Neurological Surgery, The Ohio State University Wexner Medical Center, Columbus, Ohio

**STACEY T. GRAY, MD**
Department of Otolaryngology–Head and Neck Surgery, Harvard Medical School, Department of Otolaryngology–Head and Neck Surgery, Massachusetts Eye and Ear Infirmary, Boston, Massachusetts

**SAMEAH A. HAIDER, MD, MBA**
Department of Neurological Surgery, Hermelin Brain Tumor Center, Henry Ford Hospital, Detroit, Michigan

**WAYNE D. HSUEH, MD**
Department of Otolaryngology–Head and Neck Surgery, Department of Neurological Surgery, Rutgers New Jersey Medical School, Newark, New Jersey

**ERION JUNIOR DeANDRADE, MD**
Department of Neurological Surgery, Cleveland Clinic Lerner College of Medicine of Case Western Reserve University, Section of Skull Base Surgery, Rose Ella Burkhardt Brain Tumor and Neuro-Oncology Center, Neurological Institute, Cleveland Clinic, Cleveland, Ohio

**RUPA GOPALAN JUTHANI, MD**
Assistant Professor, Department of Neurological Surgery, Weill Cornell Medicine, New York, New York

**JINU KIM, MD**
Department of Anesthesia, Assistant Clinical Professor, Albert Einstein College of Medicine, Bronx, New York

**DANIEL KREATSOULAS, MD**
Department of Neurological Surgery, The Ohio State University Wexner Medical Center, Columbus, Ohio

**VARUN R. KSHETTRY, MD**
Department of Neurological Surgery, Cleveland Clinic Lerner College of Medicine of Case Western Reserve University, Section of Skull Base Surgery, Rose Ella Burkhardt Brain Tumor and Neuro-Oncology Center, Neurological Institute, Cleveland Clinic, Cleveland, Ohio

**SHIH-SHAN LANG, MD**
Division of Neurosurgery, Children's Hospital of Philadelphia, Department of Neurosurgery, Perelman School of Medicine at the University of Pennsylvania, Philadelphia, Pennsylvania

**STELLA E. LEE, MD**
Division of Otolaryngology–Head and Neck Surgery, Brigham and Women's Hospital, Harvard Medical School, Boston, Massachusetts

**SHIRI LEVY, MD**
Division of Endocrinology, Diabetes, and Bone and Mineral Disorder, Henry Ford Hospital, Detroit, Michigan

**JAMES K. LIU, MD, FACS, FAANS**
Department of Otolaryngology–Head and Neck Surgery, Department of Neurological Surgery, Center for Skull Base and Pituitary Surgery, Professor of Neurological Surgery, Director, Cerebrovascular/Skull Base and Pituitary Surgery, Co-Director, Endoscopic Skull Base Surgery Program, Director, Surgical Neuro-Oncology and Brain Tumor Center, Departments of Neurological Surgery and Otolaryngology–Head and Neck Surgery, Rutgers Neurological Institute of New Jersey, Rutgers New Jersey Medical School, RWJBarnabas Health, Newark, New Jersey; Saint Barnabas Medical Center, RWJ Barnabas Health, Livingston, New Jersey

**CHRISTOPHER M. LOW, MD**
Department of Otolaryngology–Head and Neck Surgery, Mayo Clinic, Rochester, Minnesota

**PETER J. MADSEN, MD**
Division of Neurosurgery, Children's Hospital of Philadelphia, Philadelphia, Pennsylvania

**DALJIT MANN, MD**
Department of Otolaryngology–Head and Neck Surgery, University of Oklahoma Health Sciences Center, Oklahoma City, Oklahoma

**ERIN L. McKEAN, MD, MBA**
Associate Professor of Otolaryngology–Head and Neck Surgery and Neurosurgery, University of Michigan, Department of Otolaryngology, Ann Arbor, Michigan

**KIBWEI A. McKINNEY, MD**
Assistant Professor, Department of Otolaryngology–Head and Neck Surgery, University of Oklahoma Health Sciences Center, Oklahoma City, Oklahoma

**ESTHER NIMCHINSKY, MD, PhD**
Chief, Division of Neuroradiology, Assistant Professor, Department of Radiology, Rutgers New Jersey Medical School, Newark, New Jersey

**MAXIMILIANO NUNEZ, MD**
Department of Neurosurgery, Stanford University School of Medicine, Palo Alto, California

**BRADLEY OTTO, MD**
Department of Otolaryngology–Head and Neck Surgery, The Ohio State University Wexner Medical Center, Columbus, Ohio

**NELSON M. OYESIKU, MD, PhD, FACS**
Department of Neurosurgery, Semmes Murphy Clinic, Memphis, Tennessee; Department of Neurosurgery, University of North Carolina School of Medicine, Chapel Hill, North Carolina

**JAMES N. PALMER, MD**
Division of Neurosurgery, Children's Hospital of Philadelphia, Department of Otorhinolaryngology and Head and Neck Surgery, Perelman School of Medicine at the University of Pennsylvania, Philadelphia, Pennsylvania

**ZARA M. PATEL, MD**
Departments of Neurosurgery and Otolaryngology–Head and Neck Surgery, Stanford University School of Medicine, Palo Alto, California

**GUSTAVO PRADILLA, MD**
Department of Neurosurgery, Emory University School of Medicine, Atlanta, Georgia

**DANIEL PREVEDELLO, MD**
Department of Neurological Surgery, Department of Otolaryngology–Head and Neck Surgery, The Ohio State University Wexner Medical Center, Columbus, Ohio

**PABLO F. RECINOS, MD**
Department of Neurological Surgery, Section of Skull Base Surgery, Co-Director, Minimally Invasive Cranial Base and Pituitary Surgery Program, Rose Ella Burkhardt Brain Tumor and Neuro-Oncology Center, Neurological Institute, Section of Rhinology, Sinus, and Skull Base Surgery, Head and Neck Institute, Cleveland Clinic, Section Head, Skull Base Surgery, Associate Professor of Neurological Surgery and Otolaryngology–Head and Neck Surgery, Cleveland Clinic Lerner College of Medicine of Case Western Reserve University, Cleveland, Ohio

**ROBERT C. RENNERT, MD**
Fellow, Department of Neurosurgery, University of Utah, Salt Lake City, Utah

**JUAN MANUEL REVUELTA BARBERO, MD**
Department of Neurosurgery, Emory University School of Medicine, Atlanta, Georgia

**RIMA S. RINDLER, MD**
Department of Neurosurgery, Emory University School of Medicine, Atlanta, Georgia

**JACK P. ROCK, MD**
Department of Neurological Surgery, Hermelin Brain Tumor Center, Henry Ford Hospital, Detroit, Michigan

**ROSS SCOTT-MILLER, MD**
Department of Anesthesia, Anesthesia Resident, Montefiore Medical Center, Bronx, New York

**RAJ SINDWANI, MD**
Department of Neurological Surgery, Cleveland Clinic Lerner College of Medicine of Case Western Reserve University, Section of Skull Base Surgery, Rose Ella Burkhardt Brain Tumor and Neuro-Oncology Center, Neurological Institute, Cleveland Clinic, Section of Rhinology, Sinus, and Skull Base Surgery, Head and Neck Institute, Cleveland Clinic, Cleveland, Ohio

**CARL H. SNYDERMAN, MD**
Department of Otolaryngology–Head and Neck Surgery, University of Pittsburgh School of Medicine, Pittsburgh, Pennsylvania

**PHILLIP B. STORM, MD**
Division of Neurosurgery, Children's Hospital of Philadelphia, Department of Neurosurgery, Perelman School of Medicine at the University of Pennsylvania, Philadelphia, Pennsylvania

**NISHA SUDA, MD, MHA**
Assistant Professor, Department of Medicine, Endocrinology and Metabolism, Montefiore Medical Center, Albert Einstein College of Medicine, Bronx, New York

**STEPHEN E. SULLIVAN, MD**
Associate Professor of Neurosurgery and Otolaryngology, University of Michigan, Department of Neurosurgery, Ann Arbor, Michigan

**OLIVER Y. TANG, BS**
Department of Neurosurgery, Warren Alpert Medical School of Brown University, Providence, Rhode Island

**RAFAEL URIBE-CARDENAS, MD, MHS**
Department of Neurological Surgery, Weill Cornell Medical College, Resident, Department of Neurosurgery, NewYork-Presbyterian Hospital, New York, New York

**JOSHUA VIGNOLLES-JEONG, BA**
The Ohio State University College of Medicine, Columbus, Ohio

**VERA VIGO, MD**
Department of Neurosurgery, Stanford University School of Medicine, Palo Alto, California

**ALEXANDRA WHITE, MA**
Department of Neurological Surgery, Cleveland Clinic Lerner College of Medicine of Case Western Reserve University, Cleveland, Ohio

**SARAH K. WISE, MD**
Department of Otolaryngology–Head and Neck Surgery, Emory University School of Medicine, Atlanta, Georgia

**ALAN D. WORKMAN, MD, MTR**
Department of Otolaryngology–Head and Neck Surgery, Harvard Medical School,
Department of Otolaryngology–Head and Neck Surgery, Massachusetts Eye and Ear
Infirmary, Boston, Massachusetts

**KEVIN ZHAO, DO**
Department of Neurosurgery, Rutgers New Jersey Medical School, Newark,
New Jersey

# Contents

Management of patients with pituitary lesions is complex given the deli-
cate nature of the surrounding anatomy and complexity of underlying disease. The care of these patients ideally involves a multidisciplinary team
composed of endocrinologists, neuroradiologists, otolaryngologists,
neurosurgeons, critical care physicians, and anesthesiologists. The endoscopic endonasal approach to the skull base has revolutionized pituitary
and anterior skull base surgery and has gained popularity worldwide.
This article presents an overview of the diagnosis, work-up, and management of patients with pituitary lesions, with an emphasis on surgical,
perioperative, and postoperative considerations.

The pituitary gland is a small gland at the base of the skull controlling many
physiologic processes through its regulation of primary endocrine glands.
Pathologies of the pituitary gland and sellar space are wide ranging and
most commonly include pituitary adenomas but can also encompass pituitary hyperplasia, other benign nonadenomatous tumors, cysts, and
primary and metastatic malignancy. At present, the endoscopic approach
has been established as a safe and effective approach to surgical management of pituitary pathology. A detailed understanding of the sella and parasellar anatomy from an endoscopic approach is imperative to performing
safe endoscopic surgery in this area.

The pituitary gland plays a vital role in hormonal regulation. Pituitary lesions include tumors, cysts, and inflammatory processes that require
multidisciplinary care from endocrinologists, neuro-ophthalmologists,
neurosurgeons, and otolaryngologists. Treatment is typically aimed at
controlling hormonal hypersecretion, decompressing the optic apparatus, and reducing tumor volume, and surgery is a common first-line
approach. In this article, we provide a background on the function of

diagnosis. Cushing disease presents with characteristic clinical signs and symptoms associated with excess cortisol, but diagnosis is difficult and often relies on repeated and varied endocrinologic assays and neuroradiologic investigations. Gold standard treatment is surgical resection of adrenocorticotropic hormone–secreting pituitary adenoma, which is curative. Patients require close endocrinologic follow-up for maintenance of associated neuroendocrine deficiencies and surveillance for potential recurrence. Medications, radiation therapy, and bilateral adrenalectomy are alternative treatments for residual or recurrent disease.

Acromegaly results from excessive secretion of insulinlike growth factor-1 and growth hormone, which most commonly occurs because of pituitary somatotrophinoma. Diagnostic features of acromegaly include elevated insulinlike growth factor-1 and growth hormone; lesion on brain MRI; and clinically dysmorphic features, such as soft tissue swelling, jaw prognathism, and acral overgrowth. Transsphenoidal resection is the primary therapy for individuals with acromegaly, even in the cases where gross total resection is not possible because of parasellar extension and cavernous sinus involvement. For recurrent or persistent disease after resection, systemic medications and stereotactic radiosurgery are used.

Nonfunctioning pituitary lesions represent a subset of pituitary adenomas that do not manifest with clinical features of hormone hypersecretion. Because of their indolent nature, their diagnosis is elusive, often resulting in presentation after the tumors have grown large enough to cause compressive symptoms. Although they are clinically silent, the various subtypes correspond to the predominant cell line of origin and therefore are biochemically distinct from one another. This article reviews the biochemical, clinical, and histopathologic features of each of these subtypes. A rubric is provided for diagnostic work-up of these lesions and the management options available to the treating clinician.

Giant pituitary adenomas (GPAs) comprise 5% to 15% of pituitary adenomas, but have higher rates of extrasellar invasion, subtotal resection, surgical morbidity, and recurrence. With the possible exception of giant prolactinomas, GPAs require surgical decompression. This chapter reviews the clinical presentation, management, and surgical modalities for GPAs. On review of 3 decades of case series encompassing 699 microsurgical transsphenoidal (MT), 1060 endoscopic endonasal trans-sphenoidal (EET), and 513 transcranial (TC) patients, gross total resection and recurrence rates were comparable across modalities, but the EET approach had lower perioperative mortality and superior restoration of visual function. Each approach has unique indications and is an important component of the pituitay surgeon's armamentarium. Combined EET-TC approaches for minimizing residual tumor represent another area of study.

Advances in endoscopic surgical technique have ushered in a new era of pituitary surgery with improved rates of resection and minimized operative morbidity and burden. Anatomically, endoscopic transnasal transsphenoidal pituitary surgery is split into nasal, sphenoidal, and sellar stages, each with unique considerations. Recent developments in knowledge and technology seek to build on the success of the endoscope in pituitary surgery, while expanding its capabilities.

Many surgical considerations exist for an endoscopic approach for pituitary surgery for a neurosurgeon. The neurosurgical approach to endoscopic pituitary dissection requires proper surgical planning and identification of relevant anatomic structures. With the introduction of endoscopic transsphenoidal pituitary surgery, better visualization and more intricate surgical resections are achieved. Whether performing this surgery solo or with an otolaryngologist, the neurosurgeon must consider multiple aspects for this surgical approach. This article focuses on the surgical considerations involving the anatomic regions of the sphenoid sinus and sellar region for endoscopic pituitary dissections.

True pituitary surgical emergencies are rare. These events can occur throughout the perioperative period and are broadly categorized by the timing of occurrence. Acute indications for emergent pituitary surgery include pituitary apoplexy, vision loss, and severe Cushing presentation. Emergencies may also occur intraoperatively, secondary to bleeding. Postoperative emergencies include epistaxis, pneumocephalus, and intracranial bleeding. Cerebrospinal fluid (CSF) leak occurs in about 37.4% of transsphenoidal sellar surgery, yet postoperative CSF leaks are less frequent at approximately 2.6%. As they occur often during pituitary surgery, CSF leaks alone are generally not considered a true surgical emergency unless associated with symptomatic tension pneumocephalus.

Developed over 50 years ago, the microscopic transsphenoidal approach is a simple, efficient technique with proven efficacy for the surgical treatment of an array of sellar and parasellar diseases. Although utilization of fully endoscopic transsphenoidal approaches has dramatically increased recently because it offers enhanced visualization, current outcomes data do not clearly favor either approach. Potential advantages of the microscope that persist in the endoscopic era include decreased operative time; preservation of a single-surgeon, unobstructed, two-handed microsurgical technique; and limited disruption of the nasal mucosa. Endoscope-assisted microsurgical approaches can also be used to overcome limitations in visualization while preserving the aforementioned advantages.

Anesthesia for pituitary surgery is tailored to each individual patient and the type of tumor they have. Anesthetic considerations include difficult airways, hormonal and electrolyte abnormalities, cardiac abnormalities, the potential for catastrophic hemorrhage, and the importance of a smooth extubation. The anesthesiologist is able to assist the surgeons by keeping the patient motionless and lowering the blood pressure to minimize surgical bleeding. Postoperative nausea and vomiting are also of greater importance than usual, as the Valsalva movements associated with retching could cause bleeding and disruption of the surgical site.

Pituitary surgery has undergone rapid advancements in the last 30 years, secondary to improved surgical techniques and technologies, including those that allow endoscopic approaches. Although the endoscopic endonasal approach (EEA) offers minimally invasive access to the region of the pituitary gland, complications are a significant consideration for the combined otolaryngology-neurosurgery team that is preparing for a case. In this article, we discuss various complications related to the EEA in pituitary surgery and explore ways to plan for and avoid them during surgery.

Advancements in sellar floor defect reconstruction have expanded the capacity of skull base surgery complexity. Several investigators have developed grading scales for the intraoperative appearance of the sella following pituitary tumor resection. Certain repairs are unnecessary for lower-grade defects that typically involve low-flow cerebrospinal fluid (CSF) leaks and do not require complex repair techniques. Higher-grade defects that result in high-flow CSF leaks may require more advanced techniques, such as the nasoseptal flap or a combination of repair techniques. This review summarizes the current strategies for repair of the sella following pituitary tumor resection.

Postoperative care of patients undergoing endoscopic transsphenoidal pituitary surgery requires a multidisciplinary team approach, capitalizing on the complementary knowledge and skills of surgical and medical disciplines, including neurosurgery, otolaryngology, endocrinology, ophthalmology, and radiology. In the early postoperative period, endocrinologic problems and cerebrospinal fluid leak are the major drivers of morbidity and need for readmission or revision surgery. With a team-based approach, most complications can be mitigated with a low risk of serious complications and excellent quality of life. Patients often require long-term postoperative follow-up for surveillance and management of neurologic, endocrinologic, and sinonasal concerns.

Interdisciplinary teams have many potential and proven benefits, including decreased burnout, decreased medical errors, increased quality, and leveraging of competing values and skills. Pituitary Tumor Centers of Excellence must have adequate volumes and high-functioning teams in order to provide exceptional, high-value care. Organizational logistics, attentive operations management, facilitated collaboration, and clear communication are key teamwork tools in delivering that care.

Lesions of the pituitary and sellar region in children comprise a wide variety of pathologic conditions, but advances in surgical technology and techniques have enabled both biopsy and resection of such lesions despite age-dependent anatomic constraints. In this article, the authors discuss the common pathologic conditions encountered, perioperative management of these patients, surgical techniques required to address these lesions and repair the pediatric skull base, points of controversy, and future areas of work.

# OTOLARYNGOLOGIC CLINICS OF NORTH AMERICA

## SERIES OF RELATED INTEREST

*Facial Plastic Surgery Clinics*
*Available at:* https://www.facialplastic.theclinics.com/

**THE CLINICS ARE AVAILABLE ONLINE!**
Access your subscription at:
www.theclinics.com

# Foreword

# Pituitary Surgery: Then, Now, and In the Future

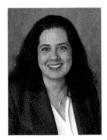

Sujana S. Chandrasekhar, MD, FACS, FAAOHNS
*Consulting Editor*

The history of pituitary surgery is one of more and more minimally invasive approaches and of better and better interspecialty collaboration.[1] This issue of *Otolaryngologic Clinics of North America*, ably edited by Drs Eloy, Fang, and Agarwal, reflects all that we have learned, what are the best current practices, and where we think we will go from here.

As with other skull base tumors, the juxtaposition of the neurosurgical and otolaryngologic approaches for pituitary lesions has led to the development of true surgical collaboration. In addition, because the pituitary gland is a "master gland" of hormonal activity, advances in endocrinology allow for proper selection of surgical candidates and those who do not need surgery, and optimal medical treatment. We continuously learn from our colleagues in radiology and ophthalmology as to how to correctly identify these tumors in a timely fashion.

The first report of pituitary surgery in western medicine was in 1893, when Paul performed a temporal decompression for acromegaly, but he didn't actually touch the tumor. In 1889, Horsley performed the first western operation on a pituitary tumor and published a series of 10 patients in 1906, initially using frontal craniotomy and then via a temporal approach. The first transsphenoidal approach to this gland was via lateral rhinotomy, turbinectomy, and removal of all the sinuses, by Schloffer in 1907. Kocher performed a somewhat less-invasive transseptal submucosal approach via a midline rhinotomy approach while avoiding the sinus resection. The first totally endonasal procedure was done in 1910 in FIVE stages under local anesthesia by Hirsch, who was the first to use a nasal speculum for this. Halstead pioneered the sublabial approach, initially as a multistage, in 1910. Cushing did his first sublabial, transseptal, transsphenoidal approach in 1909, but he then derided and abandoned it for transcranial approaches, a move that was supported by Dandy and most other neurosurgeons.

Otolaryngol Clin N Am 55 (2022) xix–xxi
https://doi.org/10.1016/j.otc.2022.01.006
0030-6665/22/© 2022 Published by Elsevier Inc.

The 1920s to the 1960s were a poor period for transsphenoidal surgery due to lack of antibiotics, lack of hormone replacement therapy, poor illumination, and Cushing's strong opinions against it. During this time, the only student of Cushing who did not abandon the transnasal approach was Dott in Edinburgh, who added two light bulbs to the speculum Cushing had designed. Dott taught Guiot in France, and Guiot taught Hardy in Montreal. The latter two men are credited with the "transsphenoidal renaissance" in the late 1960s and 1970s, with Guiot introducing intraoperative fluoroscopy and Hardy introducing operative microscopy along with the concepts of microadenoma and microsurgical resection. This corresponds to when the operative microscope was introduced into lateral skull base surgery as well. Guiot tried, but then abandoned, using an endoscope for pituitary surgery, in 1963.

The next big advancement in pituitary surgery came in the 1990s with routine use of endoscopes to further minimize the invasive nature of the procedure while allowing for excellent visibility and complete tumor removal. Agreement and collaboration between the specialties of otolaryngology, neurosurgery, endocrinology, and radiology as well as advances in biomolecular, robotic, and miniaturization technologies are taking us further forward.

I congratulate Drs Eloy, Fang, and Agarwal on compiling this thorough and enjoyable issue of *Otolaryngologic Clinics of North America* on Pituitary Surgery. It covers the subject completely, and I encourage otolaryngologists, endocrinologists, and neurosurgeons to read each article carefully and then keep the issue available as a handy reference that can be consulted quickly as needed.

Sujana S. Chandrasekhar, MD, FACS, FAAOHNS
Consulting Editor
Otolaryngologic Clinics of North America

Past President
American Academy of Otolaryngology–
Head and Neck Surgery

Secretary-Treasurer
American Otological Society

Partner, ENT & Allergy Associates LLP
18 East 48th Street, 2nd Floor
New York, NY 10017, USA

Clinical Professor, Department of Otolaryngology–
Head and Neck Surgery
Zucker School of Medicine at Hofstra-Northwell
Hempstead, NY, USA

Clinical Associate Professor
Department of Otolaryngology–
Head and Neck Surgery
Icahn School of Medicine at Mount Sinai
New York, NY, USA

*E-mail address:*
ssc@nyotology.com

http://www.ears.nyc/

**REFERENCES**

1. Cappabianca P, Cavallo LM, de Divitiis O, et al. Chapter 19—pituitary surgery. In: Jameson JL, De Groot LJ, editors. Endocrinology. 6th edition. Philadelphia: WB Saunders; 2010. p. 358–76. https://doi.org/10.1016/B978-1-4160-5583-9.00019-8.

# Preface

# Pituitary Surgery

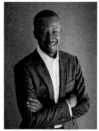 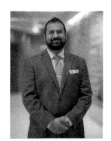

Jean Anderson Eloy, MD, FARS, FACS    Christina H. Fang, MD    Vijay Agarwal, MD
*Editors*

Advancements in surgical technology, as well as improved understanding of endoscopic skull base anatomy have revolutionized pituitary surgery in recent decades. The endoscopic transsphenoidal approach for pituitary surgery is considered by many to be state-of-the-art practice and has been shown to be safe and effective with low morbidity. Despite such innovations, practice patterns vary considerably depending on setting, location, and surgeon preference and experience. With new advances in endoscopic techniques and an enhanced ability to perform extended approaches to the sellar and parasellar region, there is the need for an updated comprehensive review of contemporary advances in pituitary surgery.

Preoperative workup and imaging modalities used for pituitary lesions are discussed in this issue, as well as common histopathologic findings. Focus is given to surgical considerations for both otolaryngologists and neurosurgeons. The endoscopic anatomy of this surgical corridor can present unique surgical challenges; thus, a detailed understanding of the sellar and parasellar anatomy from an endoscopic viewpoint is imperative. Microscopic transsphenoidal pituitary surgery, still an important and valuable approach in the pituitary surgeon's armamentarium, is discussed. Nuances in the management of functional and nonfunctional pituitary adenomas, as well as giant pituitary adenomas are examined. Meticulous reconstruction of the skull base and comprehensive postoperative care, both of which are discussed, can help mitigate patient morbidity.

The management of patients with pituitary lesions is complex and commonly involves a multidisciplinary team composed of otolaryngologists, neurosurgeons, endocrinologists, neuroradiologists, neuroophthalmologists, neuropathologists, and anesthesiologists. Development of such a pituitary care team is described, with emphasis on the organizational logistics, operations management, collaboration, and communication necessary to provide high-value patient care.

Otolaryngol Clin N Am 55 (2022) xxiii–xxiv
https://doi.org/10.1016/j.otc.2022.01.005
0030-6665/22/© 2022 Published by Elsevier Inc.                    oto.theclinics.com

In this issue of *Otolaryngologic Clinics of North America*, we present a comprehensive approach to the management of pituitary disease. It is with great honor that we guest-edit this important issue on "Pituitary Surgery." We believe that this issue will be valuable to the practicing rhinologist, comprehensive otolaryngologist, neurosurgeon, and allied health care worker involved in the care of patients with these complex pathologic conditions.

Jean Anderson Eloy, MD, FARS, FACS
Department of Otolaryngology–
Head and Neck Surgery
Department of Neurological Surgery
Department of Ophthalmology and Visual Science
Rutgers, New Jersey Medical School
Center for Skull Base and Pituitary Surgery
Neurological Institute of New Jersey
90 Bergen Street, Suite 8100
Newark, NJ 07103, USA

Department of Otolaryngology and
Facial Plastic Surgery
Saint Barnabas Medical Center–
RWJ Barnabas Health
Livingston, NJ, USA

Christina H. Fang, MD
Department of Otorhinolaryngology–
Head and Neck Surgery
Montefiore Medical Center
The University Hospital of
Albert Einstein College of Medicine
3400 Bainbridge Avenue
Medical Arts Pavilion, 3rd Floor
Bronx, NY 10467, USA

Vijay Agarwal, MD
Department of Neurological Surgery
Montefiore Medical Center
Department of Otorhinolaryngology– Head and Neck Surgery
The University Hospital of Albert Einstein College of Medicine
3316 Rochambeau Avenue
Bronx, NY 10467, USA

*E-mail addresses:*
jean.anderson.eloy@gmail.com (J.A. Eloy)
christina.fang1@gmail.com (C.H. Fang)
vagarwal@montefiore.org (V. Agarwal)

# Overview of Pituitary Surgery

Christina H. Fang, MD[a], Vijay Agarwal, MD[a,b,c], James K. Liu, MD, FAANS[d,e,f],
Jean Anderson Eloy, MD, FARS[d,e,f,g,h],*

## KEYWORDS

- Pituitary surgery • Pituitary • Skull base surgery • Pituitary adenoma
- Transsphenoidal surgery • Endoscopic surgery • Sella

## KEY POINTS

- With advancements in surgical technology and improved understanding of endoscopic skull base anatomy, pituitary surgery has rapidly evolved over the past few decades.
- A comprehensive history and physical examination should be performed to evaluate patients with pituitary lesions. A full hormone laboratory panel, including but not limited to serum prolactin, thyroid-stimulating hormone, adrenocorticotropic hormone (ACTH), and growth hormone should be obtained. Formal neuro-ophthalmologic testing should be obtained and documented.
- Magnetic resonance imaging is the imaging of choice to evaluate the sellar and suprasellar regions. The presence of a mass, thickening of the infundibulum, impingement of the optic chiasm, presence of cystic or solid areas, presence of flow voids on T2 sequence, calcification, bony destruction, enlargement of the cavernous sinus, abnormal enhancement, and mass effect on adjacent structures should be assessed on postcontrast T1-weighted imaging.
- The endoscopic transsphenoidal approach for pituitary surgery has been shown to be safe and effective with low morbidity.

[a] Department of Otorhinolaryngology – Head and Neck Surgery, Montefiore Medical Center, The University Hospital for the Albert Einstein College of Medicine, 3400 Bainbridge Street, 3rd Floor, Bronx, NY 10467, USA; [b] Department of Neurological Surgery, Montefiore Medical Center, The University Hospital of Albert Einstein College of Medicine, Bronx, NY, USA; [c] Division of Skull Base and Minimally Invasive Neurosurgery, Montefiore Medical Center, The University Hospital for the Albert Einstein College of Medicine, 3316 Rochambeau Avenue, Bronx, NY 10467, USA; [d] Department of Otolaryngology – Head and Neck Surgery, Rutgers New Jersey Medical School, Newark, NJ, USA; [e] Department of Neurological Surgery, Rutgers New Jersey Medical School, Newark, NJ, USA; [f] Center for Skull Base and Pituitary Surgery, Neurological Institute of New Jersey, Rutgers New Jersey Medical School, Newark, NJ, USA; [g] Department of Ophthalmology and Visual Science, Rutgers New Jersey Medical School, Newark, NJ, USA; [h] Department of Otolaryngology and Facial Plastic Surgery, Saint Barnabas Medical Center - RWJBarnabas Health, Livingston, NJ, USA
* Corresponding author. Department of Otolaryngology – Head and Neck Surgery, Rutgers New Jersey Medical School, 90 Bergen St., Suite 8100, Newark, NJ 07103.
E-mail address: jean.anderson.eloy@gmail.com

Otolaryngol Clin N Am 55 (2022) 205–221
https://doi.org/10.1016/j.otc.2022.01.001
0030-6665/22/© 2022 Elsevier Inc. All rights reserved.

## INTRODUCTION

The capability and utility of endoscopic pituitary surgery has significantly expanded over the past 30 years because of advancements in surgical and optical technology and increased understanding of endoscopic endonasal anatomy. Management of patients with pituitary lesions commonly involves multiple medical and surgical subspecialties, including endocrinology, otolaryngology, neurosurgery, critical care, and neuroradiology. This overview presents an up-to-date survey of the diagnosis, work-up, and management of pituitary lesions, and nuances of surgical treatment. Focus is placed on the endoscopic transsphenoidal approach, particularly its use for the treatment of functional and giant pituitary adenomas.

## ANATOMIC CONSIDERATIONS FOR ENDOSCOPIC PITUITARY SURGERY

The pituitary lies within the sella turcica of the ventral skull base, which is bordered anteriorly by the tuberculum sellae and anterior clinoid processes and posteriorly by the dorsum sellae and posterior clinoid processes. The sella turcica is bordered laterally by the cavernous sinuses, which contain the cavernous carotid arteries in their inferomedial aspect. The diaphragma sellae, a reflection of the dura, is located superior to the gland, with the infundibulum running through it. Intercommunicating sinuses beneath the diaphragma sellae connect the cavernous sinuses. The superior hypophyseal arteries, inferior hypophyseal arteries, and branches of the cavernous and ophthalmic segments of the carotid artery supply the pituitary gland. The suprasellar compartment is limited inferiorly by the diaphragma sellae, superiorly by the optic chiasm and floor of the third ventricle, anteriorly by the anterior arachnoid membrane of the chiasmatic cistern, and posteriorly by the diencephalic portion of Liliequist membrane.

Understanding the bony anatomy of the sphenoid sinus is vital in endoscopic transsphenoidal approaches to the pituitary. The prominences and depressions in the sphenoid sinus include the clival recess, sella, optic nerve, opticocarotid recesses, tuberculum, limbus sphenoidale, and planum sphenoidale (**Fig. 1**). Knowledge of the underlying structures is also important when tailoring approaches to the pituitary. (See C.M. Low, V. Vigo, M. Nunez, J.C. Fernández-Miranda, and Z.M. Patel's article, "Anatomic Considerations in Endoscopic Pituitary Surgery," in this issue.)

## DIAGNOSIS AND WORK-UP

The clinical presentation of a pituitary lesion depends on its hormonal secretory status, rate of growth, and effect on surrounding structures, such as the hypothalamic-pituitary axis (HPA) and optic chiasm. Generally, only functional pituitary adenomas cause hormonal hypersecretion. Hormonal hyposecretion is caused by mass effect of a sellar mass on the pituitary itself, HPA, or hypothalamus. Patients with sellar masses should undergo a comprehensive history and physical examination. Laboratory tests should be performed for every patient because functional adenomas may not exhibit any clinical symptoms. Hormone panels should include serum prolactin, thyroid-stimulating hormone, free thyroxine, adrenocorticotropic hormone, morning cortisol, follicle-stimulating hormone, luteinizing hormone, testosterone, and insulin-like growth factor. Additional laboratory testing includes 24-hour urinary-free cortisol, dexamethasone suppression testing, and oral glucose tolerance testing.[1] Other diagnoses, such as granulomatous disease and inflammatory processes, should be excluded because the appropriate treatment may significantly differ depending on the pathology.

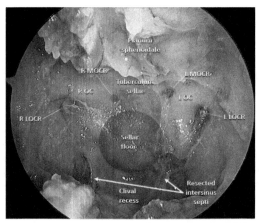

**Fig. 1.** Photograph of an endoscopic endonasal cadaveric dissection demonstrating the bony landmarks of the sphenoid sinus. Depicted is the planum sphenoidale, tuberculum sellae, sella floor, clival recess, resected intersinus septi, right optic canal (R OC), left optic canal (L OC), right medial opticocarotid recess (R MOCR), left medial opticocarotid recess (L MOCR), right lateral opticocarotid recess (R LOCR), and left lateral opticocarotid recess (L LOCR).

Visual field testing should be performed in patients who present with visual defects or whose tumors are adjacent to, or abutting against, the optic chiasm. In most cases, complete endocrinologic, ophthalmologic, neurologic, and imaging evaluation can lead to a suspected diagnosis. For surgical cases, neurosurgical and otolaryngologic consultation is recommended for preoperative planning. Sellar lesions often require a multidisciplinary approach, including medical treatment, surgery, and/or radiotherapy. Long-term follow-up consists of regular imaging, and ophthalmologic and endocrinologic evaluations.[2] (See A. White, E.J. de Andrade, V.R. Kshettry, R. Sindwani, and P.F. Recinos's article, "Preoperative Workup for Patients with Pituitary Lesions" and E. McKean and S.E. Sullivan's article, "Developing an Integrated Multidisciplinary Pituitary Management Team" in this issue.)

## IMAGING

Magnetic resonance imaging (MRI) with and without contrast is the imaging modality of choice for the sellar and parasellar region because of its superior soft tissue resolution. MRI is ideal for the diagnosis, localization, and posttreatment surveillance of pituitary lesions. Standard MRI imaging consists of T1 turbo spin-echo, postcontrast T1-weighted sequences, and T2-weighted images.[3] The postcontrast T1 coronal (**Fig. 2**A) and sagittal (**Fig. 2**B) images are best used to evaluate the size, shape, and signal homogeneity of the pituitary gland, infundibulum, optic chiasm and nerves, and cavernous sinus. The T2-weighted images are useful for evaluating lesions involving or pushing into brain parenchyma with significant edema (**Fig. 2**C) or if there is a contraindication to administration of contrast. The main role of computed tomography (CT) is to assist in preoperative planning and to assess bone involvement of tumor (**Fig. 3**). Thin sections, measuring between 0.625 and 1.33 mm, with coronal and sagittal reconstructions are used to better evaluate the bony anatomy of the sella and ventral skull base. Computed tomography angiography or MR angiogram should be performed if an aneurysm is suspected.

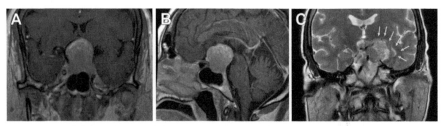

**Fig. 2.** Coronal (*A*) and sagittal (*B*) T1-weighted gadolinium-enhanced MRIs of a patient with a large pituitary macroadenoma. The contrast images are best used to evaluate the size, shape, and signal homogeneity of the pituitary gland, infundibulum, optic chiasm and nerves, cavernous sinus, and the lesion. The T2-weighted image (*C*) in this different patient is useful for evaluating potential brain parenchyma involvement. Note the edema associated with involvement of the left temporal lobe (*arrows*).

On T1-weighted MRI, the normal pituitary gland is isointense to the brain and enhances moderately and homogeneously with contrast.[4] A narrow differential diagnosis is determined by careful examination of the imaging. The presence of an enlarged sella turcica, a mass separate or arising from the gland, epicenter of the mass, thickening of the infundibulum, impingement of the optic chiasm, presence of cystic or solid areas, presence of flow void on T2 sequence, calcification, bony destruction, enlargement of the cavernous sinus, and mass effect on adjacent structures should be assessed.

Pituitary adenomas are classified into microadenomas (<10 mm), macroadenomas (>10 mm), and giant adenomas (>40 mm). Microadenomas are usually hypointense or isointense on T1 and T2-weighted images. With administration of contrast, microadenomas are often hypoenhancing relative to the normal pituitary gland (**Fig. 4**). They can also cause thickening, elevation, or displacement of the infundibulum. Pituitary macroadenomas appear as solid masses and are usually isointense on T1 and T2-weighted imaging. Macroadenomas often extend into the suprasellar space and narrow as they pass through the diaphragma sella, with a classic "snowman" type appearance (**Fig. 5**). Involvement and invasion of the cavernous sinus is evaluated on preoperative MRI. Knosp and colleagues[5] proposed a grading system to evaluate parasellar extension of the tumor based on its relationship to the intercavernous carotid artery. Detection of compression or elevation of the optic chiasm is also critical for preoperative planning (**Fig. 6**). For larger tumors, T2-weighted imaging is useful in delineating tumor margins and brain parenchymal involvement. (See K. Zhao, E. Nimchinsky, and P.K. Agarwalla's article, "Differential Diagnosis and Radiographic Imaging of Pituitary Lesions" in this issue.) Furthermore, this issue discusses the histopathology of pituitary lesions. (See A.B. deLeon's article, "Histopathology of Pituitary Lesions" in this issue.)

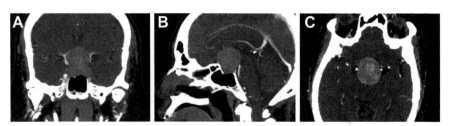

**Fig. 3.** Coronal (*A*), sagittal (*B*), and axial (*C*) CT scans of a patient after intravenous contrast demonstrating a large pituitary tumor, with suprasellar extension and thinning of the sella floor.

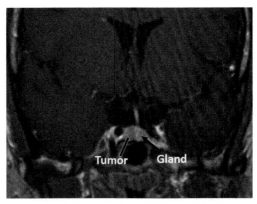

**Fig. 4.** Coronal T1-weighted gadolinium-enhanced MRI of a patient with a pituitary micro-adenoma with Cushing disease showing the typical hypoenhancing tumor relative to the normal pituitary gland.

## INDICATIONS FOR SURGERY

Prolactinomas are the most common functional adenoma and account for nearly 50% of all pituitary adenomas.[6–9] Patients can present with symptoms of hyperprolactine-mia, including impotence, infertility, decreased libido, oligo/amenorrhea, or galactor-rhea. Serum prolactin levels greater than 200 ng/mL are highly suggestive of a prolactinoma. Prolactin levels greater than 1000 ng/mL suggest cavernous sinus inva-sion.[10] It is important to remember that other sellar and parasellar pathologies that impair production or transport of dopamine from the hypothalamus can cause hyper-prolactinemia, often resulting in serum prolactin levels less than 100 ng/mL. These pa-thologies include craniopharyngiomas, head trauma, granulomatous infiltration of the hypothalamus, and large pituitary adenomas.[11–13]

The mainstay of treatment is dopamine-agonist medical therapy, with the goals of restoring normal endocrine function and reducing tumor size of macroadenomas. In-dications for treatment include infertility, bothersome galactorrhea, disturbance of pu-berty, long-standing hypogonadism, prevention of osteoporosis, and tumors with neurologic defects.[8] Dopamine agonists have demonstrated efficacy rates of 60%

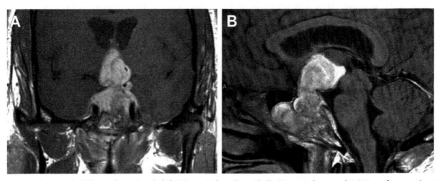

**Fig. 5.** Coronal (A) and sagittal (B) T1-weighted gadolinium-enhanced MRIs of a patient with a pituitary macroadenoma extending into the suprasellar space with narrowing at the diaphragma sella, with the classic "snowman" dumbbell-shaped appearance.

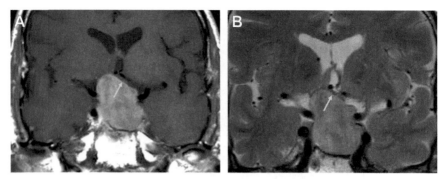

**Fig. 6.** Coronal (*A*) T1-weighted gadolinium-enhanced MRI and coronal T2-weighted (*B*) image of a patient with a pituitary macroadenoma with suprasellar extension showing compression and elevation of the optic chiasm (*arrow*).

to 80% in restoring normal prolactin levels,[14] and have been shown to significantly reduce the volume of tumors of all sizes.[15,16] Bromocriptine was first introduced in clinical practice 40 years ago. Cabergoline, a second-generation dopamine agonist, has since become a more popular choice given its improved efficacy and tolerability compared with bromocriptine.[14]

Surgical treatment of prolactinomas is reserved for patients with acute complications, such as pituitary apoplexy, resistance to or intolerance of medical treatment, young patients who do not want to undergo prolonged medical treatment, and predominantly cystic tumors.[17,18] Transsphenoidal pituitary surgery for prolactinomas has been shown to achieve high rates of postoperative normoprolactinemia.[18,19] (See N. Suda's article, "Non-Surgical Interventions for Pituitary Lesions" and S.A. Haider, S. Levy, J.P. Rock, and J.R. Craig's article, "Prolactinoma – Medical and Surgical Considerations" in this issue.)

Transsphenoidal pituitary surgery remains the primary treatment of adenomas excreting adrenocorticotropic hormone and growth hormone, with acceptable rates of biochemical remission.[20,21] Nonfunctional pituitary adenomas are common and estimated to occur in 10% to 20% of the population.[22] Nonfunctional pituitary adenomas are often diagnosed late as macroadenomas secondary to their compressive symptoms.[23] Surgery is usually reserved for patients with visual compromise or serial growth on imaging.[24] These topics are further discussed in this issue. (See D.P. Bray, R.S. Rindler, R.A. Dawoud, A.B. Boucher, and N.M. Oyesiku's article, "Cushing's Disease – Medical and Surgical Considerations"; A.M. Giantini-Larsen, R. Uribe-Cardenas, and R.G. Juthani's article, "Acromegaly – Medical and Surgical Considerations"; and B.P. Brownlee, D. Mann, C. Glenn, and K.A. McKinney's article, "Non-Functioning Pituitary Lesions" in this issue.)

## SURGICAL CONSIDERATIONS

The endoscopic transsphenoidal approach has been widely adopted for pituitary surgery, because it provides a wide panoramic view and enhanced visualization of critical anatomic structures.[25] Given the small area of the operative field and the proximity of the visualization instrument (endoscope) to the surgical site, a small amount of bleeding or pooling of blood can create significant hindrance to the surgeon.[26] Twenty-degree reverse Trendelenburg positioning, nasal mucosa decongestion and infiltration, use of irrigating endoscope sheaths, and warm saline irrigation have been shown to decrease intraoperative blood loss and improve surgical visualization.[27–29] Following exposure and resection of the sellar floor, a micro-Doppler ultrasound probe and stereotactic navigation are used to confirm the location of the parasellar carotid arteries. The dura is incised in the midline to avoid damage to the carotid arteries and intercavernous sinuses. Intracapsular debulking and decompression of the tumor and/or en bloc extracapsular resection is performed while preserving the normal gland.[30] In cases where the arachnoid membranes prolapse into the surgical field, care should be taken to dissect the tumor without violating the membranes to reduce the incidence of cerebrospinal fluid (CSF) leak. The medial cavernous sinus walls and suprasellar region can then be explored using 30- or 70-degree endoscopes. Use of intraoperative image guidance is helpful in identifying anatomic landmarks and tumor extent. (See T. Fan, A.D. Workman, and S.T. Gray's article "Surgical Considerations in Endoscopic Pituitary Approaches for the Otolaryngologist" and C.I. Eseonu's article "Surgical Considerations in Endoscopic Pituitary Dissection for the Neurosurgeon" in this issue.)

The same endoscopic techniques used in adults for pituitary surgery are also used in children.[31] The pediatric population has distinct anatomic considerations compared with adults. The sphenoid bone begins pneumatization in an inferoposterolateral direction at around 2 years until 14 years of age.[32] The medial anteroinferior margin of the sphenoid bone pneumatizes earlier, which suggests that this is the safest entry point for a transsphenoidal approach.[33] The intercarotid distance at the clivus is a limiting factor, but this has been shown to be stable by 2 to 5 years of age and does not change significantly during skull base development.[33,34] Careful review of preoperative imaging is recommended for all pediatric patients to determine the safest and most appropriate surgical approach. (See P.J. Madsen, S. Lang, N.D. Adappa, J.N. Palmer, and P.B. Storm's article, "Pediatric Pituitary Surgery" in this issue.)

### GIANT PITUITARY ADENOMAS

Giant pituitary adenomas (GPAs) are defined as adenomas greater than 4 cm in size (**Fig. 7**). Surgical management of GPAs is challenging given their size, irregular shape, invasion of the cavernous sinus and suprasellar space, and proximity to the optic pathways and carotid artery.[35] The primary goal of surgical resection of GPAs is to decompress the optic apparatus, HPA, and brainstem while minimizing the risk of morbidity and mortality. The expanded endoscopic endonasal approach is generally considered to be the first choice for resection of GPAs.[35–37] These tumors are often soft and distend the optic chiasm from below and the cavernous sinus, carotid artery, and cranial nerves from a medial to lateral direction.[38] This allows the tumor to be more

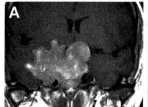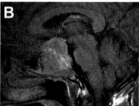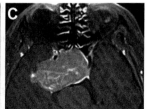

**Fig. 7.** Coronal (*A*), sagittal (*B*), and axial (*C*) T1-weighted gadolinium-enhanced MRIs of a patient with a giant pituitary adenoma with significant suprasellar and right temporal lobe extension.

radically resected from below with lower morbidity. Retrochiasmatic extension of the tumor into the ventricular system is assessed endoscopically with the use of angled endoscopes and specialized instrumentation.[35] The lateral cavernous sinus and cranial nerves form the natural lateral boundary of the endoscopic approach.[35] Several groups have reported improved efficacy and visual outcomes of the endoscopic approach for resection of GPAs when compared with transcranial or microscopic transsphenoidal approaches.[35–37,39,40]

Transcranial approaches are usually performed as a second choice in cases where the remnant suprasellar tumor does not descend into the sellar space after transsphenoidal resection.[36] A combined endoscopic and transcranial approach may also be necessary in cases of eccentric extension of the tumor into the frontal or temporal lobe or posterior fossa and in cases of a dumbbell-shaped tumor with a small intrasellar portion and a narrow neck.[36] Tumors that encase the optic nerves or intracranial arteries are also candidates for a transcranial approach.[41]

Gross total resection of GPAs often cannot be achieved, and residual tumor may be left unintentionally or intentionally to protect neurovascular structures.[35–37,39,40,42] In cases of subtotal resection, the residual tumor is at risk for postoperative hemorrhage and apoplexy.[40,42–46] Some contend that the cause of postoperative apoplexy is removal of the sellar venous drainage of the tumor, resulting in venous congestion of the suprasellar aspect and hemorrhagic conversion.[47] Thus, in cases where the transsphenoidal route is chosen as the first approach, these patients should be closely monitored in the postoperative period. Any change in neurologic condition warrants immediate imaging to rule out postoperative apoplexy. (See O.Y. Tang, W.D. Hsueh, J.A. Eloy, and J.K. Liu's article, "Giant Pituitary Adenoma – Special Considerations" in this issue.)

## RECONSTRUCTION OF SKULL BASE DEFECTS

Creation of a watertight skull base reconstruction during pituitary surgery is critical in preventing postoperative CSF leak. The challenges of endoscopic reconstruction include indirect access to the surgical site and the stresses of gravity and intracranial pressure on the repair.[48,49] Reconstruction of the sellar floor is not always necessary unless there is presence of an intraoperative CSF leak, thinning of the diaphragma sellae, or extensive arachnoid herniation.[50,51] In cases of intraoperative CSF leak, the reconstruction technique used is tailored to the location and size of the defect and characteristics of CSF leak (high vs low flow).[52,53] Reconstruction is performed using a variety of grafts, flaps, and synthetic materials in a single or multilayer closure. First described in 2006, the pedicled nasoseptal flap has become the workhorse of most endoscopic skull base reconstruction techniques.[54,55] Coverage of a sellar defect requires a shorter and narrower pedicled nasoseptal flap than other ventral skull base defects.[56] With improved endoscopic repair techniques, CSF diversion and the use of dural sealants have been shown to be unnecessary for sellar defects, except in cases of a large dural defect and high-flow intraoperative CSF leak.[56,57] (See C. Anderson, N. Akbar, and P. Colley's article, "Reconstruction of Skull Base Defects in Pituitary Surgery" in this issue.)

## POSTOPERATIVE CARE AND COMPLICATIONS

Patients are admitted postoperatively for close monitoring of neurologic status, hemodynamic stability, visual acuity, electrolyte balance, urinary output, and signs of CSF leak. To decrease the risk of postoperative CSF leak, patients are commonly placed on stool softeners and asked to avoid nose-blowing, straw-sipping, and straining. Postoperative pain is managed without narcotics to avoid oversedation and to promote early mobilization. Patients undergo regular serum sodium, urine-specific gravity, urine osmolality, serum osmolality, and serum cortisol testing to assess for diabetes insipidus (DI) and adrenal insufficiency. Perioperative antibiotics that cover *Staphylococcus* and *Streptococcus* are usually continued until nasal packing is removed.[58] Patients are typically discharged within 2 to 3 days if there is hemodynamic stability, appropriate sodium and fluid hemostasis, and resumption of ambulation and diet. Nasal endoscopy and debridement are performed at the patient's first outpatient visit on postoperative day 7 to 10.

Common postoperative complications of transsphenoidal pituitary surgery include central DI, hypopituitarism, CSF leak, and epistaxis.[59,60] Central DI may occur secondary to irritation or injury of the HPA. The risk of postoperative DI has been reported to be 0.3% to 45.6%, with lower rates reported among endoscopic cohorts.[2,35,61–64] Central DI is managed by increasing water intake. In the intubated or obtunded patient or in cases of hypernatremia, administration of desmopressin may be necessary.[59] Intraoperative CSF leaks are more common (14.2%–61%) than postoperative leaks (1.3%–5.9%), and many postoperative CSF leaks have an observed intraoperative leak.[2,65–72] Predictors of postoperative CSF leak include increased body mass index, intraoperative CSF leak, hydrocephalus, and pathology of the lesion.[67,68,73] Management of a postoperative CSF leak often times requires reoperation.[72] (See J. Vignolles-Jeong, D. Kreatsoulas, S. Godil, B. Otto, R. Carrau, and D. Prevedello's article, "Complications in Endoscopic Pituitary Surgery" in this issue.)

## ANESTHETIC CONSIDERATIONS

Endoscopic pituitary surgery presents unique challenges for the neuroanesthesiologist. The anesthetic goals include optimizing cerebral oxygenation, maintaining hemodynamic stability, managing intraoperative complications, providing optimal surgical conditions, and ensuring a rapid smooth anesthetic emergence.[74,75] Controlled normotension is necessary to maintain a bloodless surgical field. Infusion of dexmedetomidine has been shown to reduce intraoperative bleeding and improve surgeon satisfaction in these cases.[76] Infiltration of the nasal mucosa by a local anesthetic and vasoconstrictor is commonly performed for hemostasis and to blunt the cardiovascular response evoked by stimulation of the nasal mucosa.[77] The infiltration itself can evoke a strong sympathetic response, necessitating treatment with β-blockers or vasodilators.[78] Transsphenoidal pituitary surgery is associated with a considerable rate of transient DI.[79] Other causes of polyuria, such as overzealous fluid administration and osmotic diuresis, should be excluded. Vigilant monitoring of hemodynamic parameters and fluid status is key for early recognition and treatment of these potential complications. During emergence, avoidance of coughing and intermittent episodes of hypertension help maintain hemostasis and the integrity of the reconstruction site. Open communication is vital between the surgeons and anesthesiology team throughout the procedure. (See J. Kim and R. Scott-Miller's article, "Anesthetic Considerations in Endoscopic Pituitary Surgery" in this issue.)

## PITUITARY GLAND EMERGENCIES

Pituitary apoplexy is a serious acute complication of pituitary adenomas, with an incidence of 2% to 7% among these lesions (**Fig. 8**).[80–82] There is rapid expansion of an infarcted or hemorrhagic pituitary adenoma that can extend laterally into the cavernous sinus or superiorly to distend the optic nerves and chiasm. Patients present with sudden onset of bifrontal or retro-orbital headache, nausea, vomiting, and/or decreased consciousness. Decreased visual acuity, visual field impairment, or

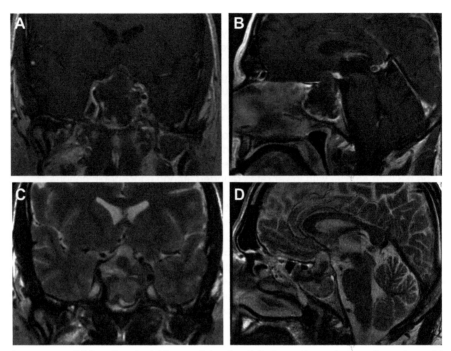

**Fig. 8.** Coronal (*A*) and sagittal (*B*) T1-weighted gadolinium-enhanced MRIs of a patient with pituitary apoplexy who presented with acute-onset headaches, nausea, vomiting, weakness, lethargy, and blurry and double vision. Coronal (*C*) and sagittal (*D*) T2-weighted images of the same patient.

diplopia also frequently occur. MRI usually reveals heterogeneous areas of hemorrhage and necrosis with an edematous pituitary gland.[80,83,84]

Hypopituitarism is frequently associated with pituitary apoplexy and can result from compression or destruction of the pituitary gland, interruption of blood supply to the gland, or pituitary stalk damage.[82,85,86] Absence of sufficient hormone production can lead to adrenal crisis and requires expeditious initiation of an intravenous glucocorticoid and thyroid hormone replacement.[85] There is controversy in the role of acute neurosurgical intervention following medical and endocrinologic stabilization.[87] Some advocate for a trial of conservative management in mild or stable cases with close clinical follow-up.[88–90] Others, however, advocate for early surgical decompression, especially in cases with visual deficits and/or cranial neuropathies.[81,85,86,91–93] In these cases, the endoscopic transsphenoidal approach is commonly used for early optic decompression and allows for improved control of vascular feeders from the anterior and middle cranial fossa.[94] (See M.A. Arnold, J.M.R. Barbero, G. Pradilla, and S.K. Wise's article, "Pituitary Gland Surgical Emergencies: The Role of Endoscopic Intervention" in this issue.)

## MICROSCOPIC TRANSSPHENOIDAL PITUITARY SURGERY

The use of the operating microscope for sublabial pituitary surgery was first described by Jules Hardy in the late 1960s.[95] In 1986, Griffith and Veerapen[96] described a direct endonasal approach using the "septum-pushover" technique, which avoids excessive dissection or removal of the nasal septum. Over the past two to three decades, however, the endoscopic transsphenoidal approach has gained popularity, particularly in large centers. In some comparative studies, the endoscopic approach has been shown to be equal or superior in terms of gross tumor resection and rates of postoperative complications.[97–99] The microscopic approach does remain a viable tool for neurosurgeons familiar with its use. Benefits of the microscopic approach include stereoscopic vision, retraction of edematous intranasal soft tissue, and in some cases, a more rapid approach.[100] (See R.C. Rennert, V.L. Fredrickson, and W.T. Couldwell's article, "Microscopic Transsphenoidal Surgery in the Era of Endoscopy: Are There any Advantages?" in this issue.)

## SUMMARY

Recent advances in technology, endoscopic skull base surgical techniques, and neuroimaging have allowed for safe and efficacious treatment of pituitary lesions. The care of these patients often involves a multidisciplinary team, consisting of an endocrinologist, neuroradiologist, otolaryngologist, critical care specialist, anesthesiologist, and neurosurgeon. This overview describes considerations essential for the diagnosis, work-up, and preoperative evaluation of patients with pituitary lesions. Surgical nuances in the adult and pediatric population, and in cases of large tumors and emergencies, are discussed.

## CLINICS CARE POINTS

---

- Patients with pituitary lesions should be evaluated with a comprehensive history and physical examination. A full hormone laboratory panel and neuro-ophthalmology evaluation is also recommended.

- MRI is the imaging modality of choice to evaluate patients with pituitary lesions.

- Thorough understanding of skull base anatomy allows surgeons to approach and resect the lesion and subsequently reconstruct the defect in a safe and efficient manner.

- Postoperative care of patients who undergo pituitary surgery involves close monitoring of neurologic status, hemodynamic stability, visual acuity, electrolyte balance, urinary output, and signs of CSF leak.

- A multidisciplinary approach to management of patients with pituitary lesions is imperative to providing high quality and high value care.

---

## REFERENCES

1. Cardinal T, Brunswick A, Strickland BA, et al. Safety and effectiveness of the direct endoscopic endonasal approach for primary sellar pathology: a contemporary case series of more than 400 patients. World Neurosurg 2021;148:e536–46.
2. Ikeda AK, Luk LJ, Patel ZM, et al. Follow-up management of patients after transsphenoidal approach for resection of pituitary adenomas. Am J Rhinol Allergy 2020;34(2):150–5.
3. Jipa A, Jain V. Imaging of the sellar and parasellar regions. Clin Imaging 2021;77:254–75.
4. Pressman BD. Pituitary imaging. Endocrinol Metab Clin North Am 2017;46(3):713–40.

5. Knosp E, Steiner E, Kitz K, et al. Pituitary adenomas with invasion of the cavernous sinus space: a magnetic resonance imaging classification compared with surgical findings. Neurosurgery 1993;33(4):610–7 [discussion: 617-8].

6. Daly AF, Rixhon M, Adam C, et al. High prevalence of pituitary adenomas: a cross-sectional study in the province of Liege, Belgium. J Clin Endocrinol Metab 2006;91(12):4769–75.

7. Fernandez A, Karavitaki N, Wass JA. Prevalence of pituitary adenomas: a community-based, cross-sectional study in Banbury (Oxfordshire, UK). Clin Endocrinol (Oxf) 2010;72(3):377–82.

8. Casanueva FF, Molitch ME, Schlechte JA, et al. Guidelines of the Pituitary Society for the diagnosis and management of prolactinomas. Clin Endocrinol (Oxf) 2006;65(2):265–73.

9. Daly AF, Beckers A. The epidemiology of pituitary adenomas. Endocrinol Metab Clin North Am 2020;49(3):347–55.

10. Molitch ME. Diagnosis and treatment of pituitary adenomas: a review. JAMA 2017;317(5):516–24.

11. Giustina A, Gola M, Doga M, et al. Clinical review 136: primary lymphoma of the pituitary: an emerging clinical entity. J Clin Endocrinol Metab 2001;86(10): 4567–75.

12. Shin JL, Asa SL, Woodhouse LJ, et al. Cystic lesions of the pituitary: clinicopathological features distinguishing craniopharyngioma, Rathke's cleft cyst, and arachnoid cyst. J Clin Endocrinol Metab 1999;84(11):3972–82.

13. Prayson RA. Biopsy proven pituitary sarcoidosis presenting as a possible adenoma. J Clin Neurosci 2016;34:217–8.

14. Webster J, Piscitelli G, Polli A, et al. A comparison of cabergoline and bromocriptine in the treatment of hyperprolactinemic amenorrhea. Cabergoline Comparative Study Group. N Engl J Med 1994;331(14):904–9.

15. Molitch ME, Elton RL, Blackwell RE, et al. Bromocriptine as primary therapy for prolactin-secreting macroadenomas: results of a prospective multicenter study. J Clin Endocrinol Metab 1985;60(4):698–705.

16. Bevan JS, Webster J, Burke CW, et al. Dopamine agonists and pituitary tumor shrinkage. Endocr Rev 1992;13(2):220–40.

17. Kreutzer J, Buslei R, Wallaschofski H, et al. Operative treatment of prolactinomas: indications and results in a current consecutive series of 212 patients. Eur J Endocrinol 2008;158(1):11–8.

18. Honegger J, Nasi-Kordhishti I, Aboutaha N, et al. Surgery for prolactinomas: a better choice? Pituitary 2020;23(1):45–51.

19. Tampourlou M, Trifanescu R, Paluzzi A, et al. Therapy of endocrine disease: surgery in microprolactinomas: effectiveness and risks based on contemporary literature. Eur J Endocrinol 2016;175(3):R89–96.

20. Starnoni D, Daniel RT, Marino L, et al. Surgical treatment of acromegaly according to the 2010 remission criteria: systematic review and meta-analysis. Acta Neurochir (Wien) 2016;158(11):2109–21.

21. Broersen LHA, Biermasz NR, van Furth WR, et al. Endoscopic vs. microscopic transsphenoidal surgery for Cushing's disease: a systematic review and meta-analysis. Pituitary 2018;21(5):524–34.

22. Molitch ME, Russell EJ. The pituitary "incidentaloma. Ann Intern Med 1990; 112(12):925–31.

23. Messerer M, De Battista JC, Raverot G, et al. Evidence of improved surgical outcome following endoscopy for nonfunctioning pituitary adenoma removal. Neurosurg Focus 2011;30(4):E11.

24. Farrell CJ, Nyquist GG, Farag AA, et al. Principles of pituitary surgery. Otolaryngol Clin North Am 2016;49(1):95–106.

25. Gondim JA, Schops M, de Almeida JP, et al. Endoscopic endonasal transsphenoidal surgery: surgical results of 228 pituitary adenomas treated in a pituitary center. Pituitary 2010;13(1):68–77.

26. Hanson M, Li H, Geer E, et al. Perioperative management of endoscopic transsphenoidal pituitary surgery. World J Otorhinolaryngol Head Neck Surg 2020; 6(2):84–93.

27. Gan EC, Habib AR, Rajwani A, et al. Five-degree, 10-degree, and 20-degree reverse Trendelenburg position during functional endoscopic sinus surgery: a double-blind randomized controlled trial. Int Forum Allergy Rhinol 2014; 4(1):61–8.

28. Higgins TS, Hwang PH, Kingdom TT, et al. Systematic review of topical vasoconstrictors in endoscopic sinus surgery. Laryngoscope 2011;121(2):422–32.

29. Gan EC, Alsaleh S, Manji J, et al. Hemostatic effect of hot saline irrigation during functional endoscopic sinus surgery: a randomized controlled trial. Int Forum Allergy Rhinol 2014;4(11):877–84.

30. Thakur JD, Corlin A, Mallari RJ, et al. Complication avoidance protocols in endoscopic pituitary adenoma surgery: a retrospective cohort study in 514 patients. Pituitary 2021. https://doi.org/10.1007/s11102-021-01167-y.

31. Kassam A, Thomas AJ, Snyderman C, et al. Fully endoscopic expanded endonasal approach treating skull base lesions in pediatric patients. J Neurosurg 2007;106(2 Suppl):75–86.

32. Scuderi AJ, Harnsberger HR, Boyer RS. Pneumatization of the paranasal sinuses: normal features of importance to the accurate interpretation of CT scans and MR images. AJR Am J Roentgenol 1993;160(5):1101–4.

33. Tatreau JR, Patel MR, Shah RN, et al. Anatomical considerations for endoscopic endonasal skull base surgery in pediatric patients. Laryngoscope 2010;120(9): 1730–7.

34. Li L, Carrau RL, Prevedello DM, et al. Intercarotid artery distance in the pediatric population: implications for endoscopic transsphenoidal approaches to the skull base. Int J Pediatr Otorhinolaryngol 2021;140:110520.

35. Koutourousiou M, Gardner PA, Fernandez-Miranda JC, et al. Endoscopic endonasal surgery for giant pituitary adenomas: advantages and limitations. J Neurosurg 2013;118(3):621–31.

36. Mortini P, Barzaghi R, Losa M, et al. Surgical treatment of giant pituitary adenomas: strategies and results in a series of 95 consecutive patients. Neurosurgery 2007;60(6):993–1002 [discussion: 1003-4].

37. Komotar RJ, Starke RM, Raper DM, et al. Endoscopic endonasal compared with microscopic transsphenoidal and open transcranial resection of giant pituitary adenomas. Pituitary 2012;15(2):150–9.

38. Schwartz TH. The endoscope and the giant macroadenoma: a match made in heaven. World Neurosurg 2014;82(1–2):e119–20.

39. de Paiva Neto MA, Vandergrift A, Fatemi N, et al. Endonasal transsphenoidal surgery and multimodality treatment for giant pituitary adenomas. Clin Endocrinol (Oxf) 2010;72(4):512–9.

40. Gondim JA, Almeida JP, Albuquerque LA, et al. Giant pituitary adenomas: surgical outcomes of 50 cases operated on by the endonasal endoscopic approach. World Neurosurg 2014;82(1–2):e281–90.

41. Youssef AS, Agazzi S, van Loveren HR. Transcranial surgery for pituitary adenomas. Neurosurgery 2005;57(1 Suppl):168–75 [discussion: 168-75].

42. Goel A, Nadkarni T, Muzumdar D, et al. Giant pituitary tumors: a study based on surgical treatment of 118 cases. Surg Neurol 2004;61(5):436–45 [discussion: 445-6].
43. de Divitiis E, de Divitiis O. Surgery for large pituitary adenomas: what is the best way? World Neurosurg 2012;77(3–4):448–50.
44. Azab WA, Nasim K, Abdelnabi EA, et al. Endoscopic endonasal excision of large and giant pituitary adenomas: radiological and intraoperative correlates of the extent of resection. World Neurosurg 2019;126:e793–802.
45. Elshazly K, Kshettry VR, Farrell CJ, et al. Clinical outcomes after endoscopic endonasal resection of giant pituitary adenomas. World Neurosurg 2018;114:e447–56.
46. Juraschka K, Khan OH, Godoy BL, et al. Endoscopic endonasal transsphenoidal approach to large and giant pituitary adenomas: institutional experience and predictors of extent of resection. J Neurosurg 2014;121(1):75–83.
47. Pezzutti DL, Magill ST, Albonette-Felicio T, et al. Endoscopic endonasal transtubercular approach for resection of giant pituitary adenomas with subarachnoid extension: the "second floor" strategy to avoid postoperative apoplexy. World Neurosurg 2021. https://doi.org/10.1016/j.wneu.2021.06.142.
48. Tabaee A, Anand VK, Brown SM, et al. Algorithm for reconstruction after endoscopic pituitary and skull base surgery. Laryngoscope 2007;117(7):1133–7.
49. Snyderman CH, Carrau RL, Kassam AB, et al. Endoscopic skull base surgery: principles of endonasal oncological surgery. J Surg Oncol 2008;97(8):658–64.
50. Couldwell WT, Kan P, Weiss MH. Simple closure following transsphenoidal surgery. Technical note. Neurosurg Focus 2006;20(3):E11.
51. Sciarretta V, Mazzatenta D, Ciarpaglini R, et al. Surgical repair of persisting CSF leaks following standard or extended endoscopic transsphenoidal surgery for pituitary tumor. Minim Invasive Neurosurg 2010;53(2):55–9.
52. Khan DZ, Ali AMS, Koh CH, et al. Skull base repair following endonasal pituitary and skull base tumour resection: a systematic review. Pituitary 2021. https://doi.org/10.1007/s11102-021-01145-4.
53. Harvey RJ, Parmar P, Sacks R, et al. Endoscopic skull base reconstruction of large dural defects: a systematic review of published evidence. Laryngoscope 2012;122(2):452–9.
54. Snyderman CH, Kassam AB, Carrau R, et al. Endoscopic reconstruction of cranial base defects following endonasal skull base surgery. Skull Base 2007;17(1):73–8.
55. Hadad G, Bassagasteguy L, Carrau RL, et al. A novel reconstructive technique after endoscopic expanded endonasal approaches: vascular pedicle nasoseptal flap. Laryngoscope 2006;116(10):1882–6.
56. Eloy JA, Marchiano E, Vazquez A, et al. Management of skull base defects after surgical resection of sinonasal and ventral skull base malignancies. Otolaryngol Clin North Am Apr 2017;50(2):397–417.
57. Zhan R, Chen S, Xu S, et al. Postoperative low-flow cerebrospinal fluid leak of endoscopic endonasal transsphenoidal surgery for pituitary adenoma: wait and see, or lumbar drain? J Craniofac Surg 2015;26(4):1261–4.
58. Moldovan ID, Agbi C, Kilty S, et al. A systematic review of prophylactic antibiotic use in endoscopic endonasal transsphenoidal surgery for pituitary lesions. World Neurosurg 2019;128:408–14.
59. Cote DJ, Iuliano SL, Catalino MP, et al. Optimizing pre-, intra-, and postoperative management of patients with sellar pathology undergoing transsphenoidal surgery. Neurosurg Focus 2020;48(6):E2.

60. Cote DJ, Dasenbrock HH, Muskens IS, et al. Readmission and other adverse events after transsphenoidal surgery: prevalence, timing, and predictive factors. J Am Coll Surg 2017;224(5):971–9.
61. Fatemi N, Dusick JR, Mattozo C, et al. Pituitary hormonal loss and recovery after transsphenoidal adenoma removal. Neurosurgery 2008;63(4):709–18 [discussion: 718-9].
62. Nomikos P, Ladar C, Fahlbusch R, et al. Impact of primary surgery on pituitary function in patients with non-functioning pituitary adenomas: a study on 721 patients. Acta Neurochir (Wien) 2004;146(1):27–35.
63. Schreckinger M, Walker B, Knepper J, et al. Post-operative diabetes insipidus after endoscopic transsphenoidal surgery. Pituitary 2013;16(4):445–51.
64. Kristof RA, Rother M, Neuloh G, et al. Incidence, clinical manifestations, and course of water and electrolyte metabolism disturbances following transsphenoidal pituitary adenoma surgery: a prospective observational study. J Neurosurg 2009;111(3):555–62.
65. Goudakos JK, Markou KD, Georgalas C. Endoscopic versus microscopic transsphenoidal pituitary surgery: a systematic review and meta-analysis. Clin Otolaryngol 2011;36(3):212–20.
66. Agam MS, Wedemeyer MA, Wrobel B, et al. Complications associated with microscopic and endoscopic transsphenoidal pituitary surgery: experience of 1153 consecutive cases treated at a single tertiary care pituitary center. J Neurosurg 2018;1:1–8.
67. Patel PN, Stafford AM, Patrinely JR, et al. Risk factors for intraoperative and postoperative cerebrospinal fluid leaks in endoscopic transsphenoidal sellar surgery. Otolaryngol Head Neck Surg 2018;158(5):952–60.
68. Karnezis TT, Baker AB, Soler ZM, et al. Factors impacting cerebrospinal fluid leak rates in endoscopic sellar surgery. Int Forum Allergy Rhinol 2016;6(11): 1117–25.
69. Berker M, Aghayev K, Yucel T, et al. Management of cerebrospinal fluid leak during endoscopic pituitary surgery. Auris Nasus Larynx 2013;40(4):373–8.
70. Berker M, Hazer DB, Yucel T, et al. Complications of endoscopic surgery of the pituitary adenomas: analysis of 570 patients and review of the literature. Pituitary 2012;15(3):288–300.
71. Zhou Q, Yang Z, Wang X, et al. Risk factors and management of intraoperative cerebrospinal fluid leaks in endoscopic treatment of pituitary adenoma: analysis of 492 patients. World Neurosurg 2017;101:390–5.
72. Parikh A, Adapa A, Sullivan SE, et al. Predictive factors, 30-day clinical outcomes, and costs associated with cerebrospinal fluid leak in pituitary adenoma resection. J Neurol Surg B Skull Base 2020;81(1):43–55.
73. Ivan ME, Iorgulescu JB, El-Sayed I, et al. Risk factors for postoperative cerebrospinal fluid leak and meningitis after expanded endoscopic endonasal surgery. J Clin Neurosci 2015;22(1):48–54.
74. Dunn LK, Nemergut EC. Anesthesia for transsphenoidal pituitary surgery. Curr Opin Anaesthesiol 2013;26(5):549–54.
75. Prabhakar H, Mahajan C, Kapoor I. Anesthesia for minimally invasive neurosurgery. Curr Opin Anaesthesiol 2017;30(5):546–50.
76. Salimi A, Sharifi G, Bahrani H, et al. Dexmedetomidine could enhance surgical satisfaction in trans-sphenoidal resection of pituitary adenoma. J Neurosurg Sci 2017;61(1):46–52.

77. Abou-Madi MN, Trop D, Barnes J. Aetiology and control of cardiovascular reactions during trans-sphenoidal resection of pituitary microadenomas. Can Anaesth Soc J 1980;27(5):491–5. https://doi.org/10.1007/BF03007050.

78. Chelliah YR, Manninen PH. Hazards of epinephrine in transsphenoidal pituitary surgery. J Neurosurg Anesthesiol 2002;14(1):43–6.

79. Nemergut EC, Zuo Z, Jane JA Jr, et al. Predictors of diabetes insipidus after transsphenoidal surgery: a review of 881 patients. J Neurosurg 2005;103(3):448–54.

80. Verrees M, Arafah BM, Selman WR. Pituitary tumor apoplexy: characteristics, treatment, and outcomes. Neurosurg Focus 2004;16(4):E6.

81. Bills DC, Meyer FB, Laws ER Jr, et al. A retrospective analysis of pituitary apoplexy. Neurosurgery 1993;33(4):602–8 [discussion: 608-9].

82. Wakai S, Fukushima T, Teramoto A, et al. Pituitary apoplexy: its incidence and clinical significance. J Neurosurg 1981;55(2):187–93.

83. Dulipsingh L, Lassman MN. Images in clinical medicine. Pituitary apoplexy. N Engl J Med 2000;342(8):550.

84. Piotin M, Tampieri D, Rufenacht DA, et al. The various MRI patterns of pituitary apoplexy. Eur Radiol 1999;9(5):918–23.

85. Arafah BM, Harrington JF, Madhoun ZT, et al. Improvement of pituitary function after surgical decompression for pituitary tumor apoplexy. J Clin Endocrinol Metab 1990;71(2):323–8.

86. Randeva HS, Schoebel J, Byrne J, et al. Classical pituitary apoplexy: clinical features, management and outcome. Clin Endocrinol (Oxf) 1999;51(2):181–8.

87. Rajasekaran S, Vanderpump M, Baldeweg S, et al. UK guidelines for the management of pituitary apoplexy. Clin Endocrinol (Oxf) 2011;74(1):9–20.

88. Ayuk J, McGregor EJ, Mitchell RD, et al. Acute management of pituitary apoplexy: surgery or conservative management? Clin Endocrinol (Oxf) 2004;61(6):747–52.

89. Maccagnan P, Macedo CL, Kayath MJ, et al. Conservative management of pituitary apoplexy: a prospective study. J Clin Endocrinol Metab 1995;80(7):2190–7.

90. Shepard MJ, Snyder MH, Soldozy S, et al. Radiological and clinical outcomes of pituitary apoplexy: comparison of conservative management versus early surgical intervention. J Neurosurg 2021;1–9.

91. Tu M, Lu Q, Zhu P, et al. Surgical versus non-surgical treatment for pituitary apoplexy: a systematic review and meta-analysis. J Neurol Sci 2016;370:258–62.

92. Turgut M, Ozsunar Y, Basak S, et al. Pituitary apoplexy: an overview of 186 cases published during the last century. Acta Neurochir (Wien) 2010;152(5):749–61.

93. Zhang X, Fei Z, Zhang W, et al. Emergency transsphenoidal surgery for hemorrhagic pituitary adenomas. Surg Oncol 2007;16(2):115–20.

94. Romano A, Ganau M, Zaed I, et al. Primary endoscopic management of apoplexy in a giant pituitary adenoma. World Neurosurg 2020;142:312–3.

95. Hardy J. Transphenoidal microsurgery of the normal and pathological pituitary. Clin Neurosurg 1969;16:185–217.

96. Griffith HB, Veerapen R. A direct transnasal approach to the sphenoid sinus. Technical note. J Neurosurg 1987;66(1):140–2.

97. Yu SY, Du Q, Yao SY, et al. Outcomes of endoscopic and microscopic transsphenoidal surgery on non-functioning pituitary adenomas: a systematic review and meta-analysis. J Cell Mol Med 2018;22(3):2023–7.

98. Li A, Liu W, Cao P, et al. Endoscopic versus microscopic transsphenoidal surgery in the treatment of pituitary adenoma: a systematic review and meta-analysis. World Neurosurg 2017;101:236–46.
99. Guo-Dong H, Tao J, Ji-Hu Y, et al. Endoscopic versus microscopic transsphenoidal surgery for pituitary tumors. J Craniofac Surg 2016;27(7):e648–55.
100. Singh H, Essayed WI, Cohen-Gadol A, et al. Resection of pituitary tumors: endoscopic versus microscopic. J Neurooncol 2016;130(2):309–17.

# Anatomic Considerations in Endoscopic Pituitary Surgery

Christopher M. Low, MD[a], Vera Vigo, MD[b],
Maximiliano Nunez, MD[b], Juan C. Fernández-Miranda, MD[b],
Zara M. Patel, MD[a],*

## KEYWORDS

- Anatomy - Pituitary - Endoscopic endonasal - Sella - Skull base

## KEY POINTS

- The endoscopic endonasal approach for pituitary surgery presents unique surgical challenges.
- Detailed understanding of the anatomy of the nasal cavity, sphenoid sinuses, cavernous sinuses, and their variations is key to optimizing surgical exposure to pituitary and other skull base pathology.
- The pituitary gland is composed of 2 anatomically and functionally distinct lobes—the anterior and posterior lobes.
- Four parasellar ligaments are ligamentous duralike trabeculae that connect the medial cavernous sinus wall with the internal carotid artery, anterior cavernous sinus wall, the interclinoid ligament, and the anterior clinoid process.
- The cavernous sinuses surround the pituitary gland laterally and house key neurovascular structures.

## INTRODUCTION

The pituitary gland is a small gland located at the base of the skull that controls many physiologic processes through its regulation of primary endocrine glands. Pathologic conditions of the pituitary gland and sellar space are wide ranging and most

Financial material & support: Internal departmental funding was used without commercial sponsorship or support.
Conflicts of interest to declare: None.
[a] Department of Otolaryngology-Head and Neck Surgery, Stanford University School of Medicine, 801 Welch Road, Palo Alto, CA 94305, USA; [b] Department of Neurosurgery, Stanford University School of Medicine, 213 Quarry Road, Palo Alto, CA 94304, USA
* Corresponding author. Division of Rhinology–Sinus and Skull Base Surgery, Department of Otolaryngology-Head and Neck Surgery, Department of Neurosurgery, Stanford University School of Medicine, 801 Welch Road, Palo Alto, CA 94305.
E-mail address: zmpatel@stanford.edu

Otolaryngol Clin N Am 55 (2022) 223–232
https://doi.org/10.1016/j.otc.2021.12.014
0030-6665/22/© 2022 Elsevier Inc. All rights reserved.

commonly include pituitary adenomas but can also encompass pituitary hyperplasia, other benign nonadenomatous tumors, cysts, and primary and metastatic malignancy.[1,2] These lesions can present with symptoms of hormonal dysregulation or compression of nearby anatomic structures including the optic apparatus and nerves controlling extraocular movements.[3,4]

For most of the twentieth century, the microsurgical approaches, pterional or sublabial, to the sella were the preferred approaches for surgical management of the pituitary gland and surrounding anatomy.[5,6] As endoscopic sinus surgery was being widely adopted, the early 1990s was the time of application of the endoscope to the anterior skull base for benign pathologic condition, specifically the pituitary gland. Jankowski and colleagues[6] reported the first 3 cases of endoscopic pituitary tumor surgery in 1992. Three years later, Carrau and colleagues[7] described successful pituitary surgery in a larger series of 27 patients, thus helping to launch endoscopic pituitary tumor surgery. The endoscopic approach to pituitary tumors has become an invaluable option to surgically manage pathology of the pituitary gland and sella.[8] Because of the critical surrounding neurovascular structures, a detailed understanding of the sella and parasellar anatomy from an endoscopic approach is imperative. Herein, we review this anatomy with emphasis on the endonasal endoscopic perspective.

## NASAL CAVITY

The nasal cavity is the passageway for airflow and forms the corridor through which pituitary pathology may be accessed. The nasal cavity is bounded by the nasal septum in the midline, the nasal turbinates laterally, the floor of the nose inferiorly, and the anterior skull base superiorly. At the posterior superior aspect of the nasal cavity lies the sphenoid ostium and just beyond, the sphenoid sinus.

The nasal septum is a midline structure, composed largely of the quadrangular cartilage, vomer, and perpendicular plate of the ethmoid, with minor contributions from the maxilla and palatine bones inferiorly. The nasal septum can be deviated to one side or the other, sometimes necessitating a limited septoplasty to facilitate access to the sella. The nasal septum and nasal cavity are lined by ciliated respiratory epithelium. It is this mucosa that covers the nasal septum that is the workhorse for local vascularized reconstruction of skull base defects. The posterior septal branch of the sphenopalatine artery is the vascular pedicle for the nasoseptal flap, but the anterior and posterior ethmoidal arteries and the labial artery anteriorly also supply blood to the nasal septum.

The turbinates lie along the lateral wall of the nasal cavity (**Fig. 1**). These structures increase the surface area of the mucosa of the nose and are thought to be involved in filtration, warming, and humidification of airflow. The bony inferior turbinate is composed of extensions of the maxillary and palatine bones, whereas the bony middle turbinate is made up of the ethmoid bone. When approaching the pituitary gland from a transnasal endoscopic approach, the middle turbinate may either be preserved by lateralization or resected to provide improved surgical access. Resection is only needed when far lateral, transpterygoid access is necessary. Consideration should be given to the risks of paradoxic congestion and potential loss of a portion of the olfactory epithelium when considering removal, and whether the benefit of improved access outweighs these potential risks.[9]

## SPHENOID SINUS

The sphenoid sinus is located at the posterior superior aspect of the nasal cavity and is the next space to traverse to reach the pituitary gland from an endoscopic approach.

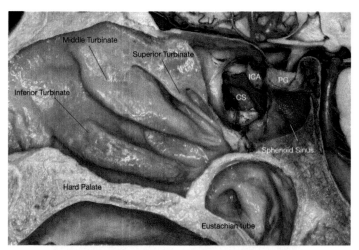

**Fig. 1.** Nasal turbinates. CS, cavernous sinus; PG, pituitary gland; ICA, internal carotid artery.

The sphenoid bone undergoes progressive pneumatization during adolescence to form the sphenoid sinus. There are different pneumatization patterns of the sphenoid sinus, which include conchal, presellar, and sellar types. A conchal sphenoid has little to no pneumatization, whereas a presellar pattern pneumatizes anterior to the plane of the tuberculum sellae, and a sellar pattern pneumatizes posterior to the plane of the tuberculum sellae. The natural opening of the sphenoid sinus is the sphenoid ostium, which is located medial to the superior turbinate in the inferomedial aspect of the sphenoethmoidal recess. In pituitary surgery, the sphenoid sinuses are widely opened to provide access and visualization of the sellar areas.

In well-pneumatized sphenoid sinuses, sellar landmarks can be easily visualized with thin layers of bone or sometimes just mucosa covering them (**Fig. 2**).[10] The sella turcica and the face of the pituitary gland are located in the center of the sphenoid. Superior to the sella turcica, the tuberculum sellae and the prechiasmatic sulcus are located. Superolateral to the sella, the optic nerves are identified. Lateral to the sella, the prominence of the paraclinoid internal carotid artery (ICA) is visualized, which runs along the roof of the cavernous sinus (CS). Between the parasellar ICA and the optic nerve in this area is often a depression called the lateral opticocarotid recess (LOCR), which represents a pneumatized optic strut of the anterior clinoid. The LOCR is essential in identifying the ICA and optic nerve right in its most susceptible point, entering the optic canal. Medially to the parasellar ICA, the middle clinoid process can be identified, as a bone depression that can vary in length and pneumatization. This landmark delimits the level of the roof of the CS and the transition between the cavernous and paraclinoid ICA segments. The depression immediately inferior to the sella is the clival recess. The paraclival segments of the ICA run lateral to the clival recess. Behind the lateral walls of the sphenoid sinus, the CS is located. In the lateral portion of the sphenoid sinus floor, the vidian nerve can be identified running in the vidian canal.

Inside the sphenoid sinus, a variable number of septa can be present. In some patients who have an Onodi cell, all relevant landmarks may not be fully located in the sphenoid sinuses. An Onodi cell is a posterior ethmoid cell that pneumatizes superolateral to the sphenoid sinus. Depending on the patient's specific anatomy, the optic nerve, OCR, and part of the sellar face may be located within the Onodi cell and not within the sphenoid sinus (**Fig. 3**).

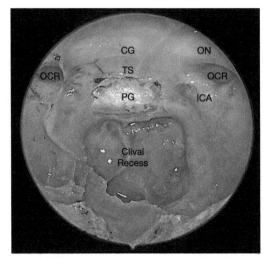

**Fig. 2.** Sellar landmarks in the sphenoid sinus. CG, chiasmatic groove; ICA, internal carotid artery; OCR, opticocarotid recess; ON, optic nerve; PG, pituitary gland; TS, tuberculum sella.

## PITUITARY GLAND

The pituitary gland is composed of 2 anatomically and functionally distinct lobes—the anterior and posterior lobes. These lobes are anatomically and functionally separate. The anterior lobe is also known as the adenohypophysis and produces and secretes prolactin, growth hormone, adrenocorticotropic hormone, thyroid-stimulating hormone, follicle-stimulating hormone, and luteinizing hormone. The posterior lobe is also called the neurohypophysis and is an extension of the hypothalamus that stores and secretes vasopressin and oxytocin. The posterior gland is thought to have a lighter, more whitish color compared with the anterior gland.

The blood supply of the anterior pituitary gland is the superior hypophyseal arteries, whereas the supply of the posterior pituitary gland is the inferior hypophyseal arteries and potentially from the superior hypophyseal system as well. The superior hypophyseal arteries arise from the medial aspect of the supraclinoidal segment of the ICA. The superior hypophyseal artery typically has 3 branches, the descending branch, which supplies the diaphragma sella[11] and the lower infundibulum; the anastomotic branch, which supplies the undersurface of the optic chiasm and the upper infundibulum; and

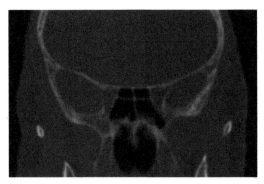

**Fig. 3.** Onodi cells.

the recurrent branch, which supplies the optic nerve. The inferior hypophyseal artery originates from the posterior bend of the cavernous ICA as a direct branch or as a branch of the meningohypophyseal trunk, which includes the dorsal meningeal artery and the tentorial artery. The inferior hypophyseal artery supplies the posterior lobe of the pituitary gland and its capsule.[12,13] Venous outflow is via a portal venous system that drains into the CS, which allows release of hypothalamic hormones to regulate anterior pituitary hormone production. The terminal hypophyseal veins drain into the CS.

The dura that covers the pituitary gland consists of 2 layers except for the lateral and superior aspects, which are composed of just one layer. The 2 layers are an inner meningeal layer and an outer periosteal layer with venous connections between the 2 CSs located between the 2 leaflets.[14] Laterally, the 2 layers separate to form different walls of the CS. The inner meningeal layer continues to hug the pituitary gland and dorsum sella and forms the medial wall of the CS. The outer layer continues laterally at the anterior aspect to form the anterior wall of the CS. Superior to the gland, the dura that forms the roof of the sella is called the diaphragma sellae and has an opening that provides passage for the infundibular stalk. There is typically no cerebrospinal fluid (CSF) within the sella because the arachnoid layer is located just above the diaphragma sellae.

## CAVERNOUS SINUS

The pituitary gland is bounded by the CSs laterally. The CS is a venous lake that contains multiple important neurovascular structures and transmits venous blood. The veins and venous spaces that the CS communicates with are numerous and include the deep middle cerebral vein; superficial sylvian vein; the superior and inferior petrosal sinuses, basilar plexus, superior and inferior ophthalmic veins; veins of foramen rotundum, foramen ovale, foramen spinosum, and the foramen of Vesalius; and the contralateral CS.[15]

### Cavernous Sinus Walls

The CS is bounded by 5 walls of dura. The walls are the anterior wall, medial wall, posterior wall, roof, and lateral wall. The roof of the CS is continuous with the roof of the sella or the diaphragma sellae, whereas the posterior wall forms a boundary with the posterior cranial fossa. The lateral wall is continuous with the outer periosteal dura of the middle fossa and is adherent with the inner meningeal layer lining the temporal lobe; it forms the lateral aspect of the CS and joins with the medial wall inferiorly at the maxillary division (V2) of the trigeminal nerve.

### Medial Wall of the Cavernous Sinus

The lateral wall of the sella is formed by the medial wall of the CS. The 2 layers of dura mater that cover the sella split in 2 at the level of the junction between the sellar floor and the carotid sulcus. The inner layer remains attached to the pituitary gland to form the medial wall of the CS, whereas the outer layer forms the anterior wall of the CS. The medial CS wall is separate from the pituitary gland by its capsule and by variable and irregular arachnoidlike bands of connective tissue. Anatomy of the medial CS wall and associated parasellar ligaments is important to understand because careful mobilization of the medial CS wall can provide access to the posterior CS wall, dura of the oculomotor triangle, and lateral interpeduncular cistern.

Four parasellar ligaments exist on the lateral aspect of the medial CS wall and are ligamentous duralike trabeculae.[14,16] These ligaments connect the medial CS wall with the ICA, anterior CS wall, the interclinoid ligament, and the anterior clinoid process (**Fig. 4**). The caroticoclinoid ligament is the strongest ligament and suspends the upper portion of the medial CS wall to the anterior ICA genu, forming the medial aspect of the proximal dural ring. The carotidoclinoid ligament joins with the interclinoid ligament to form the lateral aspect of the proximal dural ring; this is the most constant ligament, present in 97.5% of cases. The superior parasellar ligament connects the superior and posterior medial CS wall with the horizontal portion of the ICA and/or the lateral CS wall. Present in about 57% of cases, it separates the superior and inferior compartments of the CS. The inferior parasellar ligament is the first ligament to be encountered after opening the anterior CS wall; it provides an attachment from the medial CS wall to the anterior CS wall or vertical portion of the cavernous ICA and is present in 95% of cases. The posterior parasellar ligament connects the posterior aspect of the medial CS wall with the posterior aspect of the vertical portion of the cavernous ICA; it is the least constant ligament, being identified in 45% of cases. When present, it is often related to the inferior hypophyseal artery.

### Cavernous Compartments

The cavernous carotid separates the CS into 4 compartments: lateral, superior, inferior, and posterior (**Fig. 5**).[17] The lateral compartment is lateral to the horizontal segment and contains the third and fourth cranial nerves, the first division of the trigeminal nerve, and the distal cavernous segment of the abducens nerve. Moreover, branches of the inferolateral trunk can be identified in this region. The superior compartment is located between the roof of the CS superiorly and the horizontal segment of the ICA inferiorly. Three structures can be found in this compartment, the interclinoidal ligament, the dura of the oculomotor triangle, and the inferior aspect of the paraclinoidal ICA. The inferior compartment is bounded by the horizontal segment of the carotid superiorly, the anterior wall of the CS, and comprises the space located anterior to the posterior vertical carotid. This space contains the sympathetic plexus that encases the carotid as well as the abducens nerve that travels inferolateral

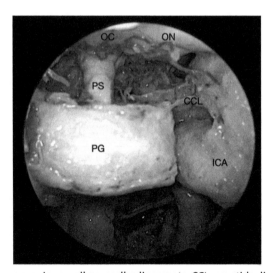

**Fig. 4.** Medial cavernous sinus wall parasellar ligaments. CCL, carotidoclinoid ligament; OC, optic chiasm; ON, optic nerve; ICA, internal carotid artery; PG, pituitary gland; PS, pituitary stalk.

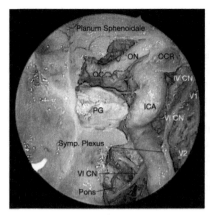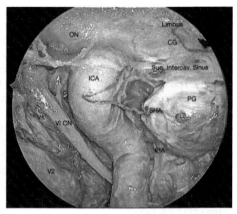

**Fig. 5.** Cavernous sinus compartments. CG, chiasmatic groove; ICA, internal carotid artery; IHA, inferior hypophyseal artery; OC, optic chiasm; OCR, opticocarotid recess; ON, optic nerve; PG, pituitary gland; SHA, superior hypophyseal artery.

to the horizontal segment. The posterior compartment is posterior to the posterior vertical ICA. This segment contains the dorsal meningeal artery and the abducens nerve as it passes through Dorello canal to enter the CS.

### Neurovascular Cavernous Sinus Contents

The ICA has 3 segments within the CS: the posterior vertical segment, horizontal segment, and anterior vertical segment or paraclinoidal segment. Separating the segments are 2 genua, the posterior and anterior genu. The branches of the ICA in the CS include the meningohypophyseal trunk and inferolateral trunk. The meningohypophyseal trunk takes off on the posterior aspect of the posterior genu and is the first branch of the cavernous carotid. The 3 branches of the meningohypophyseal trunk are the inferior hypophyseal artery, the tentorial artery, and the dorsal meningeal artery. The inferior hypophyseal artery supplies the posterior pituitary, the tentorial artery supplies the trochlear nerve and oculomotor nerve in addition to the tentorium, and the dorsal meningeal artery supplies the abducens nerve and upper clivus. The inferior lateral trunk is the second branch of the carotid in the CS and provides blood supply to the ophthalmic (V1) and maxillary (V2) branches of the trigeminal nerve. The trunk branches off the lateral or inferior aspect of the horizontal segment. The course is at first superior to the abducens and then runs between the abducens and ophthalmic division (V1) of the trigeminal nerve.

The nerves of the CS include the oculomotor, trochlear, ophthalmic division of the trigeminal nerve, abducens nerve, and sympathetic plexus. The oculomotor, trochlear, and ophthalmic divisions of the trigeminal nerve travel within the lateral CS wall, whereas the abducens nerve and sympathetic plexus run entirely within the sinus and not in a wall. After leaving the pontomedullary junction, the abducens nerve enters the dura of the clivus and continues to travel superiorly. To enter the CS, it must travel through Dorello canal and the posterior CS wall. Within the CS, it travels medially to V1 in the lateral compartment and exits at the superior orbital fissure. The oculomotor nerve exits the midbrain and courses anteriorly between the posterior cerebral artery and the superior cerebellar artery. At the oculomotor triangle, the oculomotor nerve enters the roof of the CS at the posterior aspect. The oculomotor triangle is defined by the anterior and posterior petroclinoidal folds and the interclinoidal fold. The interclinoidal fold runs between the anterior and posterior clinoids, whereas the posterior fold runs between the petrous apex and the posterior clinoid and the anterior fold runs between the petrous apex and the anterior clinoid. The oculomotor nerve runs in the oculomotor cistern, just parallel and lateral to the interclinoidal fold. The oculomotor cistern is a CSF-filled space that is variable in size and is formed by a small cuff of arachnoid-lined dura that runs with the oculomotor nerve as it enters the oculomotor triangle. The end of the cistern is the clinoidal triangle, which is at the anterior aspect of the roof. Here, the oculomotor nerve enters and travels in the lateral CS wall and exits at the superior orbital fissure. Similarly, the trochlear nerve travels in the lateral CS wall, by first entering the oculomotor triangle at the confluence of the anterior and posterior clinoidal folds. The ophthalmic division of the trigeminal nerve travels inferior to the trochlear nerve in the lateral wall. The relationships of the neural structures in the lateral wall form the supratrochlear triangle bounded by the oculomotor and trochlear nerves and the infratrochlear triangle bounded by the trochlear nerve and V1.

## SUPRASELLAR SPACE

Superior to the sella is the suprasellar space, which can house extensions of pituitary or pituitary stalk lesions (**Fig. 6**). This space starts at the diaphragma sella and extends superior to the floor of the third ventricle; it is divided into 3 sections: the infrachiasmatic, retrochiasmatic, and suprachiasmatic spaces. For surgical access, the posterior planum sphenoidale, prechiasmatic sulcus, and tuberculum sellae may either all, or selectively, need to be removed.

The infrachiasmatic space is composed of the inferior aspect of the optic chiasm and infundibulum. From the optic chiasm, the optic nerves continue in an anterior and lateral direction through the optic canal. Posterior to the infundibulum is the membrane of Liliequist, whereas suprasellar cistern arachnoid covers the infundibulum anteriorly. Branches of the supraclinoidal carotid artery course through this space. The first branch of the supraclinoidal carotid is the ophthalmic artery, which enters the optic canal inferior to the optic nerve. The next branch that arises from the supraclinoidal carotid is the superior hypophyseal artery.[18]

Superior to the optic chiasm is the suprachiasmatic space. Immediately superior to the chiasm are olfactory striae, divisions of the olfactory tract running above each

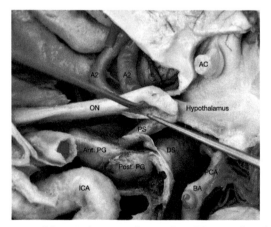

**Fig. 6.** Suprasellar space. AC, anterior commissure; Ant. PG, anterior pituitary gland; BA, basilar artery; DS, diaphragma sella; ICA, internal carotid artery, ON, optic nerve; PCA, posterior cerebral artery; Post. PG, posterior pituitary gland; PS, pituitary stalk.

optic nerve. Also, running just above the optic chiasm are the A1 segments of the anterior cerebral arteries and the anterior communicating artery. The anterior cerebral arteries continue as the A2 segments and enter the interhemispheric fissure. Two arterial branches that occupy this space are the recurrent artery of Heubner, which arise from the A1-A2 junction and travel to the anterior perforated substance, and the fronto-orbital artery, which is the first branch of the A2 segment.

The retrochiasmatic space is bounded anteriorly by the infundibulum and posteriorly by the cerebral peduncles and posterior perforated substance. The superior limit is the floor of the third ventricle. The Liliequist membrane is an arachnoid membrane that is a route for access to the interpeduncular cistern. In the interpeduncular cistern, the posterior communicating arteries run in the lateral recess and the basilar apex is at the posterior aspect.

## SUMMARY

The endoscopic approach has been established as a safe and effective approach to the surgical management of pituitary pathology. A comprehensive understanding of the endoscopic anatomy of this surgical corridor is imperative to fully realize the benefits of increased patient safety and decreased patient morbidity.

## CLINICS CARE POINTS

- As endoscopic sinus surgery was being widely adopted, the early 1990s was the time of application of the endoscope to the anterior skull base for benign pathology, specifically the pituitary gland.

- At present, the endoscopic approach has been established as a safe and effective approach to the surgical management of pituitary pathology.

- Because of its critical surrounding neurovascular structures, a detailed understanding of the sella and parasellar anatomy from an endoscopic approach is imperative to performing safe endoscopic surgery in this area.

## REFERENCES

1. Freda PU, Post KD. Differential diagnosis of sellar masses. Endocrinol Metab Clin North Am 1999;28(1):81–117.
2. Asa SL. Tumors of the pituitary gland. Amer Registry of Pathology; 1998.
3. Levy A. Pituitary disease: presentation, diagnosis, and management. J Neurol Neurosurg Psychiatr 2004;75(suppl 3):iii47–52.
4. Kim SH, Lee KC, Kim SH. Cranial nerve palsies accompanying pituitary tumour. J Clin Neurosci 2007;14(12):1158–62.
5. Liu JK, Das K, Weiss MH, et al. The history and evolution of transsphenoidal surgery. J Neurosurg 2001;95(6):1083–96.
6. Jankowski R, Auque J, Simon C, et al. How i do it: Head and neck and plastic surgery: Endoscopic pituitary tumor surgery. The Laryngoscope 1992;102(2): 198–202.
7. Carrau RL, Jho HD, Ko Y. Transnasal-transsphenoidal endoscopic surgery of the pituitary gland. Laryngoscope 1996;106(7):914–8.
8. Tabaee A, Anand VK, Barrón Y, et al. Endoscopic pituitary surgery: a systematic review and meta-analysis. J Neurosurg 2009;111(3):545–54.

9. Choby GW, Hobson CE, Lee S, et al. Clinical effects of middle turbinate resection after endoscopic sinus surgery: a systematic review. Am J rhinology Allergy 2014;28(6):502–7.

10. Rhoton AL. Anatomy of the pituitary gland and sellar region. In: Thapar, et al, editors. Diagnosis and management of pituitary tumors. Totowa, NJ: Springer; 2001. p. 13–40.

11. Campero A, Martins C, Yasuda A, et al. Microsurgical anatomy of the diaphragma sellae and its role in directing the pattern of growth of pituitary adenomas. Neurosurgery 2008;62(3):717–23.

12. Reisch R, Vutskits L, Patonay L, et al. The meningohypophyseal trunk and its blood supply to different intracranial structures. Minim Invasive Neurosurg 1996;39(03):78–81.

13. Fernandez-Miranda JC, Gardner PA, Rastelli MM, et al. Endoscopic endonasal transcavernous posterior clinoidectomy with interdural pituitary transposition. J Neurosurg 2014;121(1):91–9.

14. Truong HQ, Lieber S, Najera E, et al. The medial wall of the cavernous sinus. Part 1: Surgical anatomy, ligaments, and surgical technique for its mobilization and/or resection. J Neurosurg 2018;131(1):122–30.

15. Harris FS, Rhoton AL. Anatomy of the cavernous sinus: a microsurgical study. J Neurosurg 1976;45(2):169–80.

16. Cohen-Cohen S, Gardner PA, Alves-Belo JT, et al. The medial wall of the cavernous sinus. Part 2: Selective medial wall resection in 50 pituitary adenoma patients. J Neurosurg 2018;131(1):131–40.

17. Fernandez-Miranda JC, Zwagerman NT, Abhinav K, et al. Cavernous sinus compartments from the endoscopic endonasal approach: anatomical considerations and surgical relevance to adenoma surgery. J Neurosurg 2017;129(2):430–41.

18. Truong HQ, Najera E, Zanabria-Ortiz R, et al. Surgical anatomy of the superior hypophyseal artery and its relevance for endoscopic endonasal surgery. J Neurosurg 2018;131(1):154–62.

# Preoperative Workup for Patients with Pituitary Lesions

Alexandra White, MA[a], Erion Junior de Andrade, MD[a,b],
Varun R. Kshettry, MD[a,b], Raj Sindwani, MD[a,b,c],
Pablo F. Recinos, MD[a,b,c],*

## KEYWORDS

- Macroadenoma • Microadenoma • Meningioma • Hypopituitarism
- Craniopharyngioma • Functional pituitary tumors

## KEY POINTS

- The preoperative assessment of pituitary lesions is of utmost importance as it impacts indications for surgery, preoperative optimization, and perioperative management.
- Key steps in the assessment of pituitary lesions include a thorough history and physical examination to identify any symptoms related to mass effect or hormonal imbalance, brain magnetic resonance imaging and additional imaging if needed, formal vision testing if needed, and a laboratory assessment of pituitary hormone function to screen for underproduction or overproduction of hormones.
- Despite recent pharmacologic and radiotherapy advances, surgery remains the treatment of choice for most pituitary adenomas and other tumors involving the sellar region.

## INTRODUCTION

Despite its small size, the pituitary gland exerts regulatory control over virtually all organ systems in the body. This prominent role is even more evident when its function is disrupted. Some neoplasms produce hormones at pathologic levels (functional pituitary adenomas), resulting in classical clinical syndromes. Other tumors are hormonally inactive (eg, nonfunctioning pituitary adenomas, craniopharyngiomas, meningiomas, ectopic germinomas) but can become symptomatic due to local mass effect. Sellar

[a] Department of Neurological Surgery, Cleveland Clinic Lerner College of Medicine of Case Western Reserve University, 9500 Euclid Avenue, CA-51, Cleveland, OH 44195, USA; [b] Section of Skull Base Surgery, Rose Ella Burkhardt Brain Tumor and Neuro-Oncology Center, Neurological Institute, Cleveland Clinic, 9500 Euclid Avenue, CA-51, Cleveland, OH 44195, USA; [c] Section of Rhinology, Sinus, & Skull Base Surgery, Head and Neck Institute, Cleveland Clinic, 9500 Euclid Avenue, CA-51, Cleveland, OH 44195, USA
* Corresponding author. 9500 Euclid Avenue, CA-51, Cleveland, OH 44195.
*E-mail address:* recinop@ccf.org

Otolaryngol Clin N Am 55 (2022) 233–246
https://doi.org/10.1016/j.otc.2021.12.001
0030-6665/22/© 2022 Elsevier Inc. All rights reserved.
oto.theclinics.com

and parasellar tumors form a unique group of intracranial neoplasms, whose management is influenced by endocrinological, oncological, and neurologic aspects. Despite
recent advances in pharmacology and radiotherapy, surgery remains the treatment of
choice for most pituitary adenomas and other tumors involving the sellar space.[1–3]

The therapeutic approach differs according to whether the aim of the treatment is to
control hormone hypersecretion (functional microadenoma), to reduce tumor volume,
and alleviate mass effect (nonfunctional pituitary macroadenoma, craniopharyngiomas, meningiomas, and so forth), or both (functional macroadenoma). In most secretory pituitary adenomas, with the exception of prolactinomas, surgery is the initial
treatment of choice. In cases whereby remission is not achieved with surgery, adjunctive treatment is needed.[1–3] Medical therapy and radiotherapy/radiosurgery are adjuvant options. Radiotherapy options, in particular, can result in panhypopituitarism.
Given the importance of understanding the baseline pretreatment pituitary function
as well as diagnosing functional adenomas, the preoperative assessment of pituitary
lesions is essential. In this paper, we aim to provide a background on the function of
the pituitary gland, common pituitary lesions, and their clinical presentations, as well
as a summary of the history and physical, laboratory testing, and imaging required for
the workup of these lesions.

### Background

#### Differential diagnosis of pituitary lesions

While pituitary adenomas are by far the most common intrasellar tumors, there are a
number of differential diagnoses that must be considered when a patient presents with
a pituitary lesion.[4] In the case of cystic, purely intrasellar lesions, Rathke's cleft cysts,
and arachnoid cysts are the most common. Less commonly, dermoid or epidermoid
cysts can form in this area.[5] Craniopharyngiomas have purely cystic, solid, and mixed
forms. Their exact location is most commonly suprasellar, arising from the infundibulum with possible extension into the third ventricle, but they can also be purely intrasellar or parasellar.[6–8] Pituitary carcinomas are defined by the presence of metastasis
and represent only 0.1% of pituitary tumors. Other tumors that can arise in the immediate vicinity of the sellar region include meningiomas, chordomas, and chondromas/
chondrosarcomas, but these usually show a distinct growth pattern and can be differentiated radiographically from the pituitary gland.[9] These tumors also have a different
clinical and hormonal presentation that will be discussed further in specific sections.

#### Pituitary Physiology

The pituitary gland consists of 2 components—anterior and posterior, which have
distinct embryologic origins, structure, and function.[10] The anterior pituitary (adenohypophysis) originates from Rathke's pouch, a component of oral ectoderm that invag-
inates into the sella turcica on contact with neuroectoderm.[1,11] Rathke's pouch
ultimately closes, separating itself from oral ectoderm.[10] The anterior pituitary contains 5 cell types, each of which produces a trophic hormone, which in turn acts on
a downstream endocrine gland in the body to regulate hormone production.[12] The pituitary hormones and functions are summarized in **Table 1**.[13] These hormones are
produced by distinct cell types that usually respect a characteristic topological
arrangement, with somatotrophs occupying the anterior portion of the lateral glandular
wing, lactotrophs the posterior face of this lateral wing, and corticotrophs its central
portion.[1] Knowledge of this arrangement becomes useful to the neurosurgeon when
looking for a microadenoma. Pituitary hormones are produced in response to trophic
hormones released by the hypothalamus, which are delivered to the pituitary via the
hypothalamic-hypophyseal portal system in the pituitary stalk. Uniquely, prolactin

| Table 1<br>Summary of pituitary hormones and their functions | | | |
|---|---|---|---|
| **Hormone** | **Target Organ** | **Hormone Function** | **Metabolic Function** |
| ACTH | Adrenal Gland | Cortisol Secretion | Metabolism regulation; resistance to physiologic stress; maintenance of vascular tone |
| GH | Liver and Skeleton | IGF-1 secretion (from liver); growth and regulation of nutrient metabolism | GH stimulates growth, IGF-1 is primary effector of growth |
| LH/FSH | Ovaries/Testes | Testosterone or estrogen/progesterone secretion | Fertility, secondary sexual characteristics, and bone density |
| Prolactin | Breast, Ovaries/Testes | Lactation, gonadal inhibition | Breast milk production, Testosterone/Estrogen/Progesterone inhibition |
| TSH | Thyroid | T3/T4 secretion | Metabolism regulation |

*Abbreviations:* ACTH, adrenocorticotropic hormone; GH, growth hormone; LH, luteinizing hormone; FSH, follicle-stimulating hormone; TSH, thyrotropin; IGF-1, insulin growth factor-1.

(PRL) secretion is under tonic inhibitory control by dopamine, which is also delivered via the pituitary stalk. The secretion of pituitary hormones is tightly controlled by the hypothalamus, from negative feedback via downstream organs, and complex biochemical and neural input. Neoplastic transformation is far more common in the anterior pituitary, with pituitary adenomas being most common.[14]

The posterior pituitary (neurohypophysis) is derived from the downgrowth of the diverticulum of the floor of the third ventricle. The posterior pituitary contains the axonal terminals of 2 types of hypothalamic neurons, which release vasopressin (a.k.a antidiuretic hormone) and oxytocin.[10] Vasopressin plays a key role in maintaining serum osmolality, while oxytocin is important in lactation and labor, as well as emotional bonding, stress response, and regulation of other social behaviors. Primary tumors of the neurohypophysis are rare, and are usually hamartomas, gliomas, or granular cell tumors.[15] Notably, intrasellar, nondural-based metastases are usually found in the neurohypophysis.[15]

Altogether, the hormones produced by the pituitary gland are essential for sodium and water regulation, hemodynamic stability, reproduction, growth, cardiac function, and metabolism.[1,10]

### History and Physical Examination

Although pituitary lesions are often asymptomatic, they can cause significant neurologic and endocrine dysfunction due to mass effect on surrounding structures, including the pituitary gland and the optic chiasm. Common presenting symptoms of pituitary adenomas include headache, visual loss, and hypopituitarism. These symptoms are largely dependent on tumor size and local invasion, as well as the hormone-secreting profile of the tumor cells.[1,11,14] Pituitary tumors usually have a slow growth pattern; however, they may present with more acute symptoms (eg, neuropathies related to cranial nerves in the cavernous sinus) indicative of more aggressive behavior as the tumor grows out of the sella and compresses the surrounding structures.[3] On physical examination, a comprehensive cranial nerve evaluation with particular focus on visual acuity, visual fields, extraocular movements, and facial sensation is essential. This is typically done in conjunction with a neuro-ophthalmologist. A thorough nasal endoscopic evaluation also assists in surgical planning both for structural evaluation and to rule out any underlying sinus infection.

## Ophthalmologic Symptoms

Generally, patients with large tumors extending superiorly have symptoms resulting from mass effect on the optic chiasm.[16,17]

## Bitemporal Hemianopsia

The most common chiasmal syndrome associated with pituitary adenomas is bitemporal hemianopsia.[1,16,17] This is a visual field deficit in which bilateral vision in the temporal fields is affected, leaving only the nasal fields to be perceived. This usually occurs when the tumor displaces the visual pathways by more than 3 mm (**Fig. 1**). Visual deficits associated with pituitary lesions depend on the suprasellar extension, lesion volume, and location of the lesion, as well as the position of the chiasm as it relates to the sella turcica.[10,17]

## Other Visual Abnormalities

Pituitary adenomas and other lesions of the sellar and suprasellar region may lead to a wide range of visual disturbances, including monocular or homonymous defects as well. In a study by Lee and Colleagues, 40 of 89 patients (44.9%) with visual field defects secondary to pituitary macroadenoma had nontemporal defects.[16] Thus, it is relatively common to have extrachiasmal optic pathway involvement along with compression of the chiasm, rather than just chiasm compression alone. Any pattern of vision loss is possible, as asymmetric loss results from chiasm ischemia produced by vessel occlusion.[16] The visual abnormality (optic nerve, chiasm, or tract deficit) is correlated with the innate anatomy of the chiasm, with a prefixed chiasm lesion more likely to result in a tract deficit and a postfixed chiasm lesion more likely to result in nerve/monocular vision loss.

## Cranial Nerve Palsies

An understanding of the anatomy of the sellar region can help clarify the most common presenting symptoms of pituitary lesions. The pituitary gland is located in the sella turcica in the anterior skull base, wrapped in dura, which forms the diaphragma sellae overlying the gland. The dural anatomy of this region is covered by a double layer of dura with the exception of its lateral wall, which is flanked bilaterally by the single-layered medial wall of the cavernous sinus which makes those regions less resistant and prone to tumor extension.[18–20]

With lateral (parasellar) growth of pituitary tumors and cavernous sinus invasion, the tumor can cause compression or invasion of the cavernous sinuses, sometimes affecting cranial nerves III, IV, VI, V1, and V2 (**Fig. 2**). Thus, compression or invasion of the cavernous sinus can result in oculomotor palsies, as well as facial numbness in the V1 and V2 distribution.[20] A thorough neurologic examination can help identify cranial nerve palsies. Aside from cranial nerve palsies, the patient may present with diplopia and postganglionic Horner syndrome.[1] Notably, it is not common for slow, growing benign tumors to cause cranial neuropathies despite invading the cavernous sinus, whereas malignant tumors or inflammatory processes involving the cavernous sinus are much more likely to cause precipitous cranial neuropathies.

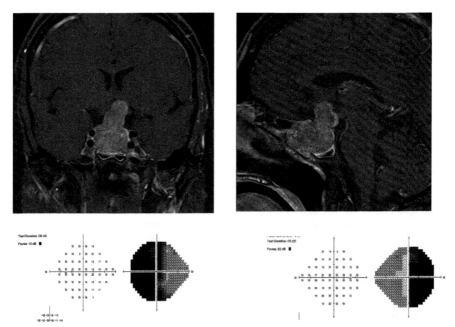

**Fig. 1.** Coronal and Sagittal T1 postcontrast MRI of a patient with progressive loss of vision, especially in the lateral fields. Humphrey visual field test showing complete bitemporal defects (bitemporal hemianopsia).

### Neurologic Symptoms

Headaches occur in 10% to 40% of patients due to the stretching of the diaphragma sellae and adjacent dural structures. Headaches related to sellar pathologies are more likely to be unilateral, retro-orbital, and neuralgiform in nature. However, many incidental sellar pathologies may be discovered in the setting of imaging for distinct headache syndromes such as migraines, cluster, and tension headaches among others. Female patients are more likely to experience headaches. Intracranial pressure is generally normal. When there is the elevation of intracranial pressure, it is likely secondary to compression of the third ventricle. This results in obstructive hydrocephalus and leads to nausea, vomiting, and headache, all of which are more severe in the morning.[11,14,21]

Rarely, the extension of the mass into cerebral structures can result in hypothalamic obesity or frontal syndrome (disinhibition, presence of primitive reflexes, executive dysfunction). Disruption of the hypothalamus by a tumor can lead to the dysregulation of sleep, appetite, and temperature, as well as autonomic dysfunction.[1]

### Endocrine Symptoms

Pituitary disorders can be broadly categorized into disorders of overproduction by a functional tumor and underproduction or disruption of normal inhibitory pathways due to mass effect from a nonfunctional tumor.[10] In addition, family history is an important component of the interview as it can help address the risk of multiple endocrine neoplasia-1, a hereditary syndrome characterized by pituitary adenomas, parathyroid hyperplasia, and pancreatic neuroendocrine tumors.[11,14]

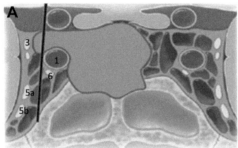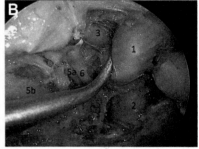

Fig. 2. (A) Artist's drawing showing the parasellar growth of a pituitary tumor above the right parasellar internal carotid artery (ICA) (1) into the cavernous sinus (CS) and its relationship with the nerves in the CS: Oculomotor nerve (3), Abducens (6), V1 (5a) and V2 (5b). *Copyright Center for Art and Photography, Cleveland Clinic Foundation.* (B) Endoscopic view of anatomic dissection of the right cavernous sinus showing the relationship of the cavernous ICA (1) with the abducens nerve (6), the only nerve that is in fact inside the cavernous sinus, and the nerves on the lateral wall of the cavernous sinus: oculomotor (3), V1 segment of the trigeminal nerve (5a) that runs immediately lateral to the abducens and the V2 segment (5b). Copyright Cleveland Clinic Skull Base Laboratory.

### Hypopituitarism

The most frequent symptoms of hypopituitarism are asthenia, reduced libido, impotence, and menstrual disorders (present in 50% of cases). The gonadal axis is the most affected (77%), followed by adrenal and thyroid hormones (28% and 22%). Growth hormone (GH) secretion has been reported to be compromised in up to 77% of patients. It should be noted that patients are often asymptomatic or have mild symptoms, which prevents them from seeking care. Hypocortisolism is potentially the most life-threatening pituitary insufficiency given the key role of cortisol in maintaining mean arterial pressure, especially under stress such as surgery or critical illness.[22]

### Hyperprolactinemia

Prolactin excess can result in infertility and symptoms of hypogonadism in both sexes, as well as galactorrhea in women and gynecomastia in men.[3] In addition, mild hyperprolactinemia can be the result of mass effect, as compression of the pituitary stalk interrupts the tonic inhibition of PRL secretion by dopamine. Elevated PRL can also be caused by pregnancy, polycystic ovarian syndrome, hypothyroidism, and prolactin-elevating drugs (eg, antipsychotics), so obtaining a thorough history is important.[23]

### Acromegaly

Excess GH and consequently elevated insulin-like growth factor-1 (IGF-1) causes gigantism when the hormonal excess occurs before the fusion of the long bone epiphysis. In adults, GH excess results in the enlargement of hands and feet, frontal bossing, jaw enlargement, as well as heart failure, obstructive sleep apnea, hypertension, and insulin resistance.[11]

### Cushing Syndrome

Hypercortisolism secondary to adrenocorticotropic hormone (ACTH) production by a pituitary adenoma is termed Cushing's disease, which is the most common cause of endogenous excess cortisol. It can present with weight gain (especially in the neck and face), fatigue, hypertension, skin fragility (accompanied by characteristic purple striae), diabetes, myopathy, and osteoporosis.

### Hyperthyroidism

Secondary hyperthyroidism is a rare cause of excess thyroid hormone. It can result in weight loss, tachycardia and tachyarrhythmias, insomnia, and heat intolerance.[22]

### Diabetes Insipidus

Central diabetes insipidus (DI) is the result of a lack of vasopressin release by the posterior pituitary. This leads to elevated urine output and hypernatremia that is correctable via the administration of vasopressin.[3] It is unusual for DI to be a presenting sign of benign pathology. Thus, patients with DI at presentation should be worked-up for other pathologies, such as inflammatory disorders, more aggressive tumors such as craniopharyngioma, and malignancies.[4]

### Laboratory Testing

The first step in biochemical workup is to differentiate between adenomas and nonadenomas. If the tumor is not a pituitary adenoma, key goals in the workup are to evaluate for hypopituitarism, replace hormones as necessary, and determine the need for perioperative stress dose corticosteroids. If the tumor is a pituitary adenoma, the key step is to identify if it is secreting or nonfunctional by ordering a pituitary hormone panel (**Table 2**). Another important step is to assess for hypopituitarism by evaluating adrenal function (morning serum cortisol), thyroid function (Free T4, thyroid-stimulating hormone (TSH)), gonadal function (luteinizing hormone (LH)/follicle-stimulating hormone (FSH), testosterone, or estradiol), GH and its downstream hormone IGF-1, and serum PRL as depicted in **Table 2**. In the case of pituitary–adrenal axis investigation, 2 out of 3 positive screening tests (24-h urinary-free cortisol (UFC), midnight salivary cortisol, and overnight low dose dexamethasone suppression test) will confirm hypercortisolism.

### Tumor-Specific Diagnostic Workup

The surgical evaluation and management of a pituitary lesion on magnetic resonance imaging (MRI) depend on its functional status and clinical presentation (**Fig. 3**).

### Cushing's Disease

Cushing's disease is a clinical syndrome of hypercortisolism produced by an ACTH producing pituitary adenoma, also called corticotropic adenoma.[11,23] Corticotropic adenomas comprise 15% of pituitary adenomas, with 20% of these lacking clinical evidence of Cushing's syndrome.

The first step in the assessment of Cushing's disease is the confirmation of Cushing's syndrome (hypercortisolism). As mentioned above, the patient with clinical suspicion of hypercortisolism should be screened and positive in 2 of 3 tests: 24-h UFC, midnight salivary cortisol, and low-dose dexamethasone suppression test. With the confirmation of Cushing's syndrome, the next step is to determine whether it is ACTH-dependent or ACTH-independent. If ACTH-dependent Cushing syndrome is confirmed, Cushing's disease is the most common cause.[25] Given that the focus of this article is workup of known pituitary lesions, it is worth mentioning that Cushing's disease can occur despite a nonvisible radiographic lesion, which is termed MRI-negative Cushing's disease.[25] However, this entity and its workup are beyond the scope of this article.

| Table 2 Pituitary hormone panel to evaluate the five hormonal axes of pituitary function | |
|---|---|
| Hormone | Laboratory Test |
| TSH | TSH, free T4 |
| ACTH | Morning Cortisol Salivary Cortisol Fasting AM Cortisol 24-h Urinary-Free Cortisol Dexamethasone Suppression Test |
| GH | Morning GH IGF-1 |
| LH/FSH | Male: Testosterone Female: Estradiol, Progesterone |
| Prolactin | Prolactin |

If a patient has an incidentally discovered pituitary lesion on magnetic resonance imaging (pituitary incidentaloma), it should be evaluated if it is greater than 1 cm in size. If is it less than 1 cm, only prolactin can be measured unless the patient is exhibiting clinical symptoms, as was demonstrated in a cost-effectiveness analysis[24]

## ACROMEGALY

Acromegaly is a clinical syndrome of elevation of GH and IGF-1 produced by a GH-secreting pituitary adenoma, also known as somatotrophic adenoma.[26] Acromegaly usually presents in patients 40 to 60 years of age and is associated with high morbidity and mortality when untreated due to cardiovascular complications, such as systemic hypertension, cardiomyopathy, and cerebrovascular disease.[1,11,22,26]

The first step in the assessment of acromegaly is the confirmation of elevated GH and IGF-1. Random serum GH levels are rarely useful due to high variability, so a serum IGF-1 and an Oral Glucose Tolerance Test (OGTT) are the most commonly used examinations. A diagnosis of acromegaly necessitates a demonstration of lack of GH suppression to <1 ng/mL after the oral ingestion of 75 g of glucose. In addition, elevated serum IGF-1 levels are generally indicative of active acromegaly, except in patients with poorly controlled diabetes, elderly patients, and patients with evidence of starvation, all of whom have reduced IGF-1 production).[11,23,26]

## PROLACTINOMAS

Prolactinomas (a.k.a. lactotrophic adenomas or PRL-secreting pituitary adenomas) represent 30% to 50% of pituitary adenomas and are thus the most common type of functioning pituitary adenoma.[23,27,28]

A key step in investigating hyperprolactinemia is discerning between a prolactinoma and stalk compression (effect), that is the loss of negative feedback by dopamine on PRL secretion, which is delivered through the pituitary stalk (Table 3). Serum PRL levels can help rule out both a prolactinoma and investigate potential stalk compression. Serum PRL greater than 200 is essentially diagnostic of a macroprolactinoma, and PRL less than 80 excludes the diagnosis of macroprolactinoma (Table 4). This is a key step, given that prolactinomas may be treated medically with dopamine agonists, making them unique among pituitary tumors. Another important laboratory scenario is the Hook effect, in which high levels of PRL binding to laboratory antibodies result in clumping and thus interfere with results, leading to false negatives or

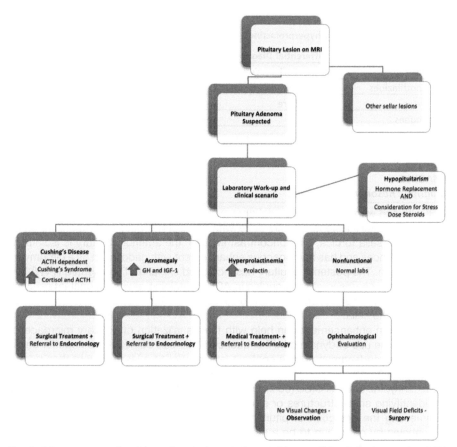

**Fig. 3.** Management algorithm of a pituitary lesion and its possible clinical scenarios. MRI, magnetic resonance imaging; ACTH, adrenocorticotropic hormone; GH, growth hormone; IGF-1, insulin growth factor-1.

inaccurately low results, an issue that can be resolved by diluting the blood sample. Today, this is done automatically by most laboratories.[3,27]

## RARE FUNCTIONING ADENOMAS

Usually, tumors arising from TSH- or LH/FSH-secreting cell lineages are clinically silent, but they can occasionally cause symptoms due to oversecretion. Replacement of each hormonal axis affected by the adenoma (TS4/T4/testosterone/estrogen) should be performed and medically managed if necessary.[14,29]

## NONFUNCTIONING ADENOMAS

Nonfunctioning pituitary adenomas make up most pituitary tumors and generally present with mass effect symptoms, such as visual disturbances or cranial nerve palsies. The hormonal workup is mainly the assessment of pituitary function to rule out hypopituitarism as mentioned above.[24]

| Table 3 Differential diagnosis for hyperprolactinemia | | | |
| --- | --- | --- | --- |
| Differential Diagnosis for Elevated Prolactin | | | |
| **Drugs** | **Metabolic Disorders** | **Tumors** | **Miscellaneous** |
| Phenothiazines | Kidney Failure | Craniopharyngioma | Sarcoidosis |
| Opiates | Liver Failure | Sellar/Suprasellar tumors | Tuberculosis |
| Estrogens | | Spinal Cord tumors | Histiocytosis |
| Antihypertensives | | | |

## IMAGING
### Magnetic Resonance Imaging

MRI with and without gadolinium enhancement is the gold standard radiological evaluation of pituitary lesions, usually done with thin cuts (1 mm) and magnified views through the sella turcica. On noncontrast images, the anterior pituitary is isointense on all sequences and has homogenous enhancement with gadolinium as a circumventricular organ. The posterior pituitary has increased signal on T1-weighted (T1W) MRI (representing neurosecretory granules in ADH-containing axons). Signal intensity on MRI will assist in distinguishing lesions originating from the pituitary gland from lesions occupying the sella.[10,11,22]

Gadolinium enhancement can help with the visualization of pituitary microadenomas. With the use of dynamic MRI sequences, one can demonstrate superior sensitivity as microadenomas uptake contrast later and/or to a lesser extent than normal pituitary tissue.[30,31]

Recently, the utility of CISS (constructive interference in steady state, which is useful for identifying small structures or structures surrounded by CSF) MRI sequences in augmenting the detection of pituitary adenomas in patients with Cushing disease was shown by our group to be a useful adjuvant to T1W pituitary protocols and an appropriate alternative for patients with gadolinium contraindications.[32] CISS sequences can also be used to determine the extent of parasellar invasion for macroadenomas, especially into the cavernous sinus with better correlation with intraoperative findings than T1W with gradient-echo techniques.[19]

## COMPUTED TOMOGRAPHY

Computed tomography (CT) or magnetic resonance (MR) angiography is used to rule out a parasellar aneurysm and chart the course of the internal carotid arteries. It is important to obtain these images with the goal of using intraoperative navigation. CT scan also be an important tool in the evaluation of cystic masses as it displays calcifications that can help differentiate from other sellar/suprasellar lesions as craniopharyngiomas that more commonly present with calcifications.[8,33,34] Thin-cut CT sella protocol is also an imaging option for patients who cannot undergo MRIs.

### Anesthesia Considerations

#### Central adrenal insufficiency
Patients with hypopituitarism may present with undiagnosed central hypercortisolism and/or hypothyroidism that needs hormonal repletion preoperatively to avoid life-threatening adrenal insufficiency that may present with hypotension or even cardiovascular shock.[22,35,36] Patients with proven ACTH deficiency preoperatively (based on response to ACTH test) should have supraphysiological glucocorticoid therapy

| Table 4 | |
| --- | --- |
| Correlation between Serum Prolactin Levels and MRI findings | |
| Prolactin Levels (ng/mL) | MRI Findings |
| <25 | Normal |
| 25–100 | Adenomas in 50% of patients |
| 100–200 | Adenomas in 75% of patients |
| >200 | Adenomas in 100% of patients |
| >1000 | Invasive Adenoma (especially Cavernous sinus) |

preoperatively (eg, stress dose hydrocortisone) to prevent adrenal insufficiency that may lead to hypotension and shock.[3,37]

### Central Hypothyroidism

Patients with hypothyroidism should receive hormone repletion if they have moderate hypothyroidism (elevated TSH and T4 >5ug/dL) before surgery. In cases of severe hypothyroidism (myxedematous coma or free T4 <0.5 ng/dL), patients should be put on hormone replacement therapy immediately with intravenous levothyroxine if surgery is urgent. Patients with severe hypothyroidism are at increased risk of cardiovascular complications, including reduced cardiac output (by as much as 30%–50%), intraoperative hypotension, coronary events, bradycardia, arrhythmias, and prolonged QT interval resulting in ventricular tachycardia and Torsades de Pointes.[35,38]

### SLEEP APNEA

Obstructive sleep apnea syndrome is characterized by recurrent episodes of partial or complete obstruction of the upper airway during sleep and its incidence in patients with acromegaly ranges from 45% to 80%.[39,40] The proliferation of soft tissue in the upper airway contributes to airway narrowing and may lead to partial or complete airway obstruction during sleep, especially at the level of the oropharynx.[40] These subsets of patients are vulnerable to the development of respiratory obstruction and postoperative respiratory failure. Thus, spirometry and indirect laryngoscopy have a central role in the preoperative evaluation of the respiratory and airway dynamics to formulate a plan for difficult airway management.[39] Awake oral fiberoptic intubation is indicated in patients with high Friedman score (difficult airway) and sedation premedication is usually avoided. In addition, the assessment of the need to resume postoperative continuous positive airway pressure (CPAP) devices can impact the decision on intraoperative reconstruction.

### SUMMARY

Pituitary tumors require a multidisciplinary care approach. Detailed preoperative workup can help minimize complications and maximize optimal therapeutic outcomes with sustained results. Active collaboration between the neurosurgeons, otorhinolaryngologists, endocrinologists, ophthalmologists, anesthesiologists, and pathologists is important. When evaluating a patient with pituitary tumors, the team must understand the clinical presentation, physical examination, and broad endocrine manifestations corresponding with the various clinicopathological entities. It is also important to differentiate between the management of nonfunctional adenomas and functional adenomas and how they differ in perioperative assessment to optimize patient outcomes.

## CLINICS CARE POINTS

- Differentiating between pituitary adenomas and nonadenoma pituitary lesions is a key first step in the workup of pituitary lesions.

- Presenting symptoms of pituitary lesions include hormone under- or over-production, visual field abnormalities, and symptoms related to neoplasm mass effect.

- Evaluating patients for hypopituitarism, repleting hormones if necessary, and determining a need for perioperative stress-dose steroids are key steps in the workup of all pituitary masses.

- If the patient has an adenoma, additional biochemical workup must be conducted to identify the cell lineage giving rise to the tumor and to determine its function.

- MRI is the primary imaging modality for the evaluation of pituitary lesions.

## REFERENCES

1. Alencastro LC, et al. Chapter 46: Adenomas Hipofisarios. In: Siqueira MG, editor. *Tratado de Neurocirurgia SBN.* 1st ed. Manole; 2016. p. 435–57.
2. De Divitiis E, Cavallo LM, Cappabianca P, et al. Extended endoscopic endonasal transsphenoidal approach for the removal of suprasellar tumors: Part 2. Neurosurgery 2007;60(1):46–58.
3. Pereira O, Bevan JS. Preoperative assessment for pituitary surgery. Pituitary 2008;11(4):347–51.
4. Hlaváč M, Sommer F, Karpel-Massler G, et al. Differential diagnosis and treatment of pituitary adenomas. HNO 2019;67(4):307–18.
5. Vaz-Guimaraes F, Koutourousiou M, de Almeida JR, et al. Endoscopic endonasal surgery for epidermoid and dermoid cysts: a 10-year experience. J Neurosurg 2019;130(2):368–78.
6. Radovanovic I, Dehdashti AR, Turel MK, et al. Expanded endonasal endoscopic surgery in suprasellar craniopharyngiomas: a retrospective analysis of 43 surgeries including recurrent cases. Oper Neurosurg 2019;17(2):132–42.
7. Dhandapani S, Singh H, Negm HM, et al. Endonasal endoscopic reoperation for residual or recurrent craniopharyngiomas. J Neurosurg 2017;126(2):418–30.
8. Momin AA, Recinos MA, Cioffi G, et al. Descriptive epidemiology of craniopharyngiomas in the United States. Pituitary 2021;24(4):517–22.
9. Fernandez-Miranda JC, Gardner PA, Rastelli MM, et al. Endoscopic endonasal transcavernous posterior clinoidectomy with interdural pituitary transposition: technical note. J Neurosurg 2014;121(1):91–9.
10. Kaiser U, Ho K. Chapter 8: Pituitary Physiology and Diagnostic Evaluation. In: Melmed S, Auchus RJ, Goldfine AB, et al, editors. *Textbook of Endocrinology.* 14th ed. Saunders/Elsevier; 2020. p. 184–235. https://doi.org/10.1016/B978-0-323-55596-8.00008-5.
11. Laws ER, Ezzat S, Asa SL, et al. *Pituitary disorders: Diagnosis and Management.* 1st ed. Wiley-Blackwell; 2013. https://doi.org/10.1002/9781118559406.
12. Hong GK, Payne SC, Jane JA. Anatomy, Physiology, and Laboratory Evaluation of the Pituitary Gland. Otolaryngol Clin North Am 2016;49(1):21–32.
13. Cheung CC, Lustig RH. Pituitary development and physiology. Pituitary 2007;10(4):335–50.
14. Cote DJ, Iuliano SL, Catalino MP, et al. Optimizing pre-, intra-, and postoperative management of patients with sellar pathology undergoing transsphenoidal surgery. Neurosurg Focus 2020;48(6):1–9.

15. Guerrero-Pérez F, Vidal N, Marengo AP, et al. Posterior pituitary tumours: the spectrum of a unique entity. A clinical and histological study of a large case series. Endocrine 2019;63(1):36–43.
16. Lee IH, Miller NR, Zan E, et al. Visual defects in patients with pituitary adenomas: The myth of bitemporal hemianopsia. Am J Roentgenol 2015;205(5):W512–8.
17. Lee JP, Park IW, Chung YS. The volume of tumor mass and visual field defect in patients with pituitary macroadenoma. Korean J Ophthalmol 2011;25(1):37–41.
18. Fernandez-Miranda JC, Zwagerman NT, Abhinav K, et al. Cavernous sinus compartments from the endoscopic endonasal approach: Anatomical considerations and surgical relevance to adenoma surgery. J Neurosurg 2018;129(2):430–41.
19. Lang M, Silva D, Dai L, et al. Superiority of constructive interference in steady-state MRI sequencing over T1-weighted MRI sequencing for evaluating cavernous sinus invasion by pituitary macroadenomas. J Neurosurg 2019; 130(2):352–9.
20. Lee JH, Lee HK, Park JK, et al. Cavernous sinus syndrome: Clinical features and differential diagnosis with MR imaging. Am J Roentgenol 2003;181(2):583–90.
21. Rizzoli P, Iuliano S, Weizenbaum E, et al. Headache in Patients with Pituitary Lesions: A Longitudinal Cohort Study. Neurosurgery 2016;78(3):316–23.
22. Nemergut EC, Dumont AS, Barry UT, et al. Perioperative management of patients undergoing transsphenoidal pituitary surgery. Anesth Analg 2005;101(4): 1170–81.
23. Mehta GU, Lonser RR. Management of hormone-secreting pituitary adenomas. Neuro Oncol 2017;19(6):762–73.
24. Arita K, Tominaga A, Sugiyama K, et al. Natural course of incidentally found nonfunctioning pituitary adenoma, with special reference to pituitary apoplexy during follow-up examination. J Neurosurg 2006;104(6):884–91.
25. Lonser RR, Nieman L, Oldfield EH. Cushing's disease: Pathobiology, diagnosis, and management. J Neurosurg 2017;126(2):404–17.
26. Lawrence L, Alkwatli K, Bena J, et al. Acromegaly: a Clinical Perspective. Clin Diabetes Endocrinol 2020. https://doi.org/10.21203/rs.3.rs-30352/v1.
27. Schlechte JA. Approach to the patient: Long-term management of prolactinomas. J Clin Endocrinol Metab 2007;92(8):2861–5.
28. Zada G, Kelly DF, Cohan P, et al. Endonasal transsphenoidal approach for pituitary adenomas and other sellar lesions: An assessment of efficacy, safety, and patient impressions. J Neurosurg 2003;98(2):350–8.
29. Santos CP, Sandouk Z, Yogi-Morren D, et al. Tsh-staining pituitary adenomas: Rare, silent, and plurihoromonal. Endocr Pract 2018;24(6):580–8.
30. Boxerman JL, Rogg JM, Donahue JE, et al. Preoperative MRI evaluation of pituitary macroadenoma: Imaging features predictive of successful transsphenoidal surgery. Am J Roentgenol 2010;195(3):720–8.
31. Chaudhary V, Bano S. Imaging of the pituitary: Recent advances. Indian J Endocrinol Metab 2011;15(7):216.
32. Lang M, Habboub G, Moon D, et al. Comparison of constructive interference in steady-state and T1-Weighted MRI sequence at detecting pituitary adenomas in cushing's disease patients. J Neurol Surgery B Skull Base 2018;79(6):593–8.
33. Shah J, Cappello ZJ, Roxbury C, et al. Prevalence and Clinical Significance of Radiographic Sinus Disease on Preoperative Computed Tomography Imaging in the Endoscopic Skull Base Surgery Population. Am J Rhinol Allergy 2021; 35(2):239–44.

34. García-Garrigós E, Arenas-Jiménez JJ, Monjas-Cánovas I, et al. Transsphenoidal approach in endoscopic endonasal surgery for skull base lesions: What radiologists and surgeons need to know. Radiographics 2015;35(4):1170–85.

35. Himes CP, Ganesh R, Wight EC, et al. Perioperative evaluation and management of endocrine disorders. Mayo Clin Proc 2020;95(12):2760–74.

36. Tien DA, Stokken JK, Recinos PF, et al. Comprehensive postoperative management after endoscopic skull base surgery. Otolaryngol Clin North Am 2016; 49(1):253–63.

37. Inder WJ, Hunt PJ. Glucocorticoid replacement in pituitary surgery: Guidelines for perioperative assessment and management. J Clin Endocrinol Metab 2002;87(6): 2745–50.

38. Hanson M, Li H, Geer E, et al. Perioperative management of endoscopic transsphenoidal pituitary surgery. World J Otorhinolaryngol Head Neck Surg 2020; 6(2):84–93.

39. Bajwa S, Bajwa S. Anesthesia and Intensive care implications for pituitary surgery: Recent trends and advancements. Indian J Endocrinol Metab 2011; 15(7):224.

40. Scapuccin M, Thamboo A, Rashid N, et al. Transsphenoidal pituitary surgery effects on obstructive sleep apnea in patients with acromegaly: a systematic review and meta-analysis. J Otolaryngol Res 2018;10(6). https://doi.org/10.15406/joentr. 2018.10.00368.

# Differential Diagnosis and Radiographic Imaging of Pituitary Lesions
## An Integrated Approach

Kevin Zhao, DO[a], Esther Nimchinsky, MD, PhD[b],
Pankaj K. Agarwalla, MD[a,c],*

## KEYWORDS

- Magnetic resonance imaging • Computed tomography • Sella • Pituitary
- Differential diagnosis

## KEY POINTS

- It is essential to understand the imaging characteristics of normal pituitary structures.
- Neuroimaging is relied on heavily in formulating a differential diagnosis for lesions in the sellar or parasellar region.
- Dynamic MRI of the pituitary gland is sometimes required to identify small pituitary microadenomas.
- It is important to integrate all available noninvasive information when formulating a differential diagnosis for lesions in this region.

## INTRODUCTION

The sellar and parasellar region of the brain represents a unique and complex area of the skull base that can harbor a wide range of pathologic conditions. These lesions can be neoplastic, infectious, inflammatory, developmental, or vascular in nature. In this article, the authors emphasize an integrated approach for narrowing the differential diagnosis of sellar lesions, focusing on all noninvasive tools available. A targeted clinical history and physical examination are essential first steps in the diagnosis process. Because of their proximity to the pituitary gland, a multitude of endocrine and

[a] Department of Neurosurgery, Rutgers, New Jersey Medical School, Doctor's Office Center, 90 Bergen Street, Room 8100, Newark, NJ 07103, USA; [b] Department of Radiology, Rutgers, New Jersey Medical School, MSB F-506, 185 South Orange Avenue, Newark, NJ 07103, USA; [c] Rutgers, New Jersey Medical School, Doctor's Office Center, 90 Bergen Street Room 8100, Newark, NJ 07103, USA
* Corresponding author. Rutgers, New Jersey Medical School, Doctor's Office Center, 90 Bergen Street, Room 8100, Newark, NJ 07103.
E-mail address: pka23@njms.rutgers.edu

Otolaryngol Clin N Am 55 (2022) 247–264
https://doi.org/10.1016/j.otc.2021.12.002
0030-6665/22/© 2022 Elsevier Inc. All rights reserved.
oto.theclinics.com

metabolic laboratory derangements can occur. With modern technologies and image resolution, radiographic modalities are necessary to narrow the differential diagnosis.

A sound clinician with a keen eye toward history, physical examination, and testing data can often make the diagnosis without surgery, an important skill for any physician treating lesions of the sella and anterior skull base.

### Imaging Modalities

Magnetic resonance imaging (MRI) with and without contrast is the most useful imaging modality when evaluating lesions in the sellar and parasellar region. Computed tomography (CT) imaging is often used as the initial diagnostic modality because of its availability, cost, and short examination time. CT angiography or conventional digital subtraction angiography can be used to assess vascular lesions.

To understand the radiographic characteristics of lesions in this region, it is imperative to recognize the normal MR characteristics of the pituitary gland (**Fig. 1**A–C). First, the neurohypophysis, or posterior pituitary gland, is usually visible on noncontrast T1-weighted imaging, presumably because of the T1-shortening effects of vasopressin, which is concentrated in the gland. It varies in size with age and is sometimes not visible if the MRI spatial resolution is inadequate.[1] The normal anterior pituitary gland ranges from 6 to 9 mm in height, although its shape and size vary considerably with age and gender, as discussed later.[2] Most pituitary glands exhibit a flat or convex upper border. However, some normal women can have upward convexity of the gland, particularly at periods and ages when it is enlarged.[3,4] It is ellipsoid in shape, with intensity like that of white matter.[2] The anterior lobe of the pituitary gland enhances slightly later than the posterior lobe and the infundibulum owing to its indirect blood supply from the pituitary portal system.[5] A dynamic sellar protocol may be used to enhance visualization of

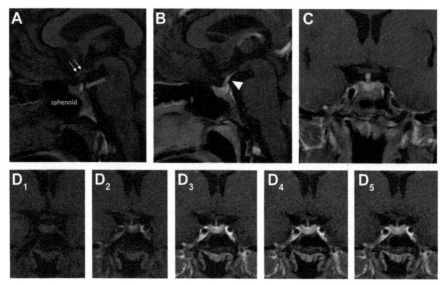

**Fig. 1.** Normal pituitary gland on MRI. Posterior pituitary gland (*pituitary white spot, arrow* in panel *A*) is often visible on noncontrast T1-weighted imaging. The optic chiasm (*double arrows* in *A*) lies superior to the pituitary stalk (*arrowhead* in panel *B*). On coronal imaging (*C*), the pituitary stalk enhances avidly and should be midline. On dynamic postcontrast imaging (*D1-5*), the stalk and central gland enhance first (*D2*), followed by the remainder of the gland (*D3–D5*).

certain lesions. With this technique, the sellar region is scanned at high-spatial resolution repeatedly during the administration of contrast (**Fig. 1**D).

MR characteristics of the normal pituitary gland may vary according to age and sex. Height of the pituitary gland increases with puberty and is found to reach its maximal measurement between 20 and 29 years of age. The height of the pituitary gland is generally greater in women of childbearing age.[3] It subsequently declines with age in both genders. However, in women, the pituitary gland shows a significant increase in size in the 50- to 59-years age group presumably owing to loss of steroid feedback due to declining hormone levels.[6,7]

An "empty sella" can be described as a sella partially or completely devoid of pituitary tissues and replaced with cerebrospinal fluid (CSF).[7] The incidence of an "empty sella" is around 2% of all brain MRI scans.[8] Causes of this phenomenon can be due to congenital malformation, increased intracranial pressure, postpartum (Sheehan syndrome), obesity, cranial trauma, or radiotherapy.[8,9] These findings can be completely incidental or result in neurologic disturbances, such as headaches, nausea, vomiting, rhinorrhea, dizziness, cranial nerve deficits, or seizures.[9] In CT or MRI, CSF that is continuous with the overlying subarachnoid space fills the sella. The pituitary gland can appear absent or flattened at the bottom of the sella. The sellar space often appears enlarged, and the pituitary stalk appears thinned. The intrasellar fluid signal is consistent with normal CSF.[9]

Chiasmal herniation is a phenomenon whereby the optic chiasm herniates into the sella after transsphenoidal surgery or following dopamine-agonist treatment of large prolactinomas. Patients with this imaging finding can be either asymptomatic or experience visual loss.[10]

## PRIMARY LESIONS OF THE PITUITARY GLAND
### Pituitary Adenoma

Pituitary adenomas are benign tumors of the pituitary gland. They are situated within the sella and can be categorized as microadenomas if they are less than 10 mm in greatest dimension or macroadenomas if they are more than 10 mm.

Because the pituitary gland is the primary regulator of hormones, tumors of the pituitary can produce a wide range of clinical abnormalities depending on the hormones they secrete. A detailed history and physical examination are essential to elicit the clinical manifestations. Functional pituitary adenomas can secrete a surplus of prolactin, growth hormone (GH), adrenocorticotropic hormone (ACTH), thyroid-stimulating hormone (TSH), follicle-stimulating hormone (FSH), or luteinizing hormone (LH).[11]

Prolactinomas are functioning pituitary adenomas that secrete an excess level of prolactin. They generally manifest clinically as amenorrhea with galactorrhea.[12] Affected prepubescent adolescents usually experience delay in development in their reproductive systems. Premenopausal women can also suffer from infertility. In men, reduced libido, impotence, infertility, and galactorrhea may be present.[11] GH-secreting pituitary adenomas present with gigantism before epiphyseal closure and acromegaly after puberty. They can cause significant alterations in connective tissues affecting multiple systems in the body. Visceromegaly, changes in facial features, frontal skull bossing, macroglossia, increased shoe size, painful osteoarthritis, barrel chest, glucose intolerance, and a wide range of systemic impairments can occur as a result of excess GH production.[13] ACTH-secreting pituitary adenomas are the cause of Cushing disease. These patients present with clinical symptoms owing to chronic glucocorticoid excess. Symptoms typically involve weight gain, moon facies, buffalo hump, hirsutism, hyperpigmentation, and purple striae. TSH-secreting pituitary adenomas are very rare. They can manifest clinically as hyperthyroidism or hypothyroidism. Functional gonadotrophic adenomas secrete FSH and LH. Patients can have polycystic ovarian syndrome, infertility, irregular menses, testicular hypertrophy, and ovarian hyperstimulation syndrome. Precocious puberty can be seen in children.[14]

Large sellar and parasellar lesions, such as nonfunctioning pituitary adenomas, can exhibit mass effects on the surrounding anatomic structures. Headache is generally an early nonspecific symptom. With the optic chiasm situated superiorly, compression often leads to bitemporal hemianopsia, as well as alteration in visual acuity. With continued growth superiorly, compression on the hypothalamus can cause disorders of sleep, behavior, and emotion. Some large sellar or parasellar lesions can extend into the ventricular system through the floor of the third ventricle. These lesions can eventually cause hydrocephalus. With lateral growth of these large lesions, the cavernous sinus can be invaded, and various cranial nerve palsies can ensue.

Pituitary apoplexy is a result of intralesional hemorrhage and causes sudden-onset headaches and visual impairments. The symptoms then progress to impaired mental state and hypopituitarism, which can include diabetes insipidus and adrenal crisis.[15,16]

### Pituitary Adenoma Laboratory Findings

Patients with prolactinomas will generally have a serum level exceeding 200 ng/mL.[17] When interpreting the prolactin result, stalk effect and hook effect should be taken into consideration. Stalk effect is a phenomenon caused by the mass effect of any sellar mass on the pituitary stalk. This results in impairment of dopamine secretion, which in turn increases prolactin secretion owing to loss of inhibition. This typically results in a moderate increase in serum prolactin level (<150 ng/mL).[11] Hook effect is a phenomenon whereby high true serum concentrations of prolactin produce a falsely low laboratory readout owing to oversaturation of the laboratory assay.[18] This can be overcome by a diluted prolactin study.

GH-secreting pituitary adenomas are diagnosed with failure of suppression of GH on oral glucose tolerance testing (<2 ng/mL) as well as an elevation in serum insulin growth factor 1 level. The basal GH level in these patients can also be elevated (>5 ng/mL).[11]

Diagnosing Cushing disease biochemically requires multiple, often complementary laboratory tests. Multiple elevated midnight salivary cortisol laboratory tests are often a reliable, early clinical indicator in suspected Cushing disease.[19] An elevated 24-hour urine-free cortisol can verify the presence of hypercortisolemia. A low-dose dexamethasone (1 mg) suppression test is warranted in suspected hypercortisolemia to establish a failure of the negative feedback loop . Next, an elevated serum ACTH level will provide evidence of primary ACTH-dependent pathologic condition (vs ACTH-independent pathologic condition, such as adrenal tumor or exogenous corticosteroid use).

To differentiate from an ectopic lesion, ACTH is generally suppressed in corticotroph pituitary adenomas with a high-dose dexamethasone (8 mg) challenge.[20] Inferior petrosal sinus sampling is an invasive technique that can also be used to differentiate a pituitary versus an ectopic source of ACTH and/or to help lateralize the location of a functional microadenoma. Catheter angiography is performed with catheters situated in the inferior petrosal sinuses. ACTH levels are measured from the sinuses as well as peripherally after corticotropin-releasing hormone stimulation. A 3-fold central-to-peripheral ratio after stimulation indicates Cushing disease.[21]

TSH-secreting pituitary adenomas generally have high serum TSH levels in combination with high levels of circulating thyroid hormones. Some patients will have concurrent high levels of GH or prolactin.[11] Gonadotrophs secrete excess levels of serum FSH and LH.[11]

For any sellar pathologic condition, it is prudent to obtain a full endocrine laboratory panel, and an astute clinician should be able to integrate the history, physical examination, and laboratory data to get close to a diagnosis, particularly in functional adenomas.

### Pituitary Adenoma Radiographic Findings

Although macroadenomas, because of their size, may be relatively easy to identify, microadenomas often require specialized techniques. Some microadenomas may be visible only with dynamic postcontrast imaging, where the sella is scanned rapidly and repeatedly before and during administration of contrast. The delayed enhancement of the microadenoma contrasts with the early and vivid enhancement of the stalk and normal pituitary gland (**Fig. 2**). On MRI, they are typically hypointense on T1-weighted sequence and of variable intensity on T2-weighted sequence. These lesions exhibit delayed and less contrast enhancement compared with the normal anterior pituitary gland. Displacement of the pituitary stalk can be observed because of local mass effect. Deformation of the sellar floor and convexity of the diaphragma sellae can be subtle indications of pituitary adenomas.[4,22]

Macroadenomas can sometimes extend superiorly causing compression on the hypothalamus and optic chiasm and may extend into the third ventricle, causing hydrocephalus (**Fig. 3**). The signal intensity of macroadenomas may be heterogeneous, especially on T2-weighted sequences.[22] They can also extend laterally into the cavernous sinus compressing on the cranial nerves and the cavernous segment of the internal carotid artery. Careful evaluation of the lateral extent of a macroadenoma and the degree to which it encases the cavernous segment of the internal carotid artery is necessary for preoperative assessment of the likelihood of cavernous sinus

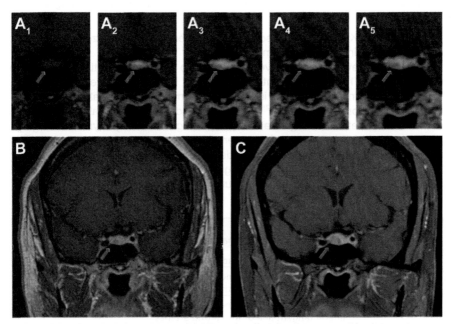

Fig. 2. Pituitary microadenoma. A small adenoma may be seen best on dynamic postcontrast T1-weighted imaging. Here, it appears as a hypoenhancing nodule in the inferior gland (*A*). This microadenoma grew significantly in the 7 years between panels (*A, B*) and (*C*).

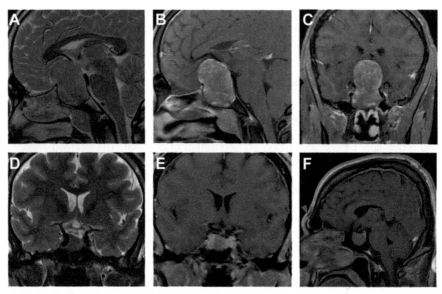

**Fig. 3.** (*A–C*) Pituitary macroadenoma. A large adenoma arises from a markedly enlarged sella. It may be intermediate or hyperintense on T2-weighted imaging (*A*) and demonstrates characteristic slightly granular enhancement (*B, C*). It often has a "waist" at the level of the diaphragma sella (*arrows* in panel *C*), creating a "snowman" appearance on coronal images. (*D, E*) Secreting macroadenoma. A macroadenoma in the right side of the sella is hypointense on T2-weighted imaging (*D*) deviates the stalk to the left (*arrows* in panels *D–E*). The sella is enlarged (*F*). Note calvarial thickening (*arrows* in panel *F*) and frontal bossing (*arrowhead* in panel *F*) in this patient with acromegaly because of a GH-secreting adenoma.

invasion.[23] The Knosp grading scale was created to characterize the degree of cavernous sinus invasion from a macroadenoma[24] (**Table 1**).

There is some evidence of an inverse relationship between prolactin level and T2 intensity on MRI. The more hyperintense the tumor is on T2-weighted sequence, the lower the prolactin levels are. The inverse also seems to hold true, although T2 hypointense prolactinomas are rare.[22,25] Corticotroph adenomas are challenging because of their size sometimes being smaller than radiological visibility. Dynamic imaging is often used, and 3-T MRI has shown superior visualization than lower field MRI.[26]

Invasive pituitary adenomas refer to adenomas that exhibit extrasellar expansion. They are classified as and behave as benign lesions, but they infiltrate the surrounding sellar bone, cavernous sinus, clivus, or dura[27] (**Fig. 4**A–C).

| Table 1 | |
|---|---|
| **The Knosp grading scale of pituitary adenomas[24]** | |
| Grade 0 | The adenoma does not invade the cavernous sinus |
| Grade 1 | The adenoma invades the medial tangent line of the carotid arteries but does not extend beyond the intercarotid line |
| Grade 2 | The adenoma extends beyond the intercarotid line but does not go past the lateral tangent line of the carotid arteries |
| Grade 3 | The adenoma extends beyond the lateral tangent line of the carotid arteries |
| Grade 4 | The adenoma encases the intracavernous carotid artery |

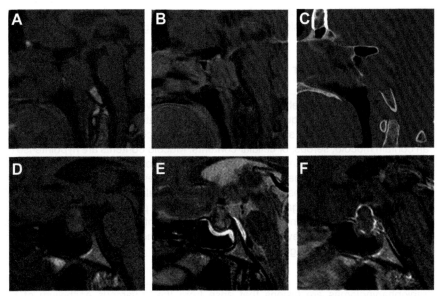

**Fig. 4.** (*A–C*) Invasive pituitary adenoma. This patient presented with meningitis and a CSF leak. Mass replacing the bone marrow of the clivus (*A*) enhances in a manner reminiscent of a pituitary adenoma (*B*), although it does not extend above the sella. Noncontrast CT demonstrates destruction of the clivus and walls of the sphenoid sinus (*C*) by this invasive mass, which proved to be a pituitary adenoma. (*D–F*) Pituitary apoplexy. A heterogeneous mass arising from an enlarged sella is partly hyperintense on noncontrast T1-weighted imaging (*D*), and heterogeneous on T2-weighted imaging (*E*). The central portion of the mass is hemorrhagic and does not enhance, but viable tumor at the periphery enhances (*F*).

Intratumoral hemorrhage can manifest as pituitary apoplexy (**Fig. 4D–F**). T2-weighted gradient-echo MRI is very sensitive in detecting the presence of past hemorrhage.[28] Pituitary infarction is another essential element of pituitary apoplexy and can be identified via diffusion-weighted MRI.[29]

### Pituicytoma

Pituicytomas are rare World Health Organization grade 1 spindle cell tumors from the neurohypophysis and the infundibulum. These lesions are typically isointense on T1-weighted imaging, are typically isointense to hyperintense on T2-weighted imaging, and exhibit homogeneous or heterogeneous contrast enhancement.[30,31] Pituicytomas are highly vascular, therefore making surgical resection difficult. They can be accompanied by enlarged superior hypophyseal and hypothalamic vessels.[32] Recent studies have discovered that mitogen-activated protein kinase (MAPK) pathway activation is associated with pituicytoma, which lays the groundwork for possible targeted therapy.[33]

### Pituitary Carcinoma

Pituitary adenomas rarely transform into pituitary carcinoma, and there may be invasion into the brain parenchyma and spine via CSF seeding. Liver, lung, and bone involvement has also been reported.[34] Most of these lesions are macroadenomas at the time of diagnosis, which manifest clinically with mass effect in addition to endocrine abnormalities. Imaging findings are similar to those of pituitary macroadenomas, with additional features, such as sellar destruction as well as more aggressive supra-sellar and parasellar extension. Spinal and body imaging are useful to identify meta-static lesions.[35]

## CRANIOPHARYNGEAL DUCT LESIONS
### Rathke Cleft Cyst

Rathke cleft cysts are largely asymptomatic and discovered incidentally. They arise from the remnants of the squamous epithelium from Rathke pouch and are predominantly intrasellar, although suprasellar cysts are not uncommon (**Fig. 5**). These cysts can contain mucoid, serous, or cellular contents. Mucoid contents are hypointense on both T1- and T2-weighted images. Those with serous contents match the intensity of CSF. Rathke cleft cysts generally do not show contrast enhancement.[36] A fluid-debris level could be seen with those cysts that contain high cellular contents.[30] Rathke cleft cysts may have clinically significant hormonal sequelae, particularly if associated with significant mass effect. Standard of care for treatment of Rathke cleft cyst is surgical drainage or resection; however, in rare cases of recurrence, stereotactic radiosurgery is a safe and feasible salvage treatment option.[37]

### Craniopharyngioma

Craniopharyngiomas are lesions that arise from the squamous epithelium of the Rathke pouch remnant. They occur in the sella and can extend into the suprasellar region as well as the third ventricle. The adamantinomatous type is the most common and arises in children and adolescents. Adamantinomatous craniopharyngiomas are lobulated, contain cystic components, and are generally partially calcified (**Fig. 6**A–D). The cystic components are typically "motor oil"-like, exhibit variable signal

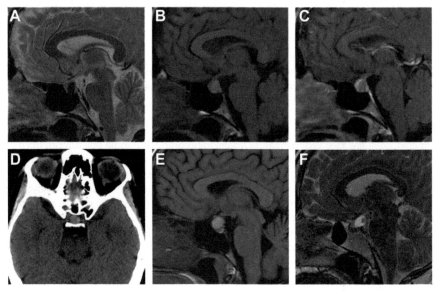

**Fig. 5.** Rathke cleft cyst. A lesion within the sella is hypointense on T2-weighted imaging (*A*) and hyperintense on noncontrast T1-weighted imaging (*B*), demonstrating no enhancement with contrast administration (*C*). Sellar-suprasellar lesion is hyperattenuating on CT (*arrows* in panel *D*) and hyperintense on noncontrast T1-weighted imaging (*E*). A suprasellar lesion, also hyperintense on T1-weighted imaging (*D*), demonstrates nonenhancing internal nodules (*arrow* in panel *F*), which when present, may be pathognomonic for Rathke cleft cyst.

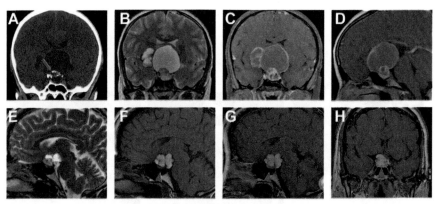

**Fig. 6.** (*A–D*) Adamantinomatous type craniopharyngioma in a 17-year-old man. Noncontrast CT (*A*), T2-weighted MRI (*B*), and T1-weighted postcontrast imaging (*C, D*). Large partly calcified (*arrow* in panel *A*) mixed cystic and solid mass within and above the sella. T2 hypointense hemosiderin rim on T2-weighted imaging (*arrows* in panel *B*) indicates prior hemorrhage. There is mass effect on the optic chiasm, which is not resolved, and on the lateral and third ventricles. (*E–H*) Papillary type craniopharyngioma in a 49-year-old woman. T2 (*E*), noncontrast T1 (*F*), and postcontrast T1-weighted imaging (*G, H*). Mixed cystic and solid mass within and above the sella is visualized. The cystic component in this case is hyperintense on T1-weighted imaging (*F*), indicating proteinaceous contents and/or hemorrhage. The normal pituitary gland is visible along the floor of the sella (*arrowheads* in panels *F-H*).

intensities on MRI, but can be hyperintense on T1-weighted imaging.[38] The solid portions can be isointense or hypointense on T1-weighted imaging and hyperintense on T2-weighted imaging.[39] CT is generally superior to MRI in the evaluation of calcification as hyperdensities. The papillary type is rarer and typically found in adults[36] (**Fig. 6**E–H).

Recent genomic characterization has found that more than 90% of adamantinomatous craniopharyngiomas harbor *CTNNB1* mutation, and more than 90% of papillary craniopharyngiomas possess *BRAF V600E* alterations, which serves as the basis for ongoing trials assessing combined BRAF/MEK inhibition in papillary subtypes.[40,41]

## LESIONS OF THE SURROUNDING TISSUES
### Meningioma

Meningiomas are benign lesions that can occur in the parasellar region. They can arise from the tuberculum sellae, planum sphenoidale, clinoid, cavernous sinus, or the sphenoid (**Fig. 7**A, B). Mass effects causing visual defects are the most common presenting symptoms. Meningiomas usually occur in adults, with higher prevalence in women.[42] Recent molecular genetic investigations have revealed an association of *POLR2A* mutations with anterior skull base meningiomas, especially in the region of tuberculum sellae.[43]

On MRI, meningiomas have notable characteristics, such as a dural tail, CSF cleft, as well as adjacent bony involvement. When invading into the cavernous sinus, they can cause narrowing of the internal carotid artery, which is not a typical feature of pituitary adenomas.[34] Homogeneous contrast enhancement is usually observed, along with variable hyperintensity on T2-weighted images.[22,34] A grading scale had been proposed to aid surgical approach decision making for tuberculum sellae meningiomas based on MRI. This grading scale takes into consideration tumor size, optic canal invasion, and carotid artery involvement.[44]

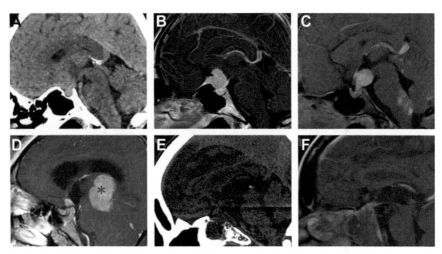

**Fig. 7.** (*A, B*) Suprasellar/planum sphenoidale meningioma. Noncontrast CT (*A*) shows a hyperdense mass above a normal-sized sella. Contrast-enhanced T1-weighted imaging (*B*) reveals an enhancing mass with a dural tail, distinct from the normal pituitary within the sella. (*C*) Enhancing mass along the infundibulum is nonspecific in appearance, but the presence of another enhancing mass in the brainstem (*asterisk*) supports the diagnosis of midline glioma. (*D*) Enhancing mass along the infundibulum (*arrow*), in the context of a larger pineal region mass. (*asterisk*) Most suggestive of bifocal germinoma. (*E–F*) Enlarged sella contains hyperdense material on CT (*E*), which on contrast enhanced T1-weighted imaging (*F*) demonstrates peripheral enhancement. This proved to be a metastatic mucinous carcinoma.

### Teratoma

Teratoma is a heterogeneous tumor that contains multiple different tissues, such as hair, muscle, tooth, and bone. These lesions are highly variable in their content and can range from benign mature teratomas to poorly differentiated immature teratomas. They can present as extra-axial lesions in the suprasellar cistern. Teratomas can cause hydrocephalus and macrocephaly in infants and often cause stillbirth in fetuses.[45] On neuroimaging, they show a mixed signal intensity consistent with their tissue contents, with soft tissue, fat signal, and calcifications.[39]

### Lipoma

Lipomas are congenital malformations that derive from the embryologic "meninx primitiva." They can occur in the suprasellar cistern and hypothalamus. On MRI, they show increased signal on T1-weighted imaging and decreased signal on T2-weighted imaging, consistent with fat signal. They lack contrast enhancement and lack calcifications on CT.[30,46,47]

### Chordoma

Chordomas are low-grade tumors that arise from notochordal remnants. They can develop anywhere along the neuraxis. Intracranially, approximately 39% of cases are situated in the clivus. These lesions can have characteristic CT findings owing to their calcifications as well as bony destruction. On MRI, they are isointense on T1-weighted sequences and heterogeneously hyperintense on T2-weighted images. Chordomas typically show contrast enhancement, and most of the time can be seen separate from a normal pituitary gland.[39,48] Physaliferous cells are typical of chordoma in histologic studies.[49] T-box-family transcription factor brachyury is an essential regulator for notochord development and is found to be overexpressed in chordomas. This discovery lays the foundation of possible future targeted therapies for treatment of chordomas.[50]

## Glioma

Gliomas can also be seen in the juxtasellar region. These gliomas usually occur in the first decade of life and originate from the visual pathway or the hypothalamus. They are sometimes grouped as a single entity and referred together as optic chiasmatic-hypothalamic glioma because of their ability to infiltrate. Gliomas in this region are usually slow growing in childhood and can present as massive lesions. They cause visual symptoms as well as hypothalamic dysfunction. Most reports have indicated that these are low-grade lesions, but they can have a malignant course. Parasellar gliomas can be associated with neurofibromatosis type 1 and have a more malignant course. These tumors are most often isointense on T1-weighted imaging, are hyperintense on T2-weighted imaging, and exhibit some degree of contrast enhancement (**Fig. 7**C). It is important to distinguish these lesions from hamartomas, which do not enhance.[36,39,51] Parasellar midline glioma can harbor histone *H3K27M* mutation and typically is indicative of poor prognosis.[52]

## Germinoma

Germinomas are the most common germ cell tumors to arise in this area. They mostly arise in the pituitary stalk, hypothalamus, and pineal region in children and young adults. These lesions can extend superiorly into the third ventricle, or inferiorly into the sella (**Fig. 7**D). They typically cause diabetes insipidus and pituitary dysfunction. Germinomas have no tumor capsule, and therefore, seeding of the CSF is common. They are usually hypointense on T1-weighted imaging, are usually hyperintense on T2-weighted imaging, and show marked homogeneous contrast enhancement.[22,47] If a germ cell tumor, such as germinoma, is suspected, serum and CSF laboratory studies, such as placental alkaline phosphatase, alpha-fetoprotein, and beta-human chorionic gonadotropin, are needed.[53]

## Hamartoma

Hypothalamic hamartomas can arise in the parasellar region from the tuber cinereum as a pedunculated mass. They are often isointense on T1-weighted imaging, and hyperintense on T2-weighted imaging, and can be distinguished from other lesions in this region by their lack of contrast enhancement on MRI. Hamartomas can cause precocious puberty owing to secretion of LH and gelastic seizures characterized by uncontrollable laughter.[30,39]

## Metastasis

Pituitary metastases are rare but sometimes may be the only metastatic focus in a patient with known malignancy. The most common malignancies are breast cancer in women and lung cancer in men. Metastatic lesions tend to affect the infundibulum and the posterior gland preferentially. Compared with other sellar lesions, they are more often associated with cranial nerve deficits and diabetes insipidus because of their involvement with the pituitary stalk.[39] Metastatic lesions are typically hypointense to isointense on T1-weighted imaging, are typically hyperintense on T2-weighted imaging, and show varying degrees of contrast enhancement (**Fig. 7**E, F). Occasionally, leptomeningeal enhancement can be evident, especially in the posterior fossa.[36]

## INFECTIOUS AND INFLAMMATORY LESIONS

Inflammation of the pituitary gland and stalk is broadly termed hypophysitis. It is a heterogeneous condition with multiple causes. Primary hypophysitis refers to inflammation confined to the gland, whereas secondary hypophysitis refers to inflammation secondary to systemic conditions, iatrogenic drugs, or other neighboring pathologic conditions.[54,55] In particular, autoimmune endocrine diseases, such as Graves disease and Hashimoto disease, as well as other autoimmune or inflammatory diseases, such as lupus, Sjogren, Behcet, or Langerhans cell histiocytosis, are known to be associated with secondary hypophysitis[56] (**Fig. 8A–C**).

On contrast-enhanced pituitary MRI, hypophysitis manifests as an enlarged homogeneously enhancing pituitary gland with a thickened pituitary stalk.[54] The degree of involvement of the stalk versus the gland may be highly variable. In patients presenting with diabetes insipidus, the absence of a posterior pituitary bright spot on T1-weighted imaging could point toward hypophysitis.[57] The presence of a dural tail or an empty sella could represent the late stages of the disease.[56] However, the imaging characteristics of different forms of hypophysitis (see later discussion) do not differ substantially or consistently enough to permit the distinction to be made on imaging alone.

Hypophysitis can also be classified based on histopathologic features, including lymphocytic, granulomatous, xanthomatous, immunoglobulin G4 (IgG4), or necrotizing.[55] Lymphocytic hypophysitis is the most common form of hypophysitis. It predominantly affects women in their fourth decade of life. Pregnancy is the strongest

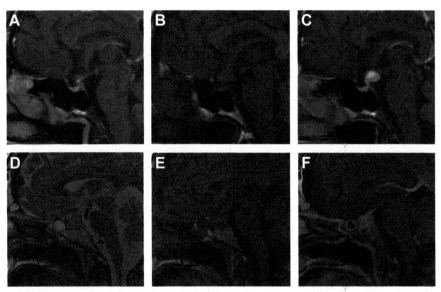

**Fig. 8.** (*A–C*) A 56-year-old woman, with prior history of presumed primary lymphocytic hypophysitis. (*A*) Surveillance MRI scan. (*B*, *C*) 2 years later, the patient presented with hyperprolactinemia. There is marked enhancement inseparable from the pituitary stalk. Biopsy of a lesion in the iliac bone yielded Langerhans cell histiocytosis. (*D–F*) Homogenous enlargement of the pituitary gland in biopsy-proven granulomatous hypophysitis owing to neurosarcoidosis in a 60-year-old female patient with previously undiagnosed sarcoidosis. (*A, C, F*) Postcontrast T1-weighted imaging. (*B, E*) Noncontrast T1-weighted imaging. (*D*) T2-weighted imaging.

association, and the cause is probably autoimmune.[54] Hypopituitarism is the most common clinical finding in lymphocytic hypophysitis. Central diabetes insipidus can also occur, as well as hyperprolactinemia owing to stalk involvement.[58]

Granulomatous hypophysitis is the second most common form of hypophysitis. It is a chronic inflammatory condition that affects women more than men.[54] Unlike lymphocytic hypophysitis, granulomatous hypophysitis does not have an association with pregnancy. Secondary granulomatous hypophysitis may be caused by other systemic granulomatous disorders, including tuberculosis, sarcoidosis, or Wegener granulomatosis.[58,59] The radiographic appearance of granulomatous hypophysitis may be indistinguishable from lymphocytic hypophysitis (**Fig. 8**D–F).

Xanthomatous hypophysitis is extremely rare and can be an inflammatory response owing to Rathke cleft cyst rupture.[54] It is more commonly seen in women and has similar clinical features as lymphocytic hypophysitis.[59]

IgG4-related hypophysitis is a recently recognized variant of hypophysitis. It can be systemic or isolated to the pituitary gland. It has a predilection for men in their seventies.[55] It is characterized by mononuclear infiltration of lymphocytes and plasma cells. Making an accurate diagnosis of IgG4-related hypophysitis is crucial because it responds well to glucocorticoid therapy.[56] Serum IgG4 level of greater than 140 mg/dL and MRI finding of a sellar mass or thickened pituitary stalk are highly suspicious for IgG4-related hypophysitis.[60]

Necrotizing hypophysitis is the rarest form of hypophysitis. Women are 3 times more commonly affected than men.[55] Its pathogenesis is not clearly understood; however, it may represent a more severe form of one of the other forms of hypophysitis. Clinically, it manifests more acutely with findings of intracranial mass effect. The pituitary has extensive areas of necrosis in histopathologic studies.[56]

Immune checkpoint inhibitors have been reported to be a cause of hypophysitis. Reported immune checkpoint inhibitors include medications that target CTLA-4, PD-1, and PD-L1.[61] They reactivate T cells to enhance detection of cancer cells.[56] It is mostly a clinical diagnosis because of its difficulty to diagnose based on radiographic findings.

Central nervous system involvement of Langerhans cell histiocytosis is rare but should also be considered. The most commonly affected region in the brain is the hypothalamic pituitary region.[62] Studies have shown that this disease process is partially driven by activating MAPK somatic mutations.[63]

## ECTODERMAL INCLUSION CYSTS

Dermoid cysts are benign, slow-growing midline lesions that present in childhood. They owe their hyperintensity on T1-weighted sequences to their sebum content within the cyst (**Fig. 9**A–C). Dermoid cysts may cause recurrent aseptic meningitis owing to spillage of their intralesional contents.[39]

Epidermoid cysts are rare benign lesions that present typically in the fourth and fifth decades. They can cause visual defects, hypopituitarism, diabetes insipidus, and cranial nerve deficits. They differ from other lesions in the parasellar region by their diffusion restriction on diffusion-weighted imaging.[39]

## VASCULAR LESIONS

Vascular lesions, especially aneurysms, in the parasellar region must be distinguished from neoplasms to avoid catastrophic intraoperative complications. Aneurysms may arise in the parasellar region and mimic neoplasms. They can arise from the cavernous and paraclinoid regions of the internal carotid artery. Large aneurysms in this region

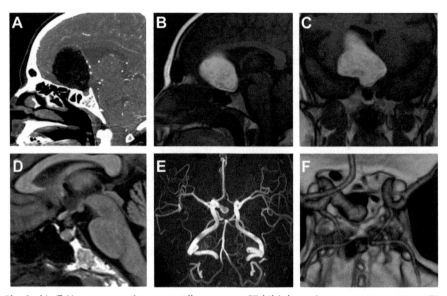

**Fig. 9.** (*A–C*) Hypoattenuating suprasellar mass on CT (*A*) is hyperintense on noncontrast T1-weighted imaging (*B, C*), compatible with a dermoid. Hypoattenuation on CT and T1 signal within a dermoid is due to the presence of sebum, not fat. (*D*) Suprasellar mass on noncontrast T1-weighted imaging in this patient being evaluated before liver transplant proved on MR angiography (*E*) to be a superior hypophyseal artery aneurysm, rendered in 3 dimensions on CT angiogram (*F*).

can cause compression on cranial nerves, causing cranial nerve palsies, as well as optic nerves or optic chiasm. They can also extend into the sella and cause endocrine dysfunctions.

Although conventional MRI is not the preferred modality to assess these lesions, they can be seen as flow voids on T2-weighted images, and the abnormal vasculature will be apparent after contrast injection. CT angiography, MR angiography, and digital subtraction angiography are used to characterize these vascular lesions (**Fig. 9**D–F). Because of the nature of these pathologic conditions, a patient's first presentation may be at the time of hemorrhage. Acute blood is well seen on CT and appears hyperdense in the subarachnoid space. Blood products can also extend into the ventricular system or brain parenchyma. On MRI, susceptibility weighted sequence may demonstrate signal dropout or blooming artifact. On neuroimaging, these aneurysms are mostly saccular in shape, but can also be fusiform. The aneurysmal wall can be calcified, which can be seen on CT.[39]

Cavernous carotid fistula can also be seen in the parasellar region. It is an abnormal connection between the carotid circulation and the cavernous sinus. It can be a direct connection as a result of trauma or an indirect connection. The most common clinical signs are proptosis, chemosis, exophthalmos, and ophthalmoplegia. Orbital bruit can sometimes be appreciated on physical examination. Neuroimaging often reveals enlarged superior ophthalmic veins. Digital subtraction angiography can show shunting from the carotid artery to the cavernous sinus and enlarged draining veins.[64]

### SUMMARY

There is a broad spectrum of pathologic conditions in the sellar and parasellar region. Neuroimaging plays a critical role in understanding and diagnosing disease in this area, but the authors emphasize a combined, integrated approach in making a differential diagnosis before any surgical intervention is planned. All patients require a complete history and physical examination as well as laboratory testing to help narrow the diagnosis. As the modern molecular classification of neoplastic and inflammatory diseases also takes hold, noninvasive genetic testing could be extremely useful in diagnosis (such as blood-based "liquid biopsies" for cancer). An astute diagnostician will put together all the information available and present patients with a cogent treatment plan based on presumed diagnosis, natural history, and severity of clinical presentation.

## CLINICS CARE POINTS

- Pathological conditions in the sellar region, particularly within and around the pituitary gland, require a multi-disciplinary expert team of neuro-radiologists, neuro-endocrinologists, neurosurgeons, and neuro-ophthalmologists to provide the most comprehensive diagnosis and treatment plan.

## CONFLICTS OF INTEREST

None.

## DISCLOSURE OF FUNDING

None.

## REFERENCES

1. Côté M, Salzman KL, Sorour M, et al. Normal dimensions of the posterior pituitary bright spot on magnetic resonance imaging. J Neurosurg 2014;120(2):357–62.
2. Glaser B, Sheinfeld M, Benmair J, et al. Magnetic resonance imaging of the pituitary gland. Clin Radiol 1986;37(1):9–14.
3. Swartz JD, Russell KB, Basile BA, et al. High-resolution computed tomographic appearance of the intrasellar contents in women of childbearing age. Radiology 1983;147(1):115–7.
4. Sage MR, Blumbergs PC, Mulligan BP, et al. The diaphragma sellae: its relationship to the configuration of the pituitary gland. Radiology 1982;145(3):703–8.
5. Sakamoto Y, Takahashi M, Korogi Y, et al. Normal and abnormal pituitary glands: gadopentetate dimeglumine-enhanced MR imaging. Radiology 1991;178(2):441–5.
6. Yadav P, Singhal S, Chauhan S, et al. MRI evaluation of size and shape of normal pituitary gland: age and sex related changes. J Clin Diagn Res 2017. https://doi.org/10.7860/jcdr/2017/31034.10933.
7. Tsunoda A, Okuda O, Sato K. MR height of the pituitary gland as a function of age and sex: especially physiological hypertrophy in adolescence and in climacterium. AJNR Am J Neuroradiol 1997;18(3):551–4.
8. Auer MK, Stieg MR, Crispin A, et al. Primary empty sella syndrome and the prevalence of hormonal dysregulation. Dtsch Arztebl Int 2018;115(7):99–105.
9. De Marinis L, Bonadonna S, Bianchi A, et al. Primary empty sella. J Clin Endocrinol Metab 2005;90(9):5471–7.
10. Purvin VA, Kawasaki A. Non-compressive disorders of the chiasm. Curr Neurol Neurosci Rep 2014;14(7):455.

11. Bi WL, Smith TR, Nery B, Dunn IF, Laws ER Jr. 150 - pituitary tumors: functioning and nonfunctioning. Youmans and Winn Neurological Surgery, 4-Volume Set.:1155-1182.e7.

12. Forbes AP, Henneman PH, Griswold GC, et al. Syndrome characterized by galactorrhea, amenorrhea and low urinary FSH: comparison with acromegaly and normal lactation. J Clin Endocrinol Metab 1954;14(3):265–71.

13. Colao A, Ferone D, Marzullo P, et al. Systemic complications of acromegaly: epidemiology, pathogenesis, and management. Endocr Rev 2004;25(1):102–52.

14. Ntali G, Capatina C, Grossman A, et al. Clinical review: functioning gonadotroph adenomas. J Clin Endocrinol Metab 2014;99(12):4423–33.

15. Wakai S, Fukushima T, Teramoto A, et al. Pituitary apoplexy: its incidence and clinical significance. J Neurosurg 1981;55(2):187–93.

16. Jho DH, Biller BMK, Agarwalla PK, et al. Pituitary apoplexy: large surgical series with grading system. World Neurosurg 2014;82(5):781–90.

17. Molitch ME. Pathologic hyperprolactinemia. Endocrinol Metab Clin North Am 1992;21(4):877–901.

18. St-Jean E, Blain F, Comtois R. High prolactin levels may be missed by immunoradiometric assay in patients with macroprolactinomas. Clin Endocrinol 1996; 44(3):305–9.

19. Yaneva M, Mosnier-Pudar H, Dugué M-A, et al. Midnight salivary cortisol for the initial diagnosis of Cushing's syndrome of various causes. J Clin Endocrinol Metab 2004;89(7):3345–51.

20. Kaye TB, Crapo L. The Cushing syndrome: an update on diagnostic tests. Ann Intern Med 1990;112(6):434–44.

21. Molitch ME. Diagnosis and treatment of pituitary adenomas: a review. JAMA 2017;317(5):516–24.

22. Bonneville J-F. Magnetic resonance imaging of pituitary tumors. Front Horm Res 2016;45:97–120.

23. Cottier JP, Destrieux C, Brunereau L, et al. Cavernous sinus invasion by pituitary adenoma: MR imaging. Radiology 2000;215(2):463–9.

24. Knosp E, Steiner E, Kitz K, et al. Pituitary adenomas with invasion of the cavernous sinus space: a magnetic resonance imaging classification compared with surgical findings. Neurosurgery 1993;33(4):610–7 [discussion: 617-618].

25. Raverot G, Wierinckx A, Dantony E, et al. Prognostic factors in prolactin pituitary tumors: clinical, histological, and molecular data from a series of 94 patients with a long postoperative follow-up. J Clin Endocrinol Metab 2010;95(4):1708–16.

26. Erickson D, Erickson B, Watson R, et al. 3 Tesla magnetic resonance imaging with and without corticotropin releasing hormone stimulation for the detection of microadenomas in Cushing's syndrome. Clin Endocrinol 2010;72(6):793–9.

27. Scheithauer BW, Kovacs KT, Laws ER Jr, et al. Pathology of invasive pituitary tumors with special reference to functional classification. J Neurosurg 1986;65(6): 733–44.

28. Tosaka M, Sato N, Hirato J, et al. Assessment of hemorrhage in pituitary macroadenoma by T2*-weighted gradient-echo MR imaging. AJNR Am J Neuroradiol 2007;28(10):2023–9.

29. Rogg JM, Tung GA, Anderson G, et al. Pituitary apoplexy: early detection with diffusion-weighted MR imaging. AJNR Am J Neuroradiol 2002;23(7):1240–5.

30. Go JL, Rajamohan AG. Imaging of the sella and parasellar region. Radiol Clin North Am 2017;55(1):83–101.

31. Covington MF, Chin SS, Osborn AG. Pituicytoma, spindle cell oncocytoma, and granular cell tumor: clarification and meta-analysis of the world literature since 1893. AJNR Am J Neuroradiol 2011;32(11):2067–72.
32. Gibbs WN, Monuki ES, Linskey ME, et al. Pituicytoma: diagnostic features on selective carotid angiography and MR imaging. AJNR Am J Neuroradiol 2006;27(8): 1639–42.
33. Viaene AN, Lee EB, Rosenbaum JN, et al. Histologic, immunohistochemical, and molecular features of pituicytomas and atypical pituicytomas. Acta Neuropathol Commun 2019;7(1):69.
34. Rennert J, Doerfler A. Imaging of sellar and parasellar lesions. Clin Neurol Neurosurg 2007;109(2):111–24.
35. Lopes MBS, Scheithauer BW, Schiff D. Pituitary carcinoma: diagnosis and treatment. Endocrine 2005;28(1):115–21.
36. Kucharczyk W, Truwit CL. Diseases of the Sella Turcica and Parasellar Region. In: Hodler J, Kubik-Huch R, von Schulthess G, editors. Diseases of the Brain, Head and Neck, Spine 2020–2023. Springer; Cham (Switzerland). IDKD Springer Series. p. 3-9.
37. Agarwalla PK, Koch MJ, Royce TJ, et al. Stereotactic radiation as salvage therapy for recurrent rathke cleft cysts. Neurosurgery 2020;87(4):754–60.
38. Connor SEJ, Penney CC. MRI in the differential diagnosis of a sellar mass. Clin Radiol 2003;58(1):20–31.
39. Freda PU, Post KD. Differential diagnosis of sellar masses. Endocrinol Metab Clin North Am 1999;28(1):81–117, vi.
40. Brastianos PK, Santagata S. Endocrine tumors: BRAF V600E mutations in papillary craniopharyngioma. Eur J Endocrinol 2016;174(4):R139–44.
41. Brastianos PK, Taylor-Weiner A, Manley PE, et al. Exome sequencing identifies BRAF mutations in papillary craniopharyngiomas. Nat Genet 2014;46(2):161–5.
42. Johnsen DE, Woodruff WW, Allen IS, et al. MR imaging of the sellar and juxtasellar regions. Radiographics 1991;11(5):727–58.
43. Clark VE, Harmancı AS, Bai H, et al. Recurrent somatic mutations in POLR2A define a distinct subset of meningiomas. Nat Genet 2016;48(10):1253–9.
44. Magill ST, Morshed RA, Lucas C-HG, et al. Tuberculum sellae meningiomas: grading scale to assess surgical outcomes using the transcranial versus transsphenoidal approach. Neurosurg Focus 2018;44(4):E9.
45. Isaacs H Jr. Fetal intracranial teratoma. A review. Fetal Pediatr Pathol 2014; 33(5–6):289–92.
46. Truwit CL, Barkovich AJ. Pathogenesis of intracranial lipoma: an MR study in 42 patients. AJR Am J Roentgenol 1990;155(4):855–64 [discussion: 865].
47. Hershey BL. Suprasellar masses: diagnosis and differential diagnosis. Semin Ultrasound CT MR 1993;14(3):215–31.
48. Pamir MN, Ozduman K. Analysis of radiological features relative to histopathology in 42 skull-base chordomas and chondrosarcomas. Eur J Radiol 2006;58(3): 461–70.
49. Walcott BP, Nahed BV, Mohyeldin A, et al. Chordoma: current concepts, management, and future directions. Lancet Oncol 2012;13(2):e69–76.
50. Sharifnia T, Wawer MJ, Chen T, et al. Small-molecule targeting of brachyury transcription factor addiction in chordoma. Nat Med 2019;25(2):292–300.
51. Alshail E, Rutka JT, Becker LE, et al. Optic chiasmatic-hypothalamic glioma. Brain Pathol 1997;7(2):799–806.
52. Mosaab A, El-Ayadi M, Khorshed EN, et al. Histone H3K27M mutation overrides histological grading in pediatric gliomas. Sci Rep 2020;10(1):8368.

53. Osorio DS, Allen JC. Management of CNS germinoma. CNS Oncol 2015;4(4): 273–9.
54. Kluczyński Ł, Gilis-Januszewska A, Rogoziński D, et al. Hypophysitis - new insights into diagnosis and treatment. Endokrynol Pol 2019;70(3):260–9.
55. Angelousi A, Alexandraki K, Tsoli M, et al. Hypophysitis (including IgG4 and immunotherapy). Neuroendocrinology 2020;110(9–10):822–35.
56. Gubbi S, Hannah-Shmouni F, Verbalis JG, et al. Hypophysitis: an update on the novel forms, diagnosis and management of disorders of pituitary inflammation. Best Pract Res Clin Endocrinol Metab 2019;33(6):101371.
57. Saiwai S, Inoue Y, Ishihara T, et al. Lymphocytic adenohypophysis: skull radiographs and MRI. Neuroradiology 1998;40(2):114–20.
58. Fukuoka H. Hypophysitis. Endocrinol Metab Clin North Am 2015;44(1):143–9.
59. Joshi MN, Whitelaw BC, Carroll PV. Hypophysitis – diagnosis and treatment. European Journal of Endocrinology Sept 2018;179(3):R151–63.
60. Lojou M, Bonneville JF, Ebbo M, et al. IgG4 hypophysitis: diagnosis and management. Presse Med 2020;49(1):104016.
61. Di Dalmazi G, Ippolito S, Lupi I, et al. Hypophysitis induced by immune checkpoint inhibitors: a 10-year assessment. Expert Rev Endocrinol Metab 2019; 14(6):381–98.
62. Grois N, Prayer D, Prosch H, et al, CNS LCH Co-operative Group. Neuropathology of CNS disease in Langerhans cell histiocytosis. Brain 2005;128(Pt 4): 829–38.
63. Allen CE, Merad M, McClain KL. Langerhans-cell histiocytosis. N Engl J Med 2018;379(9):856–68.
64. Jindal G, Miller T, Raghavan P, et al. Imaging evaluation and treatment of vascular lesions at the skull base. Radiol Clin North Am 2017;55(1):151–66.

# Histopathology of Pituitary Lesions

Ada Baisre de León, MD

## KEYWORDS

- Pituitary adenoma • Pituitary neoplasms histology • Prolactinoma • Pituicytoma
- Rathke cleft cyst • Craniopharyngioma

## KEY POINTS

- The adenohypophysis, which represents ~80% of the entire pituitary gland, is composed of 5 types of cells: somatotrophs, gonadotrophs, lactotrophs, corticotrophs, and thyrotrophs.
- The neurohypophysis is composed of pituicytes, which are modified glial cells, mixed with axons and its endings, as well as axonal swellings (Herring bodies).
- Cysts and tumorlike lesions can also involve the pituitary gland.
- Hematopoietic and metastatic tumors as well as infectious and inflammatory lesions may also involve the pituitary gland.
- Pituitary carcinoma only represents 0.2% of all pituitary tumors, and the diagnosis can only be made in the setting of a pituitary adenoma that has metastasized, noncontiguously, through the central nervous system or to other organs.

## INTRODUCTION

The pituitary gland is a neuroendocrine organ composed of the adenohypophysis (anterior pituitary) and the neurohypophysis (posterior pituitary) (**Fig. 1**). The adenohypophysis, which represents ~80% of the entire gland, is composed of 5 types of cells: somatotrophs, gonadotrophs, lactotrophs, corticotrophs, and thyrotrophs, all of which are arranged in an acinar pattern (**Fig. 2**). This pattern is highlighted by a Reticulin stain (**Fig. 3**). The neurohypophysis is composed of pituicytes, which are modified glial cells, mixed with axons and its endings, as well as axonal swellings (Herring bodies) (**Fig. 4**).[1]

The different types of cells within the adenohypophysis and embryonic nests trapped during development give rise to the most common types of pituitary lesions. Less commonly, tumors may arise from the neurohypophysis and

Department of Pathology, Immunology and Laboratory Medicine, Rutgers, New Jersey Medical School, 185 South Orange Avenue, MSB C525, Newark, NJ 07103, USA
E-mail address: baisread@njms.rutgers.edu

Otolaryngol Clin N Am 55 (2022) 265–285
https://doi.org/10.1016/j.otc.2021.12.003
0030-6665/22/© 2021 Elsevier Inc. All rights reserved.
oto.theclinics.com

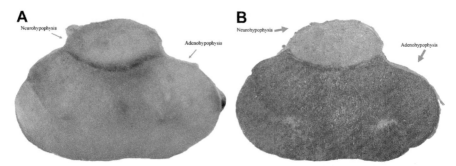

**Fig. 1.** Normal pituitary gland, gross (A) and microscopic (B) whole section, illustrating the clearly distinct neurohypophysis and adenohypophysis.

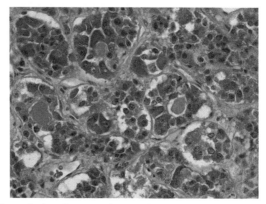

**Fig. 2.** Hematoxylin-eosin (H&E), original magnification ×200. Normal adenohypophysis. A mixture of morphologically different cell types is present in an acinar pattern.

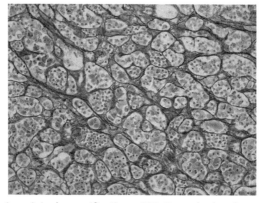

**Fig. 3.** Reticulin stain, original magnification ×200. Normal adenohypophysis with emphasized acinar pattern.

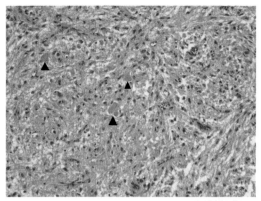

**Fig. 4.** H&E, original magnification ×200. Normal neurohypophysis. Pituicyte nuclei in a background of axons, its endings and Herring bodies (*arrowheads*).

**Box 1**
**Pituitary lesions**

Tumors of the adenohypophysis
- Pituitary adenoma
- Pituitary carcinoma
- Pituitary blastoma

Tumors of neurohypophysis
- Pituicytoma
- Spindle cell oncocytoma
- Granular cell tumor
- Sellar ependymoma

Other neoplasms, cysts, and tumorlike lesions
- Adamantinomatous craniopharyngioma
- Papillary craniopharyngioma
- Rathke cleft cyst
- Epidermoid cyst
- Arachnoid cyst
- Lymphocytic hypophysitis
- Granulomatous hypophysitis

Other miscellaneous and secondary lesions
- Germ cell tumors
- Chordoma
- Chondrosarcoma
- Plasmacytoma
- Metastatic tumors to the pituitary and surrounding structures
- Meningioma
- Schwannoma
- Erdheim-Chester disease
- Langerhans cell histiocytosis
- Hematopoietic tumors

Data from Refs.[2–4]

---

**Box 2**
**Pituitary adenomas**

- Acidophilic lineage (PIT-1)
  - Somatotroph (growth hormone [GH])
    - Densely granulated adenoma
    - Sparsely granulated adenoma
    - Mammosomatotroph adenoma
    - Mixed somatotroph-lactotroph adenoma
  - Lactotroph (prolactin)
    - Densely granulated adenoma
    - Sparsely granulated adenoma
    - Acidophilic stem cell adenoma
  - Thyrotroph (β-thyroid-stimulating hormone [β-TSH] and α-subunit)

- Corticotroph lineage (T-PIT and adrenocorticotropic hormone [ACTH])
  - Densely granulated adenoma
  - Sparsely granulated adenoma
  - Crooke cell adenoma

- Gonadotroph lineage (SF-1)
  - Sparsely granulated adenoma (β-follicle-stimulating hormone [β-FSH], β-luteinizing hormone [β-LH], and α-subunit)

- Null cell adenoma (no markers)

- Plurihormonal adenoma (PIT-1 or unusual IHC combinations)

- Double adenoma (variable)

*Data from* Refs.[2–4]

---

surrounding meninges and bone structures. Hematopoietic and metastatic tumors as well as infectious and inflammatory lesions may also involve the pituitary gland (**Box 1**).

## Tumors of the Adenohypophysis

### Pituitary adenoma

Pituitary adenomas are neoplasms of the adenohypophysis that arise from the different cell types. Adenomas represent ∼15% of all intracranial neoplasms.[2] They are classified based on their expression of hormones and transcription factors by immunohistochemistry (IHC) (**Box 2**), as somatotrophs (**Box 3**), lactotrophs (**Box 4**), thyrotrophs (**Box 5**), corticotrophs (**Box 6**), gonadotrophs (**Box 7**), null cell, plurihormonal, and double adenomas (**Box 8**). Overproduction of hormones causes clinical symptoms, occasionally in the form of dramatic syndromes, such as gigantism and acromegaly, whereas symptoms of compression of adjacent structures and headache are more common in tumors in which hormonal excess is not seen. A common histologic feature of all adenomas is the effacement of the normal acinar architecture and loss of cellular heterogeneity. The monomorphic neoplastic cells grow in several patterns, such as diffuse sheets, papillae, cords, nests, and perivascular rosettes (**Fig. 5**). These different patterns have no bearing on the diagnosis, prognosis, or classification. Cytoplasmic characteristics, although not specific, may offer a clue to the lineage. Gonadotrophs, lactotrophs, and thyrotrophs may show chromophobic cytoplasm; somatotrophs may be acidophilic, and corticotrophs may be basophilic.

*Acidophilic Lineage Adenomas (Expression of PIT-1 Transcription Factor)*

---

**Box 3**
**Somatotrophs adenomas (PIT-1 and growth hormone expression)**

| Densely granulated (**Fig. 6**) | Sparsely granulated | Mammosomatotroph | Mixed somatotroph and lactotroph (**Fig. 7**) |
|---|---|---|---|
| Most common variant | Likely chromophobic cytoplasm | Mostly eosinophilic cells | Expression of prolactin and GH |
| Likely eosinophilic cytoplasm | Cytoplasmic fibrous bodies, | Both cells express GH and prolactin | by different cells |
| Strong and diffuse expression of GH | which are cytokeratin (+) | PIT-1 (+) | PIT-1 (+) |
| PIT-1 (+) | GH expression | May express α-subunit | May express |
| May express α-subunit | is variable | Estrogen Receptor (ER) | α-subunit and ER |
|  | PIT-1 (+) | and cytokeratin (+) |  |

---

**Box 4**
**Lactotrophs adenomas (PIT-1 and prolactin expression)**

| Densely granulated (**Fig. 8**A, B) | Sparsely granulated (**Fig. 8**C, D) | Acidophilic stem cell |
|---|---|---|
| Eosinophilic cytoplasm | Most common variant | Neoplastic cells have |
| Strong and diffuse | Chromophobic cytoplasm | oncocytic features and |
| prolactin staining | Perinuclear dotlike | cytoplasmic vacuolization |
| PIT-1 (+) | Prolactin staining | Prolactin and PIT-1 (+) |
| ER (+) | PIT-1 (+) | ER (+) |
|  | ER (+) |  |

---

**Box 5**
**Thyrotroph adenomas (PIT-1, β-thyroid-stimulating hormone, and α-subunit expression)**

Polygonal or spindle cells with chromophobic cytoplasm (**Fig. 9**)

Stromal fibrosis is common

PIT-1, β-TSH, and α-subunit (+)

GATA-2 and SSTR2 also (+)

---

*Corticotroph Lineage Adenomas*

---

**Box 6**
**Corticotroph adenomas (T-PIT and adrenocorticotropic hormone expression)**

| Densely granulated (**Fig. 10**) | Sparsely granulated | Crooke cell adenoma |
|---|---|---|
| Most common variant | Weakly basophilic | Tumor cells with |
| Likely basophilic cytoplasm | Weak ACTH expression | Crooke hyaline change |
| Strong and diffuse expression of ACTH | T-PIT (+) | Ringlike expression of cytokeratin |
| T-PIT and Periodic acid–Schiff (PAS)(+) |  | T-PIT (+) |

*Gonadotroph Lineage Adenomas*

---

> **Box 7**
> **Gonadotroph adenomas (SF1, β-follicle-stimulating hormone, β-luteinizing hormone, and α-subunit expression)**
>
> Chromophobic neoplastic cells **(Fig. 11)**
>
> Perivascular pseudorosettes or trabecular pattern are common
>
> SF1 (+)
>
> Variable staining for β-FSH, β-LH, and α-subunit expression
>
> GATA-2 and SSTR2 also (+)

*Other Adenomas*

---

> **Box 8**
> **Other adenomas**
>
> | Null cell | Plurihormonal | Double adenoma **(Fig. 12)** |
> |---|---|---|
> | No expression of hormones or transcription factors | Expression of >1 hormone | Two separate tumors with 2 different cell types |
> | Occur typically in the 6th or 7th decade | Single cell producing 2 or more hormones | Silent lactotroph and another type are common |
> | Chromophobic or acidophilic cells | 2 or more cell lineage | Functioning gonadotroph are also common |
> | | Commonly PIT-1 (+) | Transcription factor is helpful in separating the tumors |

## PITUITARY CARCINOMA

Pituitary carcinoma only represents 0.2% of all pituitary tumors, and the diagnosis can only be made in the setting of a pituitary adenoma that has metastasized, noncontiguously, through the central nervous system or to other organs.[4,5] No consensus exists in predicting which adenoma will behave aggressively or become carcinoma, and this remains a challenge for neuropathologists, as cytologic atypia, necrosis, and mitosis, although worrisome, cannot be used as criteria for malignancy in a tumor that has not metastasized. Biomarkers, such as FGFR4, MMP, PTTG, Ki-67, p53, and deletions in chromosome 11 have been reported as potential candidates in predicting and managing aggressive pituitary adenomas and carcinoma.[6]

## PITUITARY BLASTOMA

First described in 2008, pituitary blastoma is a rare tumor of early childhood with a poor prognosis associated with *DICER1* mutations.[7,8] It was added to the 2017 classification of tumors of endocrine organs[2] and is one of the hallmarks of *DICER1* syndrome.[7] Morphologically, they are composed of 3 types of cells as follows: primitive cells, secretory cells, and Rathke-like columnar/cuboidal epithelium. Cushing disease is the usual presentation of most pituitary blastomas.[2]

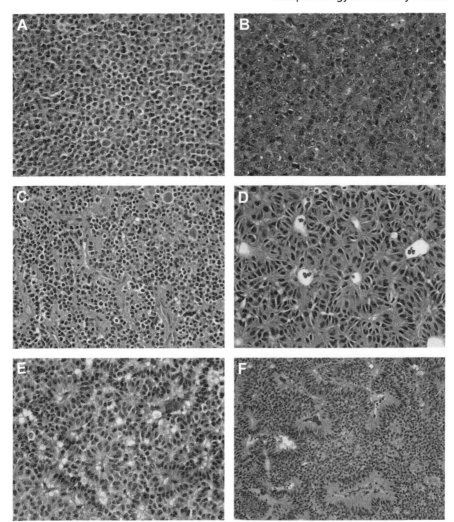

**Fig. 5.** H&E growth patterns of pituitary adenomas. (A) Original magnification ×400, sheets of chromophobic neoplastic cells. (B) Original magnification ×400, strongly eosinophilic tumor also growing in sheets. (C) Original magnification ×400, nests of chromophobic neoplastic cells. (D–E) Original magnification ×400 and (F) ×200, the neoplastic cells are arranged in a dramatic perivascular pseudorosette pattern.

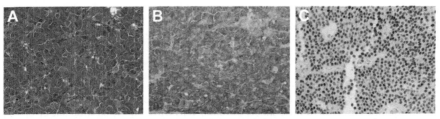

**Fig. 6.** Densely granulated somatotroph adenoma. (A) H&E, original magnification ×400, the neoplastic cells show strongly eosinophilic cytoplasm. (B) GH, original magnification ×400, strong and diffuse expression of growth hormone. (C) PIT-1, original magnification ×400, diffuse nuclear expression is identified.

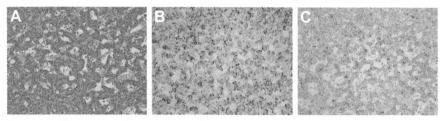

**Fig. 7.** Mixed somatotroph and lactotroph adenoma. (*A*) H&E, original magnification ×200, arranged in a trabecular pattern. (*B*) Prolactin, original magnification ×200, staining of several cells is noted. (*C*) GH, original magnification ×200, staining of a few cells within the same area.

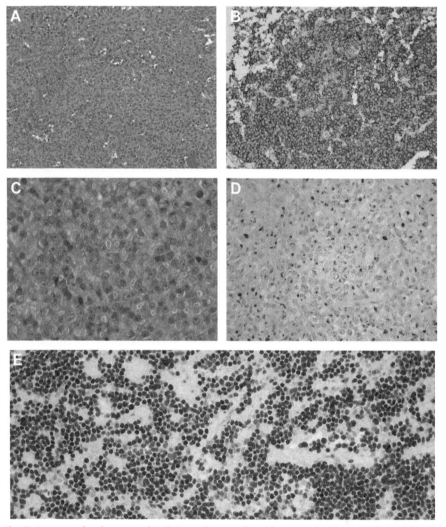

**Fig. 8.** Lactotroph adenomas. (*A, B*) Densely granulated lactotroph adenoma. (*A*) H&E, original magnification ×200, diffuse sheets of tumor cells with slightly eosinophilic cytoplasm. (*B*) Prolactin, original magnification ×400, diffuse staining. (*C, D*) Sparsely granulated lactotroph adenoma. (*C*) H&E, original magnification ×400, the neoplastic cells with pale cytoplasm displaying with prominent Golgi. (*D*) Prolactin, original magnification ×200, paranuclear dotlike reactivity. (*E*) PIT-1, original magnification ×400, both densely and sparsely granulated have strong expression of nuclear PIT-1.

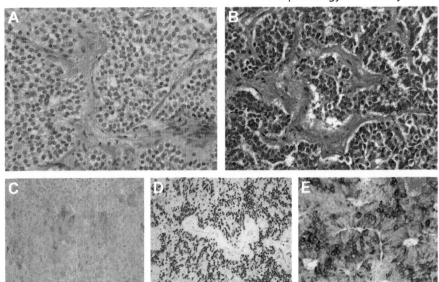

Fig. 9. Thyrotroph adenoma. (A) H&E, original magnification ×400, chromophobic cells growing in sheets separated by dense collagen septae. (B) Masson-Trichrome, original magnification ×400, highlights the fibrosis. (C) β-TSH, original magnification ×400, expression of TSH is noted in several cells. (D) PIT-1, original magnification ×200, diffuse nuclear staining is identified. (E) α-Subunit, original magnification ×400, several neoplastic cells express α-subunit.

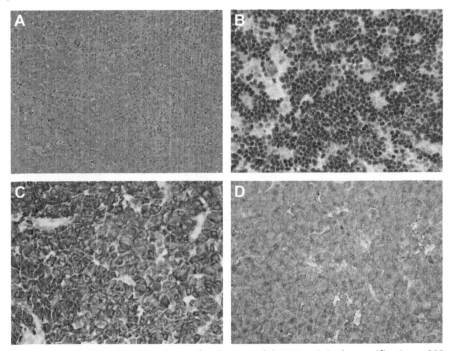

Fig. 10. Densely granulated corticotroph adenoma. (A) H&E, original magnification ×200, sheets of neoplastic cells. (B) T-PIT, original magnification ×400, strong nuclear expression is seen. (C) CK8/18 (CAM 5.2), original magnification ×400, diffuse expression is usually seen in both densely and sparsely granulated corticotrophs adenoma. (D) ACTH, original magnification ×400, diffuse expression is also seen with ACTH.

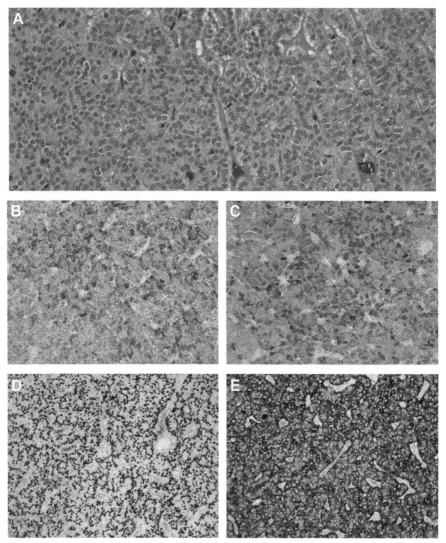

**Fig. 11.** Densely granulated gonadotroph adenoma. (*A*) H&E, original magnification ×200, the chromophobic neoplastic cells show a subtle perivascular pseudorosette pattern. (*B*) β-FSH and (*C*) β-LH, original magnification ×200, scattered cells show expression of both β-FSH and β-LH. (*D*) SF1, original magnification ×200, strong nuclear staining. (*E*) α-Subunit, original magnification ×200, strong and diffuse staining.

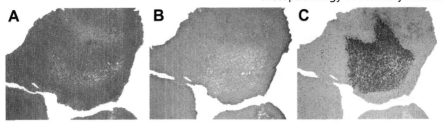

Fig. 12. Double adenoma somatotroph and lactotroph. (A) H&E, original magnification ×25, showing a distinct chromophobic adenoma in the center surrounded by a strongly eosinophilic peripheral adenoma. (B) GH, original magnification ×25, showing diffuse staining by GH of the peripheral eosinophilic adenoma and negative staining of the central chromophobic adenoma. (C) Prolactin, original magnification ×25, strongly highlights the central chromophobic adenoma and is mostly negative in the peripheral eosinophilic adenoma.

## TUMORS OF THE NEUROHYPOPHYSIS

| Box 9 |
|---|
| **Tumors of the neurohypophysis** |

| Granular cell tumor (**Fig. 13**A) | Pituicytoma (**Fig. 13**B, C) | Spindle cell oncocytoma |
|---|---|---|
| Loose polygonal cells with eccentric nuclei | Bipolar elongated cells | (**Fig. 13**D–E) |
| Characteristic abundant granular cytoplasm | Dense eosinophilic cytoplasm | Epithelioid or elongated cells |
| Arranged in sheets or nodules | Arranged in fascicles | Eosinophilic or granular cytoplasm |
| S100, TTF-1, PAS, and PAS-D (+) | TTF-1 (+) | TTF-1 and antimitochondrial antibody (+) |
|  | Variable expression of S100 and GFAP |  |

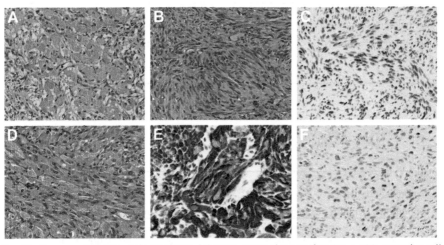

Fig. 13. Tumors of the Neurohypophysis. (A) H&E, original magnification ×400, granular cell tumor. Loose polygonal cells with very characteristic granular cytoplasm arranged in nests. (B, C) Pituicytoma. (B) H&E, original magnification ×400, fascicles of elongated cells with eosinophilic cytoplasm and bipolar nuclei. (C) TTF-1, original magnification ×400, showing characteristic nuclear expression. (D–E) Spindle cell oncocytoma. (D) H&E, original magnification ×400, epithelioid to spindle cells showing round to oval nuclei and densely eosinophilic granular cytoplasm. (E) Antimitochondrial antibody, original magnification ×400, showing strong cytoplasmic staining illustrating the abundant mitochondrial content. (F) TTF-1, original magnification ×400, showing characteristic nuclear expression. (Courtesy of Dr. Marc Rosenblum, MSKCC, New York.)

## OTHER NEOPLASMS, CYSTS, AND TUMORLIKE LESIONS

| Box 10<br>Craniopharyngiomas | |
|---|---|
| **Adamantinomatous (Fig. 14)** | **Papillary (Fig. 15)** |
| Basal layer with nuclear palisading | Mature squamous epithelium |
| Lacelike background known as stellate reticulum | Pronounced papillary structures with prominent fibrovascular cords |
| Prominent squamous whorls | *BRAF* V600E mutation |
| "Wet keratin and ghost cells" are characteristic | |
| Calcifications are common | |
| *CTNNB1* mutations | |
| Nuclear β -catenin expression | |

| Box 11<br>Common cystic lesions | | |
|---|---|---|
| **Rathke Cleft Cyst (Fig. 16)** | **Epidermoid Cyst (Fig. 17)** | **Arachnoid Cyst (Fig. 18)** |
| Lined by ciliated cuboidal/columnar epithelium with goblet cells | Lined by keratinizing squamous epithelium | Lined by meningothelial cells |
| Proteinaceous contents | "Dry" keratin contents, which are pearly white grossly | Clear "cerebrospinal fluidlike" fluid content |

| Box 12<br>Tumorlike lesions | |
|---|---|
| **Lymphocytic Hypophysitis (Fig. 19)** | **Granulomatous Hypophysitis (Fig. 20)** |
| • Destruction of the normal acinar architecture by inflammatory cells | • Destruction of the normal acinar architecture by granulomata |
| • The inflammatory infiltrate is composed of lymphocytes, plasma cells, eosinophils, and macrophages | • Granulomata can be necrotizing and nonnecrotizing |
| | • Sarcoidosis and tuberculosis have a predilection for the skull base and may involve the pituitary gland |
| | • Other infections, such as fungal, can elicit a granulomatous reaction |

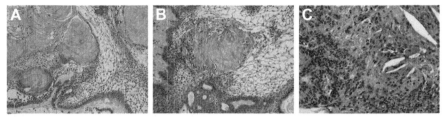

**Fig. 14.** Adamantinomatous craniopharyngioma. (*A*) H&E, original magnification ×100 and (*B*) H&E, original magnification ×200, epithelial neoplasm showing several patterns as follows: the basal layer is arranged in a picket-fence pattern with microcystic spaces and trabeculae. As this basal layer matures, it gives rise to cells with clear cytoplasm and pronounces cell membranes known as stellate reticulum. The top layer contains clumps of "wet keratin," and it may also contain calcifications. (*C*) H&E, original magnification ×400, neoplastic cell arranged in trabeculae surrounded by cholesterol clefts, responsible for the gross appearance of "machinery oil," hemosiderin-laden macrophages, and other inflammatory cells.

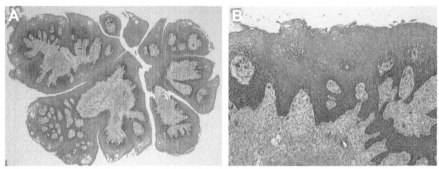

**Fig. 15.** Papillary craniopharyngioma. (*A*) H&E, original magnification ×25 and (*B*) H&E, original magnification ×200, well-formed papillae with dense fibrovascular cores are lined by well differentiated, nonkeratinizing squamous epithelium with orderly maturation.

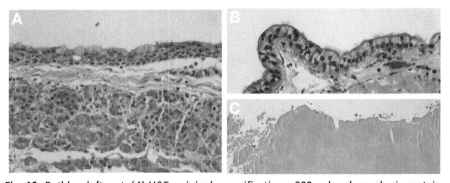

**Fig. 16.** Rathke cleft cyst. (*A*) H&E, original magnification ×200, adenohypophysis containing a cyst lined by cuboidal to columnar ciliated epithelium with goblet cells. (*B*) H&E, original magnification ×400, cystic wall with columnar epithelium with abundant goblet cells. (*C*) H&E, original magnification ×200, the contents of Rathke cleft cyst is usually dense proteinaceous material.

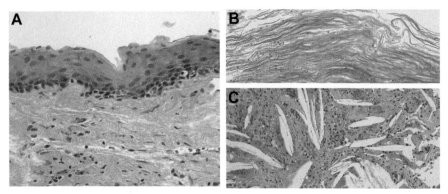

**Fig. 17.** Epidermoid cyst. (*A*) The wall of epidermoid cysts is composed of keratinizing squamous epithelium and dense collagen. (*B*) H&E, original magnification ×100, the contents of epidermoid cyst are flakes of "dry" keratin, described grossly as "pearly white." (*C*) H&E, original magnification ×200, keratin debris elicits a foreign body-giant cell reaction.

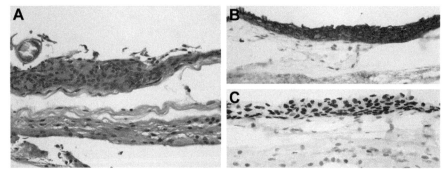

**Fig. 18.** Arachnoid cyst. (*A*) H&E, original magnification ×200, the cystic wall is lined by arachnoid/meningothelial cells, and occasional psammoma bodies can be seen. (*B*) H&E EMA, original magnification ×400, meningothelial cells diffusely express epithelial membrane antigen. (*C*) PR, original magnification ×400, strong nuclear expression of progesterone receptor is also seen in meningothelial cells.

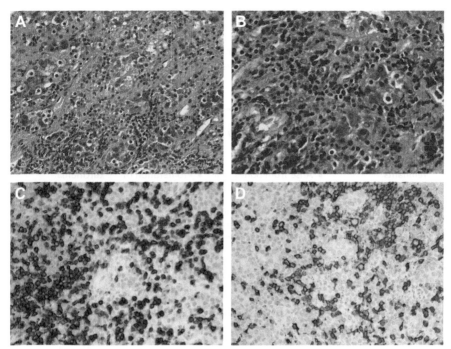

**Fig. 19.** Lymphocytic hypophysitis. (*A*) H&E, original magnification ×200 and (*B*) H&E, original magnification ×400, the adenohyophysis is heavily infiltrated by inflammatory cells, which are seen destroying the acini. (*C*) CD3, original magnification ×400 and (*D*) CD20, original magnification ×400, CD3(+) T cells and CD20(+) B cells are seen infiltrating the adenohypophysis.

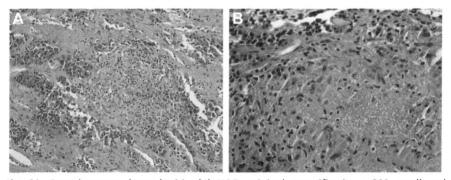

**Fig. 20.** Granulomatous hypophysitis. (*A*) H&E, original magnification ×200, small and discrete, nonnecrotizing granuloma can be seen in neurosarcoidosis, embedded within the pituitary acini. (*B*) H&E, original magnification ×400, the necrotizing granulomata typical of mycobacterial infection, particularly tuberculosis, has a predilection for the skull base, seen here involving the anterior pituitary gland.

## OTHER MISCELLANEOUS AND SECONDARY LESIONS

Other miscellaneous tumors can arise within or metastasize to the pituitary gland (**Figs. 21–28**). Other tumors, such as mesenchymal and metastatic tumors, that involve surrounding structures may involve the pituitary gland by extension (**Box 13, Table 1**).

---

**Box 13**
**Tumors from surrounding structures that may involve the pituitary gland**

| Chordoma (see **Fig. 21**) | Chondrosarcoma (see **Fig. 22**) | Plasmacytoma (see **Fig. 23**) | Metastatic mucinous carcinoma (see **Fig. 24**) |
|---|---|---|---|
| • Arise form notochord remnants<br>• Cords of tumor cells in a myxoid/mucinous background<br>• Cells have vacuolated cytoplasm known as "physaliphorous cells"<br>• Express S100, Pan-CK, EMA, and brachyury | • Arise from bones that undergo enchondral ossification[9]<br>• Chondrocytes are seen within lacunar spaces<br>• Chondroid background is usually seen<br>• Myxoid variant may show cords of tumor cells similar to chordomas<br>• Express S100 | • Proliferation of neoplastic plasma cells<br>• May be a solitary plasmacytoma or part of multiple myeloma<br>• Neoplastic plasma cells may be atypical or binucleated<br>• Express CD138 | • The neoplastic epithelial cells are arranged in cords, trabeculae, and glands in a mucinous background<br>• Express pan-CK and EMA<br>• May express other markers depending on the origin |

---

**Table 1**
**Differential diagnosis of bony lesions**

|  | S100 | Pancytokeratin | EMA | Brachyury | CD138 |
|---|---|---|---|---|---|
| Chordoma | + | + | + | + | − |
| Chondrosarcoma | + | − | − | − | − |
| Plasmacytoma | − | − | +/− | − | + |
| Carcinoma | − | + | + | − | − |

---

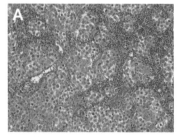 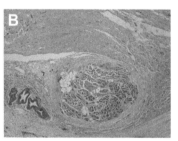

**Fig. 21.** Germ cell tumors. (*A*) H&E, original magnification ×200, germinoma showing nests of large neoplastic germ cells with large nuclei and clear cytoplasm with a lymphocytic infiltrate within the septae. (*B*) H&E, original magnification ×25, mature teratoma displaying disorganized mature elements of endodermal origin, such as gland formation, mesenchymal elements like skeletal muscle and adipose tissue, and ectodermal in origin like glioneuronal islands.

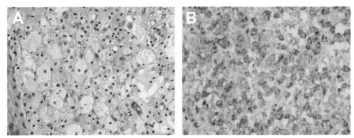

**Fig. 22.** Erdheim-Chester disease. (*A*) H&E, original magnification ×200, sheets of foamy histiocytes effacing the normal pituitary architecture. (*B*) CD68, original magnification ×200, the histiocytes express macrophage marker CD68 and are negative for CD1a (not shown).

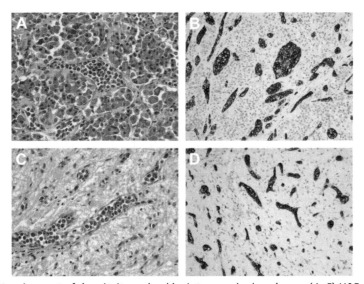

**Fig. 23.** Involvement of the pituitary gland by intravascular lymphoma. (*A, B*) H&E, original magnification ×200, the neoplastic cells are seen proliferating within (*A*) the sinusoids of the adenohypophysis and (*B*) of the capillaries of the neurohypophysis. (*C, D*) CD20, original magnification ×200, the malignant B cells are illustrated with a CD20 B-cell marker in (*A*) in the sinusoids of the adenohypophysis and (*B*) in the capillaries of the neurohypophysis.

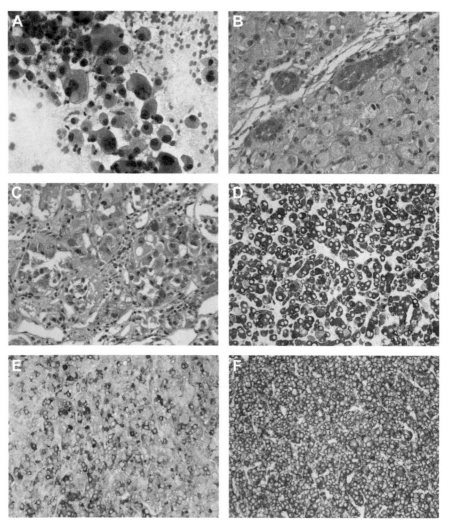

**Fig. 24.** Metastatic breast carcinoma to the pituitary gland. (*A*) H&E, original magnification ×630, smear preparation during intraoperative consultation showing the larger neoplastic cells with abundant cytoplasm containing intracytoplasmic vacuoles next to the normal adenohypophyseal cells. (*B*, *C*) Original magnification ×400; the neoplastic cells, which are large and have pale cytoplasm, have nearly obliterated the normal pituitary architecture. Remaining cells are smaller with denser eosinophilic cytoplasm. (*D*) CK7, original magnification ×200, strong and diffuse cytoplasmic expression is noted. (*E*) GCDFP-15, original magnification ×200, focal and strong expression is identified. (*F*) HER-2, original magnification ×200, 3+ expression.

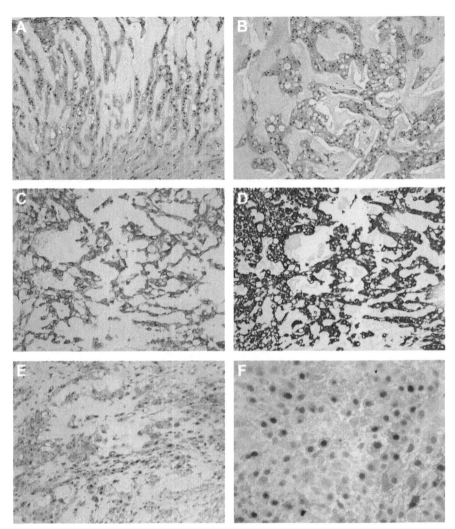

**Fig. 25.** Chordoma. (*A & B*) H&E, original magnification ×200; the tumors cells are arranged in cords and nests in a myxoid/mucinous background. The cytoplasm of many of the cells shows abundant vacuolation that earns them the name "physaliphorous" cells. (*C*) EMA, original magnification ×200, (*D*) pancytokeratin (*E*) S100, original magnification ×200; chordomas are typically diffusely positive for EMA, pancytokeratin, and S100 immunostains. (*F*) Brachyury, original magnification ×630, characteristic nuclear staining.

**Fig. 26.** Chondrosarcoma. (*A*) H&E, original magnification ×200, low to moderately cellular chondroid neoplasm where neoplastic chondrocytes are surrounded by vacuoles in a chondroid background. (*B*) H&E, original magnification ×100, myxoid chondrosarcoma may show cord arrangement of the neoplastic cells in a myxoid background similar to that of chordoma. (*C*) S100, original magnification ×200; chondrosarcomas show expression of S100, whereas keratins and EMA are generally negative (not shown).

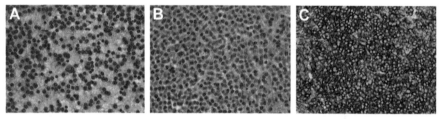

**Fig. 27.** Plasmacytoma. (*A*) Smear preparation H&E, original magnification ×400 and (*B*) H&E, original magnification ×400, proliferation of plasma cells, some of them binucleated. (*C*) CD138, original magnification ×400, strong expression of the plasma cell marker CD138.

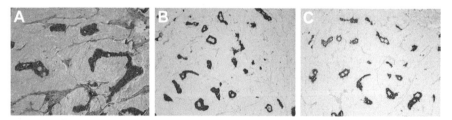

**Fig. 28.** Metastatic mucinous carcinoma from colonic origin. (*A*) H&E, original magnification ×100, rare glands and cords of neoplastic cells in a very abundant mucinous background. (*B*) CK20 and (*C*) CDX-2, original magnification ×100, strong membranous staining with CK20 and nuclear staining with CDX2 characteristic of tumors of the lower gastrointestinal tract.

## SUMMARY

Accurate histologic diagnosis and classification of the extensive assortment of benign and malignant tumors and tumorlike lesions that arise or involve the pituitary gland are critical, as their management, treatment, and prognosis differ greatly.

## CLINICS CARE POINTS

> • Understanding the histologic diagnosis and classification of primary and secondary pituitary tumors is crucial in the management of patients with such lesions.

## DISCLOSURE

The author has nothing to disclose.

## REFERENCES

1. Lopes MB, Thapar K, Horvath E, et al. Neoplasms of the sellar region. In: McLendon Roger E, Rosenblum Marc K, Bigner Darell, Russell D, et al, editors. Pathology of tumors of the nervous system. 7th edition. London: Hodder Arnold; 2006.
2. Osamura RY, Lopes MBS, Grossman A, et al. Pituitary adenoma. In: Lloyd RV, Osamura RY, Klöppel G, et al, editors. WHO classification of tumours of endocrine organs. 4th Edition. Lyon: IARC; 2017. p. 14–8.
3. Lopes MBS. The 2017 World Health Organization classification of tumors of the pituitary gland: a summary. Acta Neuropathol 2017;134:521–35.
4. Mete O, Lopes MB. Overview of the 2017 WHO classification of pituitary tumors. Endocr Pathol 2017;28(3):228–43.
5. Kaltsas GA, Nomikos P, Kontogeorgos G, et al. Clinical review: diagnosis and management of pituitary carcinomas. J Clin Endocrinol Metab 2005;90(5):3089–99.
6. Mete O, Ezzat S, Asa SL. Biomarkers of aggressive pituitary adenomas. J Mol Endocrinol 2012;49(2):R69–78.
7. Scheithauer BW, Kovacs K, Horvath E, et al. Pituitary blastoma. Acta Neuropathol 2008;116:657.
8. de Kock L, Sabbaghian N, Plourde F, et al. Pituitary blastoma: a pathognomonic feature of germ-line DICER1 mutations. Acta Neuropathol 2014;128(1):111–22. https://doi.org/10.1007/s00401-014-1285-z.
9. Rosenberg A. Chordoma and related lesions, chondrosarcoma and osteosarcoma of the cranium. In: McLendon Roger E, Rosenblum Marc K, Bigner Darell, Russell D, et al, editors. Pathology of tumors of the nervous system. 7th edition. London: Hodder Arnold; 2006.

# Non-surgical Interventions for Pituitary Lesions

Nisha Suda, MD, MHA*

## KEYWORDS

- Medical management • Nonsurgical • Hormonal • Dopamine agonists
- Somatostatin analogues • Radiotherapy

## KEY POINTS

- Many therapies for the management of pituitary tumors can be used independent of surgery, as an adjunct to surgery, and in combination with each other.
- Not all pituitary tumors require intervention.
- Cosecretion of hormones from pituitary tumors can allow for the use of multiple therapeutic agents from different medication classes.
- Hormone receptor subtyping has led to the advent of more targeted medical therapies.
- Radiotherapy can be used as an adjunct to surgical and medical therapy, but the latency of onset to achieve clinically significant outcomes remains a drawback.

## INTRODUCTION

Pituitary lesions may present with mass effect, hormonal abnormalities, or may remain clinically silent for the entirety of their existence. Pituitary lesions do not always necessitate surgical intervention, and numerous nonsurgical treatments have evolved for use as both primary and adjuvant therapies. These tumors may secrete an excess of prolactin, growth hormone (GH), thyroid-stimulating hormone (TSH), adrenocorticotrophic hormone (ACTH), and/or gonadotroph hormones, but there are also clinically silent tumors, nonsecretory tumors, and pituitary carcinomas, all of which may respond to medical and/or radiotherapy.

### Lactotroph Adenomas (Prolactin Secreting Adenomas)

First and foremost, not all prolactinomas require therapy. Indications for treatment include mass effect, premenopausal amenorrhea, male hypogonadism, bothersome galactorrhea, bothersome mastalgia, and/or gynecomastia.[1] When treatment of a prolactinoma is indicated, these lesions are highly responsive to pharmacologic therapy. Under normal physiologic conditions lactotroph cells remain under tonic inhibition by

Department of Medicine, Endocrinology & Metabolism, Montefiore Medical Center, Albert Einstein College of Medicine, Bronx, NY, USA
* Fleischer Institute for Diabetes and Metabolism, 1180 Morris Park Avenue (2nd Floor), Bronx, NY 10461,
E-mail address: nisuda@montefiore.org

Otolaryngol Clin N Am 55 (2022) 287–304
https://doi.org/10.1016/j.otc.2021.12.004
0030-6665/22/© 2021 Elsevier Inc. All rights reserved.

dopamine, thus allowing for effective utilization of dopamine agonists, such as cabergoline and bromocriptine, which can reduce both prolactinoma size in ~65% of patients and hormone production in ~80% of patients in approximately 3 months.[1–5]

Both therapies are available as oral pills, but cabergoline has greater effectiveness for normalization of prolactin, a more favorable side-effect profile, greater cost-effectiveness, and easier dosing.[1,3] Cabergoline's longer half-life allows for weekly or semiweekly administration, while bromocriptine is a daily medication. The reason for some of these differences is on account of cabergoline's selectivity for the D2 receptor, whereas bromocriptine has an affinity for both the D1 and the D2 receptors.

Because both therapies increase dopamine levels, patients may demonstrate impulse control disorders, although this has not been fully validated at standard doses. Overall, both therapies are deemed low risk with some patients experiencing side effects of nausea, nasal stuffiness, and postural hypotension.[4,6]

There remains a small subset of prolactinomas that are refractory to conventional dopamine agonist therapy, which is encountered more frequently with macroprolactinomas than microprolactinomas. Although there is no fixed definition, failure to achieve a 30% reduction in size or failure to normalize prolactin levels to achieve spontaneous menstruation within 3 to 6 months may be classified as refractory cases. Some prolactinomas may only respond hormonally, others only in size, and some may not respond in either parameter. Greater resistance occurs with bromocriptine (up to 30%) than cabergoline (10%); however, there are some subsets of patients that may respond inadequately to one but well to the other.[7] Carbergoline dosing typically starts at 0.25mg to 0.5mg twice per week and Bromocriptine dosing starts at 2.5-15mg daily. Inadequate response to conventional dosing necessitates up-titration of the dopamine agonist every 3 to 6 months, with case reports citing doses of greater than 2 mg per week of cabergoline, and one case requiring 21 mg/wk of cabergoline.[7,8] At higher doses, it is recommended that patients be screened for the development of cardiac valvopathies.[7,9]

Escalation of therapy to use of the oral alkylating agent temozolomide, typically used to treat pituitary carcinomas and neuroendocrine tumors, has been studied in a few patients. Response to therapy can be partial and carries the risk of side effects, including an increased risk of secondary malignancies.[10]

### Somatotroph Tumors (Growth Hormone-Secreting Tumors)

GH-secreting tumors account for 10% to 15% of pituitary adenomas and may cosecrete prolactin in approximately 40% of the cases on account of their shared cell lineage.[11] The incidence of GH-secreting adenomas is an estimated 3000 cases per year, with clinical manifestations ranging from subtle, such as increased sweating, to dramatic, with gigantism and cosmetically altering acromegalic features. GH secretion stimulates the production of insulin-like growth factor 1 (IGF-1), the medium through which most GH-mediated cell proliferation occurs. Because of the longer half-life of IGF-1, it can be used as a screening and disease marker. Therapeutic outcome data are presented in **Table 1**.

### Somatostatin analogues

Somatostatin (SST) is a GH inhibiting hormone, and synthetic somatostatin analogues, also called somatostatin receptor ligands (SRLs), are the initial choice of medical therapy per current Endocrine Society guidelines. They are typically used as adjuvant treatment following surgery. Although SRLs have not been shown to improve postoperative biochemical outcomes when initiated before surgery, they may be used in

**Table 1**
Medical management of somatotroph tumors with specific study outcome data

| | Medication | Mechanism | Administration | Outcome Data | Drawbacks |
|---|---|---|---|---|---|
| Somatostatin receptor ligand (SRL) | Octreotide LAR, lanreotide | Bind to SSTR-2, reducing proliferation of somatotroph cells and GH secretion | Octreotide IM, Lanreotide SC Every 4–6wk | IGF-1 normalization at 48 wk[17–19] Weighted mean percentage reduction on 37.3% in tumor volume in 66% of patients[20] | GI distress, gallstones, injection site reactions, dysglycemia |
| | Oral octreotide | Octreotide combined with an oil to facilitate opening of tight junctions in the gut to allow for system absorption | po qd-bid | Phase III: 2/3 of subjects transitioned from injectable formulations to oral maintained control of IGF-1 during dose titration phase, and 85% were able to sustain a response[21] CHIASMA OPTIMAL Trial: more stringent IGF-1 targets than phase III. At 36 wk, 58.2% maintained normal IGF-1 levels compared with 19% in placebo group. Higher satisfaction rates with oral vs injectables[22] | Must demonstrate response to injectable SRLs first GI distress, gallstones, dysglycemia |
| | Pasireotide | Bind to SSTR-3 and SSTR-5, reducing proliferation of somatotroph cells and GH secretion | SC monthly | 63% more likely to achieve biochemical control when compared with octreotide or lanreotide in patients who were previously uncontrolled on those SSTR-2 agents | Higher rates of hyperglycemia (~67% of patients) compared with other SRLs |

(continued on next page)

**Table 1**
*(continued)*

| | Medication | Mechanism | Administration | Outcome Data | Drawbacks |
|---|---|---|---|---|---|
| Growth hormone receptor antagonist | Pegvisomant | Pegylated GH analogue with affinity for GH receptor; reduces GH signaling | Daily SC injection | ACROSTUDY: normalization of IGF-1 levels in 63.2%–75% of patients after 5 y[25,26] Works independently of SSTR status Can be used in combination with SRLs[24] | No effect on tumor size, need for daily injections, transaminitis |
| D2 antagonist | Cabergoline | Acts where there is coexpression of D2 receptors | Twice weekly oral drug | Meta-analysis of 9 trials: 34% of 149 patients achieved biochemical normalization of IGF-1 levels[29,30] | Insufficient data to demonstrate IGF-1 lowering; not FDA approved for treatment of GH tumors |

*Abbreviations:* bid, twice daily; GI, gastrointestinal; IM, intramuscular; LAR, long-acting release; po, per os; qd, daily; SC, subcutaneous.

select cases to reduce the risk of GH-mediated comorbidities such as high-output heart failure, severe pharyngeal thickening, and sleep apnea.[12,13]

SRLs bind to somatostatin receptors (SSTR) to stop proliferation of somatotroph cells, thus suppressing GH secretion and blocking the synthesis of IGF-1.[14] The monthly inject-able SRLs intramuscular octreotide LAR and subcutaneous lanreotide target SSTR-2 and demonstrate equal efficacy for hormonal control and tumor shrinkage, as well as similar side-effect profiles (see **Table 1**).[15] Octreotide LAR as a first-line therapy can normalize IGF-1 to levels similar to that achieved by surgery, and tumor shrinkage can be achieved in 66% of patients. Outcome data vary based on the population being studied, with favor-able outcomes seen in patients with specific tumor receptor expression, older age, fe-male sex, dense granular pattern, and increased SSTR-2 expression, whereas high IGF-1 levels, high GH levels, sparse granular pattern, AIP gene mutation, and T2 hyper-intensity on MRI scan are predictors of poor outcomes with SRL therapy.[16] Both SSTR-2 targeting SRLs can cause diarrhea, abdominal discomfort, vomiting, hair loss, gallstones, pain at injection site, and dysglycemia.[17–20]

Oral octreotide is a once-a-day capsule that is now approved by the Food and Drug Administration (FDA) for patients with complete or partial biochemical response to the injectable SRLs. The capsule contains octreotide combined with an oil, which facili-tates the opening of tight junctions in the gut to allow for systemic absorption of octreotide. This capsule must be taken on an empty stomach for proper absorption. Both phase III trials and a subsequent large double-blinded randomized control trial demonstrated efficacy of oral octreotide therapy in achieving and maintaining normal IGF-1 levels (see **Table 1**). Furthermore, side-effect profiles between oral and inject-able SRLs were similar, and patients endorsed higher satisfaction rates with 90% of the patients choosing to continue the oral octreotide.[21,22]

Pasireotide is an SRL that targets SSTR-3 and SSTR-5 with higher affinity and has been shown to be superior in achieving biochemical control in patients who failed treatment with the SSTR-2 targeting agents.[17] Hyperglycemia-related adverse effects are more common with pasireotide compared with octreotide, with hyperglycemia occurring in approximately 67% of patients. Age younger than 40 years, normal body mass index with no dyslipidemia or diabetes, and SSTR-5 tumor expression were noted to be the major factors influencing outcomes with pasireotide.[17,23]

### Growth hormone receptor antagonists
Pegvisomant is a pegylated GH analogue with enhanced affinity for the GH receptor and acts by preventing functional GH signaling.[24] The ACROSTUDY included a large cohort of patients with acromegaly treated with pegvisomant. Normalization of IGF-1 levels was achieved in 63.2% to 75% of patients after 5 years of therapy, although there was no ef-fect on pituitary tumor size.[25,26] Pegvisomant works independently of SSTR status and can be used in combination with SRLs to achieve better hormonal control.[24] Need for daily subcutaneous injections and risk of transaminitis are the major drawbacks.[27]

### Dopamine agonists
Pituitary somatotroph tumors frequently coexpress D2 receptors. It is postulated that there is possible heterodimerization of D2 receptors and SSTR-5, thus enhancing the functional activity of both agonists; however, prolactin levels and prolactin staining of tumor tissue have not correlated with clinical response.[28] Meta-analysis has not revealed compelling data for the use of cabergoline as monotherapy in the treatment of somatotroph tumors and there remains a lack of randomized controlled trials.[29,30]

### Thyrotropin-Secreting Adenomas (Thyroid Stimulating Hormone-omas)

Elevated serum thyroxine levels with an inappropriately normal or elevated TSH may be suggestive of a TSH-oma, which accounts for less than 1% of all pituitary adenomas. Because of newer and more sensitive assays a TSH-oma can be suspected earlier and may allow for diagnosis while the lesion is still small. It is estimated that one-third of patients with TSH-omas are inadvertently treated for primary hyperthyroidism with thyroidectomy or radioactive iodine ablation, resulting in enhanced feedback to the hypothalamus and pituitary, thus stimulating growth of the TSH-oma tumor.[31]

The initial goal of therapy should be to achieve a euthyroid state in order to enable safe transition to further treatments. SRLs, such as octreotide, octreotide LAR, and lanreotide reduce intracellular cyclic adenosine monophosphate and calcium, consequently decreasing hormone secretion to achieve normalization of thyroid hormone levels in 95% of patients. A reduction in tumor size has also been observed in 50% of patients within 3 to 4 months.[31] SRLs can be used as preoperative optimization therapy and postoperative adjunctive therapy with few studies evaluating its use as primary monotherapy. Common side effects of therapy include hyperglycemia, diarrhea, cholelithiasis, and abdominal discomfort. For lesions that are not amenable to surgery or patients who are intolerant of SST analogues, dopamine agonists have also been used under the principle that cells derived from the same cell linages may share receptors, such as the dopamine receptor (D2).[32] In some instances TSH-omas with cosecretion of prolactin have demonstrated a response to dopaminergic agonist therapy, but data is limited.

### Corticotroph Tumors (Adrenocorticotrophic Hormone Secreting Tumors)

Cushing disease (CD) is excess ACTH production from a pituitary tumor. Estimated prevalence of CD is close to 40 per million, with incidence ranging from 1.2 to 2.4 per million per year.[33] The available medical treatment options for CD include pituitary-directed therapies that target excess ACTH production, inhibitors of steroidogenesis, and glucocorticoid receptor (GR) blocking agents (**Fig. 1**); however, few of these therapies are FDA approved.

#### Neuromodulators of adrenocorticotrophic hormone release

The SRL pasireotide is a multireceptor targeting SST analogue that inhibits ACTH production by pituitary adenomas through activation of the SST receptors, SSTR2 and SSTR5, which are expressed on pituitary corticotroph cells. It is the first FDA-approved medical therapy for CD and is available as a twice-daily subcutaneous formulation and a monthly intramuscular injection, with typical doses being lower than those used to treat acromegaly. The onset of action is rapid with significant reduction or normalization of urinary free cortisol (UFC) levels in $\geq$50% of patients, and a reduction in tumor size in 46% of cases, with some studies exhibiting complete tumor disappearance after 24 months of therapy.[34,35] Varying doses of pasireotide yield similar results; however, higher doses result in a greater frequency of hyperglycemia, a known side effect because pasireotide is an inhibitor of glucagon-like peptide 1, gastric inhibitory polypeptide, and insulin secretion.[35,36] Larger trials to assess durability of pasireotide are ongoing, with current phase III trials showing a significant improvement in multiple factors, including body weight, waist circumference, tumor shrinkage, total cholesterol, and improvement in quality of life in addition to the sustained reduction in UFC levels, with normalization of UFC levels in half of patients after 1 month of therapy.[37] Hyperglycemia, gastrointestinal discomfort, nausea, and cholelithiasis remain the most common side effects of therapy.

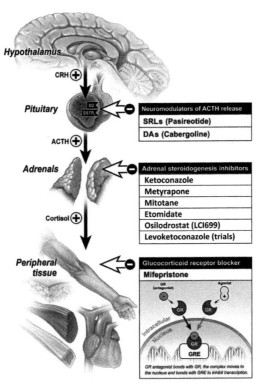

**Fig. 1.** The available medical treatment options for CD include pituitary-directed therapies that target excess ACTH production, inhibitors of steroidogenesis, and GR blocking agents. Figure abbreviations: Corticotropin Releasing Hormone (CRH), Dopamine Agonist (DA), Adrenocorticotropic Hormone (ACTH), Glucocorticoid Receptor (GR), Glucocoid Receptor Expression (GRE). (*Adapted from* Fleseriu, Medical Management of Persistent and Recurrent Cushing Disease, Neurosurgery Clinics of North America, Volume 23, Issue 4, 2012, Pages 653-668, with permission.)

D2 expression has been found in different types of pituitary tumors, including corticotroph-secreting adenomas, thus allowing for use of the D2 agonist therapy cabergoline. Cabergoline monotherapy was able to normalize UFC in approximately 36.6% of patients studied, but only 30% sustained normalization.[38,39] Furthermore, higher doses of cabergoline are required to achieve a response (5–7 mg/wk), which carries the risk of developing cardiac valvopathies. On account of the above, cabergoline is often used as an off-label add-on therapy for the treatment of CD.

Roscovitine or seliciclib, an inhibitor of cyclin-dependent kinases, has been shown to decrease ACTH secretion and cell proliferation in animal models. Clinical trials are ongoing.[11]

### Adrenal steroidogenesis inhibitors

Adrenal-directed therapies aim to decrease cortisol synthesis by inhibiting specific enzymes in the steroidogenesis pathway, as outlined in **Fig. 2**.

Osilodrostat was approved by the FDA in 2020 for the treatment of CD. It inhibits 11β-hydroxylase (CYP11B1) and aldosterone synthase (CYP11B2), thereby reducing cortisol production and the conversion of corticosterone to aldosterone, respectively. Osilodrostat is superior to placebo, with 96.4% of patients achieving at least 1 normal

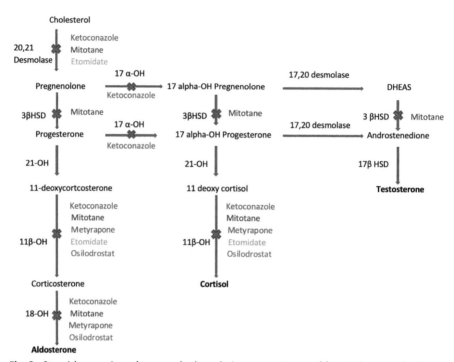

**Fig. 2.** Steroidogenesis pathway and adrenolytic agents. Figure Abbreviations: 3-β-hydroxysteroid dehydrogenase (3BHSD), Hydroxylase (OH), Dehydroepiandrosterone-sulfate (DHEAS). Levoketoconazole blocks the same enzymes as ketoconazole, but is still undergoing clinical trials, therefore it has not been added to this diagram.

UFC within 48 weeks and 66% of patients maintaining a normal UFC for 6 months.[40] Osilodrostat has a longer half-life than other steroidogenesis inhibitors, such as metyrapone and ketoconazole, thus allowing for twice-per-day oral administration with adjustments based on biweekly UFC measurements. Side effects include adrenal insufficiency, hypokalemia, hypomagnesemia, fatigue, diarrhea, headache, nausea, and an increase in androgens. Only 3% of patients demonstrated an increase in tumor size, establishing osilodrostat to be a safe and well-tolerated medical therapy for CD (**Table 2**).[40,41]

Metyrapone inhibits 11β-hydroxylase, thus inhibiting the synthesis of both cortisol and mineralocorticoids (see **Fig. 2**). Retrospective and ongoing prospective studies assessing outcomes revealed that metyrapone was able to achieve a reduction in cortisol levels in ∼75% of patients and normalize UFC after 12 weeks in nearly half of study subjects. In addition, 66% of patients had improvement in clinical signs and symptoms of hypercortisolemia (see **Table 2**).[42,43] Although it is an oral therapy, it has a wide dose range to achieve effectiveness (250 mg to 5750 mg per day) and requires 4-times-per-day dosing. Inhibition of cortisol synthesis by metyrapone induces a compensatory increase in ACTH levels, which drives an increase in glucocorticoid and mineralocorticoid precursors and adrenal androgens that are in turn responsible for the typical adverse events.[42] Although not FDA approved, it has been used off label to treat CD in patients who are pregnant.

Ketoconazole blocks multiple enzymes in the steroidogenesis pathway, thus reducing glucocorticoid, mineralocorticoid, and adrenal androgen production (see **Fig. 2**). It is an oral therapy with a short half-life, thus requiring multiple daily doses.

**Table 2**
Treatment options and outcome data for medical management of Cushing disease

| Medication | Mechanism | Administration | Outcome Data | Drawbacks |
|---|---|---|---|---|
| Pasireotide | Bind to SSTR-3 and SSTR-5 on pituitary corticotroph cells to inhibit ACTH production | SC bid injection Monthly IM (LAR) | Double-blind RCT: 50% reduction in UFC at 6 mo; 46% of patients having a demonstrable reduction in tumor volume[34] Some cases of complete tumor disappearance after 24 mo of therapy[35] | Hyperglycemia, which is linearly correlated with dosage GI discomfort, nausea, cholelithiasis |
| Cabergoline | Can act where there is coexpression of D2 receptors | 5–7 mg/wk | UFC normalization in 36.6% of patients and poor durability, with only 30% of patients sustaining UFC normalization[38,39] | High doses needed to achieve a response; therefore, side effects of mood disorders and cardiac valvulopathies may occur |
| Osilodrostat (LCI699) | Inhibits 11β-hydroxylase and 18-hydroxylase (aldosterone synthetase) | po bid Initiate 2 mg bid, slow up-titration by 1–2 mg biweekly based on UFC | Phase III: 86% of patients achieve normal UFC vs 29% in the placebo group (P<.001); 96% able to achieve normal UFC at 48 wk, and 66% of patients maintaining a normal UFC for 6 mo after the first normal UFC[40] Few cases of increase in pituitary tumor size | Adrenal insufficiency, hypokalemia, hypomagnesemia, fatigue, diarrhea, headache, nausea, and increase in androgens |

(continued on next page)

**Table 2**
*(continued)*

| Medication | Mechanism | Administration | Outcome Data | Drawbacks |
|---|---|---|---|---|
| Ketoconazole & levoketoconazole | Multiple enzymes in the steroidogenesis pathway blocked (see **Fig. 2**) | Ketoconazole, po multiday dosing Levoketoconazole po bid | Ketoconazole: 60% remission rate[44] Levoketoconazole: SONICS phase III: normalization in UFC in 42% of patients at 6 mo[47] | Ketoconazole, hepatotoxicity, numerous drug-drug interactions, hypogonadism in men Levoketoconazole, trials ongoing |
| Mitotane | Cytotoxic effect on the mitochondria of the adrenocortical cells resulting in cell death Inhibits steroidogenesis at multiple levels in the steroidogenesis pathway | | No multicenter randomized studies to assess efficacy and safety in CD | Impairs metabolism of other medications Nausea, vomiting, adrenal insufficiency, and teratogenicity |
| Metyrapone | Inhibits 11β-hydroxylase and 18-hydroxylase (aldosterone synthetase) | 4 × per day po dosing 250–5750 mg | Retrospective data with 195 patients: 75% of patients able to achieve reduction in cortisol levels[42] PROMPT prospective study: normalization of UFC after 12 wk of therapy in 23 of 49 patients (47%), and a 66% improvement in clinical signs and symptoms of hypercortisolemia[43] Has been used off label to treat CD in patients who are pregnant | Not FDA approved Inhibition of cortisol synthesis by metyrapone generally induces a compensatory increase in ACTH levels, which drives an increase in glucocorticoid and mineralocorticoid precursors[42] |

| Etomidate | Inhibits 11β-hydroxylase and 20,21 desmolase | 0.03 mg/kg bolus + 0.3 mg/kg/h IV infusion | Rapid onset of action | Requires close ICU monitoring |
|---|---|---|---|---|
| Mifepristone | Nonselective glucocorticoid receptor blocker | 300–1200 mg per day | SEISMEC clinical trial: improvement in glucose metabolism impairment in 60% of patients; 2/3 of patients had an increase in ACTH levels[51] | Inability to follow cortisol levels<br>Hypokalemia, adrenal insufficiency, antiprogestin effects (ie endometrial thickening)<br>Only FDA approved for the management of hyperglycemia associated with hypercortisolemia |

*Abbreviations:* ICU, intensive care unit; IV, intravenous; RCT, randomized controlled trial.

Therapeutic response data vary, with recent studies noting up to a 60% remission rate; however, there are numerous adverse effects of ketoconazole therapy that constrain its use.[44] Use of ketoconazole requires close liver function monitoring given the risk of hepatotoxicity, can result in hypogonadism in men, and has numerous drug interactions.[45,46] A newer twice-per-day oral formulation levoketoconazole, an enantiomer of ketoconazole, is being studied in phase III trials (SONICS). Initial data revealed normalization of UFC in 42% of patients at 6 months and a more tolerable safety profile.[47]

Mitotane is an oral adrenolytic agent that reduces cortisol production in 2 ways. First it has a cytotoxic effect on the mitochondria of the adrenocortical cells resulting in cell death, a property that lends its use to the treatment of adrenocortical carcinomas. Second, it inhibits steroidogenesis at multiple levels in the steroidogenesis pathway by blocking 11β-hydroxylase, 18-hydroxylase, and 3β-hydroxysteroid-dehydrogenase (see **Fig. 2**). Although effective for inducing a medical adrenalectomy, a large percentage of patients relapse.[48] There are no randomized studies assessing its efficacy and safety in CD; therefore, its use has remained limited. Monthly monitoring is required because it can impair the metabolism of other medications. Major adverse events include nausea, vomiting, adrenal insufficiency, and teratogenicity. Because mitotane can remain in adipose tissue long after discontinuation, ongoing monitoring is required.[48]

Etomidate is an intravenous medication that blocks CYP11B1 synthesis of cortisol and can be used in the critical care setting to rapidly control endogenous hypercortisolemia within hours. Given the requirement for intensive inpatient monitoring and adjustments, it is only used in the inpatient setting when rapid control of cortisol levels is indicated.[49]

### Glucocorticoid receptor blockers

Mifepristone, an oral nonselective GR antagonist, blocks cortisol from binding to the GR receptor, thus halting the signaling pathway for nuclear transcription and the peripheral effects of cortisol. It does not reduce cortisol secretion or levels; therefore, cortisol levels cannot be used as a marker of disease control. Instead, glycemic and metabolic markers in addition to clinicals signs and symptoms are indicators of disease control and dose titration.

Mifepristone is FDA approved for the management of hyperglycemia associated with CD and is available as a once-daily oral medication with doses ranging from 300 to 1200 mg. The SEISMIC showed an improvement of glucose metabolism in 60% patients with diabetes, and an improvement in hypertension, body weight, and waist circumference.[50] Two-thirds of patients demonstrated an increase in ACTH levels owing to GR blockade in the periphery, which bears the potential risk of an increase in pituitary tumor size. The extension study to SEISMIC found that 32 patients treated with mifepristone did not have progression of their pituitary tumor, and 3 of the 4 patients that had progression in tumor size had macroadenomas.[51] To date, there is no data indicating an increase in adrenal size in response to mifepristone therapy. Side effects include hypokalemia and adrenal insufficiency. Being a nonselective GR antagonist, it also has antiprogestin effects, which can result in abnormal vaginal bleeding and endometrial thickening for which ongoing monitoring is recommended. Relacorilant is an oral selective GR antagonist with a better safety profile than mifepristone and is currently under clinical investigation.

### Nonsecretory Pituitary Adenomas, Including Gonadotroph-Secreting Adenomas (Follicle-Stimulating Hormone/Luteinizing Hormone-omas)

Pituitary adenomas without clinically significant hormone dysfunction are often discovered once they exhibit a mass effect. The estimated prevalence of these nonsecretory adenomas is 7 to 41.2 cases per 1 million patients. They often test positive for pituitary hormones, but given the lack of hormone secretion, they are coined "silent adenomas." Most of these silent adenomas are gonadotroph (follicle-stimulating hormone/luteinizing hormone) adenomas (~80%). There is no clear correlation between the histopathologic findings and clinical behavior of these lesions; therefore, nonsurgical management remains ineffective.[52]

Gonadotropin-releasing hormone antagonists have been shown to control hormone production, but have not been shown to reduce tumor size.[53] SST analogues and dopamine agonists have also exhibited limited success in controlling hormone production and tumor size.[54,55]

### Pituitary Carcinoma

Pituitary carcinoma is by definition a pituitary mass that is noncontiguous with the pituitary gland in the sella and/or demonstrates metastatic spread. These are not cancers that metastasize to the pituitary. Pituitary carcinomas are exquisitely rare, composing 0.1% to 0.2% of all pituitary tumors, but carry a poor prognosis.[56,57] Pituitary carcinomas can begin as secretory or nonsecretory pituitary adenomas, which may initially respond to conventional therapies; however, over time, these tumors become refractory to escalating medical therapies and display aggressive growth. The timeframe over which this occurs varies significantly with data reporting intervals of 4 months to 18 years with an estimated median survival of 12 to 31 months.[57,58]

Given the rarity of pituitary carcinoma, treatment data are scant. Temozolomide has been used for aggressive pituitary lesions, and in a case series of patients with pituitary carcinoma, it reduced hormone production and tumor growth in 9 of 15 patients (60%) and increased survival by 6 months.[57,59] Further studies estimate its efficacy at ~60%.[60,61] Another alkylating agent, called lomustine, blocks DNA and RNA synthesis, and when used in combination with another DNA synthesis inhibitor 5-fluorouracil, has been shown to slow disease progression in a small case series of 4 patients, although the survival time ranged from 3 to 65 months.[57,60]

### AREAS OF INVESTIGATION

Presently, there are ongoing studies assessing the role of immunotherapies, specifically the checkpoint inhibitors targeting CTLA-4 and PD-1/PD-L1, independently and in combination with currently approved therapies.[56]

### RADIOTHERAPY

External beam radiotherapy ("fractionated") and stereotactic radiosurgery ("gammaknife") have been used as secondary or tertiary interventions for the management of residual pituitary lesions that are surgically irresectable and/or refractory to medical management. The major drawbacks to its utilization are the long latency periods necessary to achieve a clinical response and the high rates of panhypopituitarism and associated cranial nerve palsies.[62,63]

Radiotherapy has not been shown to be effective for treating prolactinomas, with less than half of cases demonstrating a reduction in prolactin levels after a median delay of 3 to 10 years.[64]

No controlled studies have evaluated radiotherapy as a sole treatment option for TSH-omas, and although few studies have shown a decrease in size of some lesions, the rate of response remains low, less than 50% in some case series.[65]

The use of radiotherapy as an adjunct therapy to treat GH tumors leads to an estimated 20% decline in IGF-1 levels per year.[66] Few patients achieve clinically significant hormonal control in the short term, and most studies demonstrate only a partial response after a long latency period. The most compelling data for the use of radiotherapy are unexceptional, showing IGF-1 normalization rates of only 69%, with 59% of the patients achieving remission after 10 years, signifying that GH tumors are particularly radio-insensitive.[62,66]

Patients with CD who are unable to attain or maintain remission may be candidates for radiotherapy. Stereotactic radiotherapy may result in faster remission rates than conventional fractionated therapy; however, up to 60% of patients may develop pan-hypopituitarism 5 years after therapy. Although tumor control can be achieved with radiotherapy, biochemical remission may not occur.[67,68]

As an adjunct to surgery, radiotherapy has been used to treat pituitary carcinomas, but the results are limited and variable given the different types of radiotherapy used and doses administered. Few case reports show some delay in tumor progression.

## SUMMARY

Advancements in non-surgical interventions for the management of pituitary lesions have allowed for a more comprehensive and multidisciplinary approach to treating these types of tumors. After assessing the need for intervention, specific therapies can be initiated based on tumor receptor subtyping. Not all effective medical therapies target the pituitary gland directly. Recognizing that there are tumors that cosecrete hormones allows for a wider selection of therapeutic options. Radiotherapy remains a treatment option, but even stereotactic therapies may take months to years to achieve hormonal or tumor volume control. Combination therapy may provide the best clinical outcomes in select cases.

## CLINICS CARE POINTS

- Pituitary tumors may cosecrete multiple hormones, often consistent with their shared cell lineages.
- Most prolactinomas respond quickly and effectively to cabergoline therapy.
- Thyroid-stimulating hormone-omas should not undergo thyroidectomy or thyroid radiation, as it may result in the growth of the primary pituitary tumor.
- Receptor subtyping may allow for the use of more targeted therapies to achieve improved clinical outcomes.
- Radiotherapy has a delayed onset of action and may result in panhypopituitarism.

## ACKNOWLEDGMENTS

The author thanks Lakshmi Priyanka Mahali, MBBS, MD.

## DISCLOSURE

The authors have nothing to disclose.

## REFERENCES

1. Melmed S, Casanueva FF, Hoffman AR, et al. Diagnosis and treatment of hyper-prolactinemia: an Endocrine Society Clinical Practice Guideline. J Clin Endocrinol Metab 2011;96(2). https://doi.org/10.1210/jc.2010-1692.

2. Melmed S. Mechanisms for pituitary tumorigenesis: the plastic pituitary. J Clin Invest 2003;112(11). https://doi.org/10.1172/JCI20401.

3. dos Santos Nunes V, el Dib R, Boguszewski CL, et al. Cabergoline versus bromocriptine in the treatment of hyperprolactinemia: a systematic review of randomized controlled trials and meta-analysis. Pituitary 2011;14(3).

4. Melmed S. Pituitary-tumor endocrinopathies. N Engl J Med 2020;(10):382. https://doi.org/10.1056/NEJMra1810772.

5. BEVAN JS, WEBSTER J, Burke CW, et al. Dopamine agonists and pituitary tumor shrinkage. Endocr Rev 1992;13(2). https://doi.org/10.1210/edrv-13-2-220.

6. Ioachimescu AG, Fleseriu M, Hoffman AR, et al. Psychological effects of dopamine agonist treatment in patients with hyperprolactinemia and prolactin-secreting adenomas. Eur J Endocrinol 2019;180(1). https://doi.org/10.1530/EJE-18-0682.

7. Maiter D. Management of dopamine agonist-resistant prolactinoma. Neuroendocrinology 2019;109(1). https://doi.org/10.1159/000495775.

8. Gillam MP, Middler S, Freed DJ, et al. The novel use of very high doses of cabergoline and a combination of testosterone and an aromatase inhibitor in the treatment of a giant prolactinoma. J Clin Endocrinol Metab 2002;87(10). https://doi.org/10.1210/jc.2002-020426.

9. Simonis G, Fuhrmann JT, Strasser RH. Meta-analysis of heart valve abnormalities in Parkinson's disease patients treated with dopamine agonists. Movement Disord 2007;22(13). https://doi.org/10.1002/mds.21639.

10. McCormack AI, Wass JAH, Grossman AB. Aggressive pituitary tumours: the role of temozolomide and the assessment of MGMT status. Eur J Clin Invest 2011;41(10). https://doi.org/10.1111/j.1365-2362.2011.02520.x.

11. Varlamov E v, McCartney S, Fleseriu M. Functioning pituitary adenomas – current treatment options and emerging medical therapies. Eur Endocrinol 2019;15(1). https://doi.org/10.17925/EE.2019.15.1.30.

12. Katznelson L, Laws ER, Melmed S, et al. Acromegaly: an Endocrine Society Clinical Practice Guideline. J Clin Endocrinol Metab 2014;99(11). https://doi.org/10.1210/jc.2014-2700.

13. Fleseriu M, Biller BMK, Freda PU, et al. A Pituitary Society update to acromegaly management guidelines. Pituitary 2021;24(1). https://doi.org/10.1007/s11102-020-01091-7.

14. Melmed S. Acromegaly. N Engl J Med 2006;355(24). https://doi.org/10.1056/NEJMra062453.

15. Auriemma RS, Pivonello R, Galdiero M, et al. Octreotide-LAR vs lanreotide-SR as first-line therapy for acromegaly: a retrospective, comparative, head-to-head study. J Endocrinol Invest 2008;31(11). https://doi.org/10.1007/BF03345632.

16. Nista F, Corica G, Castelletti L, et al. Clinical and radiological predictors of biochemical response to first-line treatment with somatostatin receptor ligands in acromegaly: a real-life perspective. Front Endocrinol 2021;12. https://doi.org/10.3389/fendo.2021.677919.

17. Colao A, Bronstein MD, Freda P, et al. Pasireotide versus octreotide in acromegaly: a head-to-head superiority study. J Clin Endocrinol Metab 2014;99(3). https://doi.org/10.1210/jc.2013-2480.

18. Colao A, Cappabianca P, Caron P, et al. Octreotide LAR vs. surgery in newly diagnosed patients with acromegaly: a randomized, open-label, multicentre study. Clin Endocrinol 2009;70(5). https://doi.org/10.1111/j.1365-2265.2008.03441.x.

19. Melmed S, Bronstein MD, Chanson P, et al. A consensus statement on acromegaly therapeutic outcomes. Nat Rev Endocrinol 2018;14(9):552–61. https://doi.org/10.1038/s41574-018-0058-5.

20. Giustina A, Mazziotti G, Torri V, et al. Meta-analysis on the effects of octreotide on tumor mass in acromegaly. PLoS ONE 2012;7(5). https://doi.org/10.1371/journal.pone.0036411.

21. Melmed S, Popovic V, Bidlingmaier M, et al. Safety and efficacy of oral octreotide in acromegaly: results of a multicenter phase III trial. J Clin Endocrinol Metab 2015;100(4). https://doi.org/10.1210/jc.2014-4113.

22. Samson SL, Nachtigall LB, Fleseriu M, et al. Maintenance of acromegaly control in patients switching from injectable somatostatin receptor ligands to oral octreotide. J Clin Endocrinol Metab 2020;105(10). https://doi.org/10.1210/clinem/dgaa526.

23. Gadelha MR, Gu F, Bronstein MD, et al. Risk factors and management of pasireotide-associated hyperglycemia in acromegaly. Endocr Connections 2020;9(12). https://doi.org/10.1530/EC-20-0361.

24. Ma L, Luo D, Yang T, et al. Combined therapy of somatostatin analogues with pegvisomant for the treatment of acromegaly: a meta-analysis of prospective studies. BMC Endocr Disord 2020;20(1). https://doi.org/10.1186/s12902-020-0545-2.

25. van der Lely AJ, Biller BMK, Brue T, et al. Long-term safety of pegvisomant in patients with acromegaly: comprehensive review of 1288 subjects in ACROSTUDY. J Clin Endocrinol Metab 2012;97(5). https://doi.org/10.1210/jc.2011-2508.

26. Tritos NA, Chanson P, Jimenez C, et al. Effectiveness of first-line pegvisomant monotherapy in acromegaly: an ACROSTUDY analysis. Eur J Endocrinol 2017; 176(2). https://doi.org/10.1530/EJE-16-0697.

27. Neggers SJCMM, Franck SE, de Rooij FWM, et al. Long-term efficacy and safety of pegvisomant in combination with long-acting somatostatin analogs in acromegaly. J Clin Endocrinol Metab 2014;99(10). https://doi.org/10.1210/jc.2014-2032.

28. Kuhn E, Chanson P. Cabergoline in acromegaly. Pituitary 2017;20(1). https://doi.org/10.1007/s11102-016-0782-6.

29. Sandret L, Maison P, Chanson P. Place of cabergoline in acromegaly: a meta-analysis. J Clin Endocrinol Metab 2011;96(5). https://doi.org/10.1210/jc.2010-2443.

30. Suda K, Inoshita N, Iguchi G, et al. Efficacy of combined octreotide and cabergoline treatment in patients with acromegaly: a retrospective clinical study and review of the literature. Endocr J 2013;60(4). https://doi.org/10.1507/endocrj.EJ12-0272.

31. Beck-Peccoz P, Giavoli C, Lania AA. 2019 update on TSH-secreting pituitary adenomas. J Endocrinol Invest 2019;42(12). https://doi.org/10.1007/s40618-019-01066-x.

32. Kienitz T, Quinkler M, Strasburger CJ, et al. Long-term management in five cases of TSH-secreting pituitary adenomas: a single center study and review of the literature. Eur J Endocrinol 2007;157(1). https://doi.org/10.1530/EJE-07-0098.

33. Nishioka Yamada. Cushing's disease. J Clin Med 2019;8(11). https://doi.org/10.3390/jcm8111951.

34. Colao A, Petersenn S, Newell-Price J, et al. A 12-month phase 3 study of pasireotide in Cushing's disease. N Engl J Med 2012;366(10). https://doi.org/10.1056/NEJMoa1105743.

35. Lacroix A, Gu F, Gallardo W, et al. Efficacy and safety of once-monthly pasireotide in Cushing's disease: a 12 month clinical trial. Lancet Diabetes Endocrinol 2018; 6(1). https://doi.org/10.1016/S2213-8587(17)30326-1.

36. Simeoli C, Auriemma RS, Tortora F, et al. The treatment with pasireotide in Cushing's disease: effects of long-term treatment on tumor mass in the experience of a single center. Endocrine 2015;50(3). https://doi.org/10.1007/s12020-015-0557-2.
37. Manetti L, Deutschbein T, Schopohl J, et al. Long-term safety and efficacy of subcutaneous pasireotide in patients with Cushing's disease: interim results from a long-term real-world evidence study. Pituitary 2019;22(5). https://doi.org/10.1007/s11102-019-00984-6.
38. Pivonello R, de Leo M, Cozzolino A, et al. The treatment of Cushing's disease. Endocr Rev 2015;36(4). https://doi.org/10.1210/er.2013-1048.
39. Godbout A, Manavela M, Danilowicz K, et al. Cabergoline monotherapy in the long-term treatment of Cushing's disease. Eur J Endocrinol 2010;163(5). https://doi.org/10.1530/EJE-10-0382.
40. Pivonello R, Fleseriu M, Newell-Price J, et al. Efficacy and safety of osilodrostat in patients with Cushing's disease (LINC 3): a multicentre phase III study with a double-blind, randomised withdrawal phase. Lancet Diabetes Endocrinol 2020;8(9). https://doi.org/10.1016/S2213-8587(20)30240-0.
41. Rasool S, Skinner BW. Osilodrostat for the treatment of Cushing's disease. Expert Opin Pharmacother 2021;22(9). https://doi.org/10.1080/14656566.2021.1897106.
42. Daniel E, Aylwin S, Mustafa O, et al. Effectiveness of metyrapone in treating Cushing's syndrome: a retrospective multicenter study in 195 patients. J Clin Endocrinol Metab 2015;100(11). https://doi.org/10.1210/jc.2015-2616.
43. Nieman LK, Boscaro M, Scaroni CM, et al. Metyrapone treatment in endogenous Cushing's syndrome: results at week 12 from PROMPT, a prospective international multicenter, open-label, phase III/IV study. J Endocr Soc 2021;5(Supplement_1). https://doi.org/10.1210/jendso/bvab048.1053.
44. Shirley M. Ketoconazole in Cushing's syndrome: a profile of its use. Drugs Ther Perspect 2021;37(2). https://doi.org/10.1007/s40267-020-00799-7.
45. Broersen LHA, Jha M, Biermasz NR, et al. Effectiveness of medical treatment for Cushing's syndrome: a systematic review and meta-analysis. Pituitary 2018;21(6). https://doi.org/10.1007/s11102-018-0897-z.
46. Castinetti F, Guignat L, Giraud P, et al. Ketoconazole in Cushing's disease: is it worth a try? J Clin Endocrinol Metab 2014;99(5). https://doi.org/10.1210/jc.2013-3628.
47. Fleseriu M, Pivonello R, Elenkova A, et al. Efficacy and safety of levoketoconazole in the treatment of endogenous Cushing's syndrome (SONICS): a phase 3, multicentre, open-label, single-arm trial. Lancet Diabetes Endocrinol 2019;7(11). https://doi.org/10.1016/S2213-8587(19)30313-4.
48. Luton JP, Mahoudeau JA, Bouchard P, et al. Treatment of Cushing's disease by O,p'DDD. Survey of 62 cases. N Engl J Med 1979;300(9). https://doi.org/10.1056/NEJM197903013000903.
49. Preda VA, Sen J, Karavitaki N, et al. Therapy in endocrine disease: etomidate in the management of hypercortisolaemia in Cushing's syndrome: a review. Eur J Endocrinol 2012;167(2). https://doi.org/10.1530/EJE-12-0274.
50. Fleseriu M, Biller BMK, Findling JW, et al. Mifepristone, a glucocorticoid receptor antagonist, produces clinical and metabolic benefits in patients with Cushing's syndrome. J Clin Endocrinol Metab 2012;97(6). https://doi.org/10.1210/jc.2011-3350.
51. Fleseriu M, Findling JW, Koch CA, et al. Changes in plasma ACTH levels and corticotroph tumor size in patients with Cushing's disease during long-term treatment with the glucocorticoid receptor antagonist mifepristone. J Clin Endocrinol Metab 2014;99(10). https://doi.org/10.1210/jc.2014-1843.

52. Esposito D, Olsson DS, Ragnarsson O, et al. Non-functioning pituitary adenomas: indications for pituitary surgery and post-surgical management. Pituitary 2019; 22(4). https://doi.org/10.1007/s11102-019-00960-0.
53. McGrath GA, Goncalves RJ, Udupa JK, et al. New technique for quantitation of pituitary adenoma size: use in evaluating treatment of gonadotroph adenomas with a gonadotropin-releasing hormone antagonist. J Clin Endocrinol Metab 1993;76(5). https://doi.org/10.1210/jcem.76.5.8496331.
54. Colao A, di Somma C, Pivonello R, et al. Medical therapy for clinically non-functioning pituitary adenomas. Endocr Relat Cancer 2008;15(4). https://doi.org/10.1677/ERC-08-0181.
55. Chanson P, Lecoq A-L, Raverot G, et al. Physiopathology, diagnosis, and treatment of nonfunctioning pituitary adenomas. In: ; 2018. doi:10.1007/978-3-319-44444-4_4.
56. Dai C, Liang S, Sun B, et al. The progress of immunotherapy in refractory pituitary adenomas and pituitary carcinomas. Front Endocrinol 2020;11. https://doi.org/10.3389/fendo.2020.608422.
57. Heaney AP. Pituitary carcinoma: difficult diagnosis and treatment. J Clin Endocrinol Metab 2011;96(12). https://doi.org/10.1210/jc.2011-2031.
58. Kontogeorgos G. Classification and pathology of pituitary tumors. Endocrine 2005;28(1). https://doi.org/10.1385/ENDO:28:1:027.
59. Pernicone PJ, Scheithauer BW, Sebo TJ, et al. Pituitary carcinoma. Cancer 1997; 79(4). https://doi.org/10.1002/(SICI)1097-0142(19970215)79:4<804::AID-CNCR1 8>3.0.CO;2-3.
60. Kaltsas GA, Mukherjee JJ, Plowman PN, et al. The role of cytotoxic chemotherapy in the management of aggressive and malignant pituitary tumors. J Clin Endocrinol Metab 1998;83(12). https://doi.org/10.1210/jcem.83.12.5300.
61. Ji Y, Vogel RI, Lou E. Temozolomide treatment of pituitary carcinomas and atypical adenomas: systematic review of case reports. Neuro-Oncology Pract 2016; 3(3). https://doi.org/10.1093/nop/npv059.
62. Ding D, Mehta GU, Patibandla MR, et al. Stereotactic radiosurgery for acromegaly: an international multicenter retrospective cohort study. Neurosurgery 2019;84(3). https://doi.org/10.1093/neuros/nyy178.
63. Liščák R, Vladyka V, Marek J, et al. Gamma knife radiosurgery for endocrine-inactive pituitary adenomas. Acta Neurochirurgica 2007;149(10). https://doi.org/10.1007/s00701-007-1253-7.
64. Chanson P, Maiter D. The epidemiology, diagnosis and treatment of prolactinomas: the old and the new. Best Pract Res Clin Endocrinol Metab 2019;33(2). https://doi.org/10.1016/j.beem.2019.101290.
65. Malchiodi E, Profka E, Ferrante E, et al. Thyrotropin-secreting pituitary adenomas: outcome of pituitary surgery and irradiation. J Clin Endocrinol Metab 2014;99(6). https://doi.org/10.1210/jc.2013-4376.
66. Jenkins PJ, Bates P, Carson MN, et al. Conventional pituitary irradiation is effective in lowering serum growth hormone and insulin-like growth factor-I in patients with acromegaly. J Clin Endocrinol Metab 2006;91(4). https://doi.org/10.1210/jc.2005-1616.
67. Tritos NA, Biller BMK. Update on radiation therapy in patients with Cushing's disease. Pituitary 2015;18(2). https://doi.org/10.1007/s11102-014-0615-4.
68. Nieman LK, Biller BMK, Findling JW, et al. Treatment of Cushing's syndrome: an Endocrine Society Clinical Practice Guideline. J Clin Endocrinol Metab 2015; 100(8). https://doi.org/10.1210/jc.2015-1818.

# Prolactinoma
## Medical and Surgical Considerations

Sameah A. Haider, MD, MBA[a], Shiri Levy, MD[b], Jack P. Rock, MD[a],
John R. Craig, MD[c],*

## KEYWORDS

- Prolactinoma • Pituitary tumor • Surgical considerations • Dopaminergic therapy
- Transsphenoidal surgery • Prolactin

## KEY POINTS

- The mainstay of prolactinoma management is medical therapy with dopamine agonists (DA).
- Surgical intervention should be considered for patients who fail to respond to DA therapy, cannot tolerate DA therapy, or have macroadenomas with a large cystic component.
- Pituitary apoplexy with sudden visual decline secondary to optic nerve compression is a surgical emergency.
- Radiation therapy is most commonly used as an adjunctive or second-line treatment.
- Whether medical or surgical interventions are pursued, long-term surveillance via endocrinologic laboratory assessment and MRI is essential.

## INTRODUCTION

Prolactinomas are the most common pathologic cause of hyperprolactinemia,[1] and the most common secretory tumor of the pituitary gland.[2] Prolactinomas are histologically benign and arise from monoclonal expansion of pituitary lactotrophs that have undergone somatic mutation. The most commonly implicated genes include pituitary tumor transforming gene and fibroblast growth factor 4.[3] Most prolactinomas arise from sporadic mutations, but they may also occur in concert with certain familial syndromes, such as multiple endocrine neoplasia type 1.

Disclosure of funding/conflict of interest: The authors have no relevant disclosures.
[a] Department of Neurological Surgery, Hermelin Brain Tumor Center, Henry Ford Hospital, 2799 West Grand Boulevard, Detroit, MI 48202, USA; [b] Division of Endocrinology, Diabetes, and Bone & Mineral Disorder, Henry Ford Hospital, 2799 West Grand Boulevard, Detroit, MI 48202, USA; [c] Department of Otolaryngology–Head and Neck Surgery, Henry Ford Hospital, 2799 West Grand Boulevard, Detroit, MI 48202, USA
* Corresponding author. Department of Otolaryngology, Henry Ford Hospital, 2799 West Grand Boulevard, Detroit, MI 48202.
E-mail address: Jcraig1@hfhs.org

Otolaryngol Clin N Am 55 (2022) 305–314
https://doi.org/10.1016/j.otc.2021.12.005
0030-6665/22/© 2021 Elsevier Inc. All rights reserved.

Symptoms at the time of presentation are either due to regional mass effect or from systemic effects of prolactin hypersecretion.[4,5] Macroadenomas, defined as greater than 10 mm, may become symptomatic via direct compression on the optic apparatus, cavernous sinus, cranial nerves, and normal pituitary gland. Microadenomas, defined as less than 10 mm, are less likely to have symptoms from direct mass effect but instead from supraphysiologic levels of prolactin that suppress the hypothalamic-pituitary (HPA) axis.

## CLINICAL PRESENTATION

Regarding macroprolactinomas, presenting symptoms are usually due to mass effect and/or hyperprolactinemia. Symptoms or sequelae related to mass effect include headaches, visual deficits, cranial neuropathies, hydrocephalus, and pituitary apoplexy. Hyperprolactinemia symptoms are generally due to hormonal dysfunction along the HPA axis. In men, this may include decreased libido and impotence. In women, one may see aberrations with menstruation, infertility, or galactorrhea. Pediatric patients may present with pubertal delay, growth arrest, or primary amenorrhea.

## DIAGNOSTIC WORKUP

Laboratory assessment for suspected prolactinoma begins with a serum prolactin level. Although prolactinoma is the most common cause of hyperprolactinemia, other causes include pregnancy, medication side effects, hypothyroidism, or other causes of mass effect on the pituitary stalk.[6] Regarding hyperprolactinemia in pregnancy and postpartum, prolactin levels normalize within about 6 months after delivery in nursing mothers, and within weeks in nonnursing mothers.[7]

For prolactinomas, although prolactin levels usually correlate with tumor volume, sometimes prolactin levels can be misleading. Prolactin levels can appear falsely low owing to the "hook effect." This occurs when extremely high serum prolactin saturates both the capture and the signal antibodies used in immunoradiometric and chemiluminescent assays, preventing the binding of the two. The artifact can be avoided by repeating the assay using a 1:100 serum dilution.[8] Macroprolactin poses another potential challenge in interpreting prolactin levels. Macroprolactin is not clinically significant but is a complex of prolactin and immunoglobulin G antibody. This can cause hyperprolactinemia through decreased prolactin clearance. Misdiagnosis can be avoided by pretreating the serum with polyethylene glycol to precipitate the macroprolactin.[9]

In addition to checking prolactin, all other pituitary hormones and other laboratory evaluations may be necessary, especially in macroprolactinomas. Because prolactin elevation can occur in primary hypothyroidism, thyroid-stimulating hormone and free thyroxine (FT4) should be assessed. Renal and hepatic function should also be evaluated, as reduced prolactin clearance may occur in renal or hepatic failure. In amenorrheic women, serum follicle-stimulating hormone should be obtained to rule out primary ovarian failure. In men, serum testosterone should be assessed. Also, of note in giant prolactinomas, cortisol, FT4, and growth hormone (GH) may be low.[10]

It is important to appreciate that a subset of functional adenomas may aberrantly cosecrete multiple hormones or induce hypopituitarism.[11,12] For example, up to 10% of prolactinomas may cosecrete excess GH.[13] Conversely, some pituitary tumors causing acromegaly may coproduce prolactin in addition to GH.[14]

Other considerations include obtaining bone density testing in patients with hypogonadism. Contrasted magnetic resonance imaging (MRI) of the sella is recommended to assess for local tumor extent. Visual field testing should also be performed to assess for compression on the optic apparatus.

## MEDICAL CONSIDERATIONS

Medical therapy for prolactinomas is indicated for macroadenomas, enlarging micro-adenomas, infertility, bothersome galactorrhea, gynecomastia, testosterone defi-ciency, oligomenorrhea or amenorrhea, acne, and hirsutism. Microprolactinomas do not always require treatment, as the risk of tumor enlargement is low if untreated.[15] Prolactin levels and tumor size on MRI can be used to monitor prolactinomas, although optimal timing of serial prolactin levels and imaging has not been estab-lished. Dopaminergic agonists (DAs) are the mainstay of medical treatment for prolac-tinomas, as most tumors are sensitive to this therapy.

### Dopamine Agonists

According to the Endocrine Society clinical guidelines for prolactinoma management, DAs are recommended to lower prolactin levels, decrease tumor size, reverse galac-torrhea, and restore gonadal function in both microprolactinomas and macroprolacti-nomas.[16] In addition, in macroprolactinomas, DAs aim to decrease or stabilize tumor size to prevent or treat optic nerve compression, cranial neuropathies, or headaches.

With some macroprolactinomas, high prolactin levels may decrease significantly without completely normalizing. As long as the tumor is stable without mass effect and other hormone levels are satisfactory or replaced, persistent prolactin elevation is generally not harmful.[17] For patients with visual field compromise, DA doses are increased rapidly with visual field monitoring every 2 to 4 weeks.[17] If visual fields do not normalize and MRI demonstrates chiasmal compression, patients should be referred for neurosurgical consultation.

Some tumors do not show a response to DA therapy despite dose increases. It is speculated that therapeutic resistance is due to reduced dopamine receptor density on the tumor; thus, changing the type of DA may lead to improvement.[18] Lactotroph cells also may express estrogen receptors and may respond to estrogen blockade.[19–21]

The 2 approved DAs in the United States are bromocriptine and cabergoline. Compared with bromocriptine, cabergoline has fewer side effects and has been more effective with longer remission rates.[22,23]

### Duration of Dopaminergic Agonist Therapy and Remission Rates

Remission rates after DA therapy withdrawal range from 15% to 80%.[23–25] The following factors are reliable predictors of success and indications for DA withdrawal: treatment duration for more than 24 months, achieving normal prolactin levels, greater than 50% reduction in tumor size, and requirement of low DA maintenance dose.[23] Treatment may also be stopped in postmenopausal women, as tumors rarely grow af-ter menopause. For patients with macroprolactinomas and extrasellar extension or persistent hyperprolactinemia, it is not advisable to stop DA therapy.

### Side Effects of Dopaminergic Agonist Therapy

Rarely, pituitary apoplexy may occur spontaneously or during DA therapy and can require surgical intervention.[26] In addition, rapid tumor shrinking on DAs can lead to cerebrospinal fluid (CSF) leak, which could necessitate surgical repair.[27]

There have also been some reports of an association between DA therapy and car-diac valvulopathy.[28] For example, tricuspid regurgitation occurred more frequently in patients taking higher doses of cabergoline than control subjects.[29] However, multiple studies have also shown no association between clinically significant valvulopathy and low-dose DA treatment.[30] Regardless, it is reasonable to obtain baseline echocardio-grams at initiation of DA therapy.[16,28]

## SURGICAL CONSIDERATIONS

Although medical therapy may be successful in normalizing prolactin levels and managing tumor growth, surgery remains an important therapeutic modality. DA treatment may require years or even lifelong therapy. Even for those who achieve endocrinologic cure, up to 50% to 80% may recur after DA withdrawal or owing to drug resistance.[24,25]

In general, surgical indications include apoplexy, DA nonresponse, or side effects of long-term medical therapy. Surgical intervention for prolactinomas is aimed at reducing tumor mass, decompressing cranial nerves, and resecting any focus of hypersecretory adenoma while preserving the native pituitary gland.

In some select situations, primary surgery may be indicated without a DA trial. First, primary surgery may be indicated for large tumors with rapidly progressing and significant visual loss, as DAs do not produce an immediate effect.[31–34] Another indication for primary surgery would be patient refusal to undergo DA therapy. A third potential indication for upfront surgery is profound hypopituitarism at clinical presentation, as some studies have demonstrated recovery of pituitary function after selective tumor debulking to decompress the pituitary gland.[10,35,36]

### Surgical Approach: Advances and Considerations

There have been significant advances in pituitary surgery that have improved surgeons' abilities to control hormonal oversecretion through precise tumor debulking, while preserving normal pituitary function. One of the greatest advancements in pituitary surgery has been the widespread adoption of endonasal endoscopic approaches to resect sellar and extrasellar tumors. Endoscopic technology allows for superior visualization through improved optical technology and angled endoscopic lenses and instrumentation. This has allowed for visualization and resection of tumors that could not be accessed or removed with straight line-of-sight microscopic approaches. For example, sellar tumors with anterior extension along the planum sphenoidale, superior extension into the third ventricle, or lateral extension into the cavernous sinus can all be visualized and resected through endonasal endoscopic approaches, whereas microscopic access to these regions would be significantly more challenging with potentially greater morbidity.[37–39] In addition to improved surgical exposure, endoscopic CSF leak repair techniques have improved significantly over the decades, with 90% to 95% success rates being achieved consistently.[40,41] The reliable success of CSF leak repair has significantly reduced the morbidity of endoscopic pituitary surgery.

The extrasellar extent of pituitary tumors also has implications on surgical approach. Microadenomas and predominantly intrasellar macroadenomas are easily approached via the transsphenoidal route. Although many macroadenomas with extrasellar extension are also resectable through a transsphenoidal approach, there are limits beyond which transcranial approaches may be necessary, depending on tumor size, shape, invasiveness, and proximity to critical neuroanatomical structures. For example, transsphenoidal approaches are limited when there is significant tumor extension lateral to the carotid artery, necessitating a frontotemporal craniotomy.[37] Large tumors encompassing sellar, suprasellar, or other extrasellar compartments may also warrant both transsphenoidal and transcranial approaches.

### Cystic Prolactinoma

Cystic prolactinomas are unique in that they are potentially more resistant to DA therapy. Some studies have demonstrated decreased DA receptor concentration in cystic portions of prolactinomas and therefore lower remission rates with DA therapy.[42] A recent case series of 30 cystic prolactinomas treated with primary medical therapy demonstrated greater than 80% reduction in cyst volume and biochemical remission, but half the patients ultimately required surgery.[43] More evidence is necessary to determine whether medical therapy can adequately reduce the volumetric burden of cystic prolactinomas. Conversely, surgery yields immediate decompression, biochemical cure, and acceptably low recurrence rates.[44,45] In a series of 212 consecutive prolactinomas, primary transsphenoidal surgery achieved an 80% remission rate for cystic prolactinomas, comparable to DA success rates reported in the literature.[31,32,46]

### Radiation Therapy

There is a paucity of literature describing radiation therapy as first-line treatment for prolactinoma given the established efficacy of medical and surgical therapy. Most series examining radiotherapy for prolactinoma have suggested its use as a second-line or adjunctive treatment for patients with suboptimal responses to medical treatment, surgery, or a combination of both.[47–49] Adjuvant radiotherapy has resulted in endocrinologic remission in one-third of cases, while causing hypopituitarism in 15% of cases.[47,50,51]

Regarding radiotherapy options for prolactinomas, conventional fractionated radiotherapy has a lower risk of adverse effects, but a slower and less complete response rate. Stereotactic radiosurgery (SRS) for prolactinoma delivers high-dose radiation in fewer fractions with a more robust treatment response, but brings an increased risk of adverse effects.[52] Patients undergoing SRS are at higher risk for developing hypopituitarism (20% of patients by 5 years and 80% by 10–15 years after treatment).[47,53] Of note, endocrinologic response to radiotherapy varies according to the hypersecretory adenoma type with adrenocorticotropic hormone and GH-secreting adenomas exhibiting a remission rate of 50% or greater, whereas remission in prolactinomas is less than 25%.[53]

In some cases, surgical debulking may be performed before radiotherapy while specifically avoiding manipulation of nearby neural tissues. In these scenarios, subtotal surgical debulking may allow for a tumor-free margin around the adjacent radiosensitive neural structures and prevent postoperative radiotherapy-induced damage to these structures (eg, optic chiasm, cranial nerves, and pituitary gland).[54]

## IMPORTANT CLINICAL SCENARIOS
### Apoplexy

Macroprolactinomas are more likely to present with visual compromise or cranial nerve palsies. When vision loss occurs acutely, as in the example of pituitary apoplexy, urgent surgical decompression is the mainstay of treatment. The hallmark of pituitary apoplexy includes the classic triad of sudden severe headache, visual changes, and altered consciousness secondary to hypopituitarism and adrenal crisis. Apoplectic signs and symptoms are due to hemorrhage and infarction of the pituitary lesion, which lead to sudden mass effect on the pituitary gland.[55] Those with subtle or gradual visual compromise may elect for a trial of medical therapy because 70% to 90% of prolactinomas exhibit some degree of involution within weeks to months after initiating DA therapy.[56] Those who suffer from progressive vision impairment or fail to demonstrate an adequate reduction in tumor size are suitable candidates for surgery. **Fig. 1** shows an MRI scan demonstrating characteristic imaging features of pituitary apoplexy in the setting of a pituitary macroadenoma.

### Dopamine Agonist-Induced Cerebrospinal Fluid Rhinorrhea

Although DA therapy remains the mainstay of primary prolactinoma treatment, approximately 6% of these patients develop CSF rhinorrhea as a consequence of

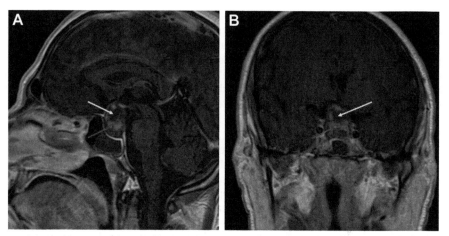

**Fig. 1.** Apoplexy case example. (*A*) Sagittal and (*B*) coronal MRI T1 scan with contrast images demonstrating a macroprolactinoma with suprasellar extension and acute hemorrhage within the tumor. The pituitary tumor extended superiorly to compress the optic chiasm and abutted the floor of the third ventricle. The sella demonstrated heterogeneous intensities, with enhancing areas of macroadenoma (*red arrows*) and isointense areas representing hemorrhage (*yellow arrows*).

tumor involution in the setting of dural and bony defects of the skull base.[5,57] Macroprolactinomas that exhibit osseous erosion through the sphenoid sinus are at higher risk for developing DA-induced CSF rhinorrhea. Interestingly, the following features have not been associated with CSF leaks after initiating DA therapy: pretreatment tumor size, rate of tumor shrinkage, serum prolactin levels, and rapidity of prolactin reduction.[5,57] The presence of CSF rhinorrhea substantially increases the risk of meningitis and pneumocephalus,[58] and patients should be educated about the signs and symptoms of CSF rhinorrhea and its complications. Importantly, clinicians should collect and test any thin clear nasal drainage for beta-2 transferrin,[59] and if CSF rhinorrhea is confirmed, high-resolution computed tomography imaging of the skull base should be obtained to localize the bony defect in the skull base. Patients should also be referred to surgeons who perform endoscopic CSF leak repair.

## SUMMARY

Prolactinomas represent the most common secretory tumor of the pituitary gland. Clinical presentation may be due to prolactin oversecretion, localized mass effect, or a combination of both. The mainstay of prolactinoma management is medical therapy with dopamine agonists, such as bromocriptine and cabergoline. Endoscopic endonasal or transcranial surgery, radiation therapy, or a combination of these is an important treatment option in select cases. Pituitary apoplexy and dopamine agonist–induced CSF rhinorrhea are important clinical considerations in the management of these lesions.

## CLINICS CARE POINTS

- Surgical intervention should be considered for patients who fail to respond to dopaminergic agonist therapy, cannot tolerate dopaminergic agonist therapy, or have macroadenomas with a large cystic component.

- Pituitary apoplexy with sudden visual decline secondary to optic nerve compression is a surgical emergency.
- Radiation therapy is most commonly used as an adjunctive or second-line treatment.
- Whether medical or surgical interventions are pursued, long-term surveillance via endocrinologic laboratory assessment and MRI is essential.
- If cerebrospinal fluid rhinorrhea is detected, high-resolution computed tomography imaging of the skull base should be obtained to localize the osseous defect.

## REFERENCES

1. Glezer A, Bronstein MD. Prolactinomas. Endocrinol Metab Clin North Am 2015; 44(1):71–8.
2. Bloomgarden E, Molitch ME. Surgical treatment of prolactinomas: cons. Endocrine 2014;47(3):730–3.
3. Passos VQ, Fortes MA, Giannella-Neto D, et al. Genes differentially expressed in prolactinomas responsive and resistant to dopamine agonists. Neuroendocrinology 2009;89(2):163–70.
4. Maiter D. Management of dopamine agonist-resistant prolactinoma. Neuroendocrinology 2019;109(1):42–50.
5. Milton CK, Lee BJ, Voronovich ZA, et al. Prolactinoma extension as a contributing factor in dopamine agonist-induced CSF rhinorrhea: a systematic review of the literature. Br J Neurosurg 2021;30:1–6.
6. Park SS, Kim JH, Kim YH, et al. Clinical and radiographic characteristics related to hyperprolactinemia in nonfunctioning pituitary adenomas. World Neurosurg 2018;119:e1035–40.
7. Nunley WC, Urban RJ, Kitchin JD, et al. Dynamics of pulsatile prolactin release during the postpartum lactational period. J Clin Endocrinol Metab 1991;72(2): 287–93.
8. Petakov MS, Damjanovic SS, Nikolic-Durovic MM, et al. Pituitary adenomas secreting large amounts of prolactin may give false low values in immunoradiometric assays. The hook effect. J Endocrinol Invest 1998;21(3):184–8.
9. Samperi I, Lithgow K, Karavitaki N. Hyperprolactinaemia. J Clin Med 2019;8(12).
10. Webb SM, Rigla M, Wagner A, Oliver B, Bartumeus F. Recovery of hypopituitarism after neurosurgical treatment of pituitary adenomas. J Clin Endocrinol Metab 1999;84(10):3696–700.
11. Lv L, Jiang Y, Yin S, et al. Mammosomatotroph and mixed somatotroph-lactotroph adenoma in acromegaly: a retrospective study with long-term follow-up. Endocrine 2019;66(2):310–8.
12. Rahman M, Jusue-Torres I, Alkabbani A, Salvatori R, Rodriguez FJ, Quinones-Hinojosa A. Synchronous GH- and prolactin-secreting pituitary adenomas. Endocrinol Diabetes Metab Case Rep 2014;2014:140052.
13. Tirosh A, Shimon I. Management of macroprolactinomas. Clin Diabetes Endocrinol 2015;1:5.
14. Melmed S, Braunstein GD, Chang RJ, Becker DP. Pituitary tumors secreting growth hormone and prolactin. Ann Intern Med 1986;105(2):238–53.
15. Schlechte J, Dolan K, Sherman B, Chapler F, Luciano A. The natural history of untreated hyperprolactinemia: a prospective analysis. J Clin Endocrinol Metab 1989;68(2):412–8.

16. Melmed S, Casanueva FF, Hoffman AR, et al. Diagnosis and treatment of hyper-prolactinemia: an Endocrine Society clinical practice guideline. J Clin Endocrinol Metab 2011;96(2):273–88.
17. Klibanski A. Clinical practice. Prolactinomas. N Engl J Med 2010;362(13):1219–26.
18. Vasilev V, Daly AF, Vroonen L, Zacharieva S, Beckers A. Resistant prolactinomas. J Endocrinol Invest 2011;34(4):312–6.
19. Molitch ME. Management of medically refractory prolactinoma. J Neurooncol 2014;117(3):421–8.
20. Choudhary C, Hamrahian AH, Bena JF, et al. The effect of raloxifene on serum prolactin level in patients with prolactinoma. Endocr Pract 2019;25(7):684–8.
21. Oh MC, Aghi MK. Dopamine agonist-resistant prolactinomas. J Neurosurg 2011;114(5):1369–79.
22. dos Santos Nunes V, El Dib R, Boguszewski CL, et al. Cabergoline versus bromo-criptine in the treatment of hyperprolactinemia: a systematic review of random-ized controlled trials and meta-analysis. Pituitary 2011;14(3):259–65.
23. Souteiro P, Belo S, Carvalho D. Dopamine agonists in prolactinomas: when to withdraw? Pituitary 2020;23(1):38–44.
24. Dekkers OM, Lagro J, Burman P, et al. Recurrence of hyperprolactinemia after withdrawal of dopamine agonists: systematic review and meta-analysis. J Clin Endocrinol Metab 2010;95(1):43–51.
25. Pereira AM. Update on the withdrawal of dopamine agonists in patients with hy-perprolactinemia. Curr Opin Endocrinol Diabetes Obes 2011;18(4):264–8.
26. Chng E, Dalan R. Pituitary apoplexy associated with cabergoline therapy. J Clin Neurosci 2013;20(12):1637–43.
27. Lam G, Mehta V, Zada G. Spontaneous and medically induced cerebrospinal fluid leakage in the setting of pituitary adenomas: review of the literature. Neuro-surg focus 2012;32(6):E2.
28. Steeds RP, Stiles CE, Sharma V, et al. Echocardiography and monitoring patients receiving dopamine agonist therapy for hyperprolactinaemia: a joint position statement of the British Society of Echocardiography, the British Heart Valve So-ciety and the Society for Endocrinology. Echo Res Pract 2019;6(1):G1–8.
29. Colao A, Galdcrisi M, Di Sarno A, et al. Increased prevalence of tricuspid regur-gitation in patients with prolactinomas chronically treated with cabergoline. J Clin Endocrinol Metab 2008;93(10):3777–84.
30. Stiles CE, Lloyd G, Bhattacharyya S, et al. Incidence of cabergoline-associated valvulopathy in primary care patients with prolactinoma using hard cardiac end-points. J Clin Endocrinol Metab 2021;106(2):e711–20.
31. Zamanipoor Najafabadi AH, Zandbergen IM, de Vries F, et al. Surgery as a viable alternative first-line treatment for prolactinoma patients. a systematic review and meta-analysis. J Clin Endocrinol Metab 2020;(3):105. https://doi.org/10.1210/clinem/dgz144.
32. Park JY, Choi W, Hong AR, et al. Surgery is a safe, effective first-line treatment modality for noninvasive prolactinomas. Pituitary 2021. https://doi.org/10.1007/s11102-021-01168-x.
33. Salvatori R. Surgical treatment of microprolactinomas: pros. Endocrine 2014;47(3):725–9.
34. Couldwell WT, Rovit RL, Weiss MH. Role of surgery in the treatment of micropro-lactinomas. Neurosurg Clin N Am 2003;14(1):89–92, vii.
35. Fatemi N, Dusick JR, Mattozo C, et al. Pituitary hormonal loss and recovery after transsphenoidal adenoma removal. Neurosurgery 2008;63(4):709–18.

36. Tritos NA, Fazeli PK, McCormack A, et al. Pituitary Society Delphi survey: an international perspective on endocrine management of patients undergoing transsphenoidal surgery for pituitary adenomas. Pituitary 2021. https://doi.org/10.1007/s11102-021-01170-3.
37. Buchfelder M, Schlaffer S. Surgical treatment of pituitary tumours. Best Pract Res Clin Endocrinol Metab 2009;23(5):677–92.
38. Cappabianca P, Cavallo LM, Esposito F, et al. Extended endoscopic endonasal approach to the midline skull base: the evolving role of transsphenoidal surgery. Adv Tech Stand Neurosurg 2008;33:151–99.
39. Cavallo LM, Prevedello DM, Solari D, et al. Extended endoscopic endonasal transsphenoidal approach for residual or recurrent craniopharyngiomas. J Neurosurg 2009;111(3):578–89.
40. Harvey RJ, Parmar P, Sacks R, et al. Endoscopic skull base reconstruction of large dural defects: a systematic review of published evidence. Laryngoscope 2012;122(2):452–9.
41. Conger A, Zhao F, Wang X, et al. Evolution of the graded repair of CSF leaks and skull base defects in endonasal endoscopic tumor surgery: trends in repair failure and meningitis rates in 509 patients. J Neurosurg 2018;130(3):861–75.
42. Bhavsar KR, Silver KD. Cystic prolactinoma: a surgical disease? AACE Clin Case Rep 2019;5(1):e66–9.
43. Faje A, Chunharojrith P, Nency J, et al. Dopamine agonists can reduce cystic prolactinomas. J Clin Endocrinol Metab 2016;101(10):3709–15.
44. Donoho DA, Laws ER Jr. The role of surgery in the management of prolactinomas. Neurosurg Clin N Am 2019;30(4):509–14.
45. Nakhleh A, Shehadeh N, Hochberg I, et al. Management of cystic prolactinomas: a review. Pituitary 2018;21(4):425–30.
46. Kreutzer J, Buslei R, Wallaschofski H, et al. Operative treatment of prolactinomas: indications and results in a current consecutive series of 212 patients. Eur J Endocrinol 2008;158(1):11–8.
47. Ding D, Starke RM, Sheehan JP. Treatment paradigms for pituitary adenomas: defining the roles of radiosurgery and radiation therapy. J Neurooncol 2014;117(3):445–57.
48. Mehta AE, Reyes FI, Faiman C. Primary radiotherapy of prolactinomas. Eight- to 15-year follow-up. Am J Med 1987;83(1):49–58.
49. Pan L, Zhang N, Wang EM, et al. Gamma knife radiosurgery as a primary treatment for prolactinomas. J Neurosurg 2000;93(Suppl 3):10–3.
50. Pouratian N, Sheehan J, Jagannathan J, et al. Gamma Knife radiosurgery for medically and surgically refractory prolactinomas. Neurosurgery 2006;59(2):255–66.
51. Sheehan JP, Pouratian N, Steiner L, et al. Gamma knife surgery for pituitary adenomas: factors related to radiological and endocrine outcomes. J Neurosurg 2011;114(2):303–9.
52. Molitch ME. Diagnosis and treatment of pituitary adenomas: a review. JAMA 2017;317(5):516–24.
53. Jagannathan J, Yen CP, Pouratian N, et al. Stereotactic radiosurgery for pituitary adenomas: a comprehensive review of indications, techniques and long-term results using the Gamma Knife. J Neurooncol 2009;92(3):345–56.
54. Forster N, Warnick R, Takiar V, et al. Debulking surgery of pituitary adenoma as a strategy to facilitate definitive stereotactic radiosurgery. J Neurooncol 2018;138(2):335–40.

55. Abbara A, Clarke S, Eng PC, et al. Clinical and biochemical characteristics of patients presenting with pituitary apoplexy. Endocr Connect 2018. https://doi.org/10.1530/EC-18-0255.

56. Venkatesh SK, Kothari D, Manchanda S, et al. Spontaneous reduction of prolactinoma post cabergoline withdrawal. Indian J Endocrinol Metab 2012;16(5):833–5.

57. Suliman SG, Gurlek A, Byrne JV, et al. Nonsurgical cerebrospinal fluid rhinorrhea in invasive macroprolactinoma: incidence, radiological, and clinicopathological features. J Clin Endocrinol Metab 2007;92(10):3829–35.

58. Daudia A, Biswas D, Jones NS. Risk of meningitis with cerebrospinal fluid rhinorrhea. Ann Otol Rhinol Laryngol 2007;116(12):902–5.

59. Zervos TM, Macki M, Cook B, et al. Beta-2 transferrin is detectable for 14 days whether refrigerated or stored at room temperature. Int Forum Allergy Rhinol 2018;8(9):1052–5.

# Cushing Disease
## Medical and Surgical Considerations

David P. Bray, MD[a],*, Rima S. Rindler, MD[a], Reem A. Dawoud, BS[b],
Andrew B. Boucher, MD[c], Nelson M. Oyesiku, MD, PhD[d]

### KEYWORDS

- Cushing disease • Adenoma • Pituitary • Endonasal • Endoscopic • Skull base
- Transnasal

### KEY POINTS

- Cushing disease is a disorder of hypercortisolemia caused by hypersecretion of adreno-corticotropic hormone (ACTH) by a pituitary adenoma.
- Patients with Cushing disease present with characteristic clinical signs and symptoms associated with excess cortisol, but diagnosis is difficult and often relies on repeated and varied endocrinologic assays and neuroradiologic investigations.
- Gold standard treatment is surgical resection of ACTH-secreting pituitary adenoma, which is curative.
- Patients require close endocrinologic follow-up for maintenance of associated neuroendocrine deficiencies and surveillance for potential recurrence.
- Medications, radiotherapy, and bilateral adrenalectomy are alternative treatments for residual or recurrent disease.

 Video content accompanies this article at http://www.oto.theclinics.com.

## INTRODUCTION

Cushing disease (CD), named for the father of modern neurosurgery, remains one of the most difficult-to-treat pathologies in neurosurgery. Twelve patients with CD were first described by Dr Harvey Cushing in 1912, and the management of the disease has evolved with the medical advances and dramatic improvement in surgical techniques over the last century.[1,2] The successful treatment of CD relies on the

Conflict of interest: None.
[a] Department of Neurosurgery, Emory University School of Medicine, 1365 Clifton Road, Atlanta, GA 30322, USA; [b] Emory University School of Medicine, 1365 Clifton Road, Atlanta, GA 30322, USA; [c] Department of Neurosurgery, Semmes Murphy Clinic, 6325 Humphreys Boulevard, Memphis, TN 38120, USA; [d] Department of Neurosurgery, University of North Carolina School of Medicine, 321 S Columbia Street, Chapel Hill, NC 27516, USA
* Corresponding author. Department of Neurosurgery, Emory University School of Medicine, 1365 Clifton Road, Atlanta, GA 30322.
E-mail address: dbray3@emory.edu

Otolaryngol Clin N Am 55 (2022) 315–329
https://doi.org/10.1016/j.otc.2021.12.006
0030-6665/22/© 2022 Elsevier Inc. All rights reserved.

strength of a multidisciplinary team, as in a Pituitary Center of Excellence; diagnosis and cure depends on a tight meshwork of endocrinologic, neurosurgical, otolaryngologic, neurointerventional, neuroradiologic, and radiation oncologic care.[3,4] Following endocrinologic diagnosis, surgical intervention is curative; therefore, a pituitary surgery team with experienced neurosurgeons and otolaryngologists is critical for care of these patients. Failure to completely treat CD subjects afflicted patients to ongoing morbidity and reduced life expectancy.[5,6]

It is critical to differentiate between Cushing syndrome (CS) and CD. CS is caused by hypercortisolism of any cause. Long-term exogenous glucocorticoid use is the most common cause of CS.[7] CD is the most common, so-called "endogenous CS." CD occurs when a functional pituitary adenoma results in hypersecretion of adrenocorticotropic hormone (ACTH), leading to overstimulation of the adrenal glands that secrete excess glucocorticoids, including cortisol. This article reviews the complex diagnostic work-up of CD, surgical treatment, postoperative management, and strategies for persistent and recurrent disease.[8]

## PREOPERATIVE EVALUATION OF CUSHING DISEASE
### Epidemiology

CD is a rare phenomenon, especially when compared with the more common clinical entity of CS. A high-index of suspicion is required to initiate a work-up for diagnosis. Epidemiologic studies estimate that CD occurs in 0.7 to 2.4 per million persons.[9–11] Given the rarity of CD, there is often a significant delay to diagnosis and treatment.[12] Although there is little sex preference of CD in children, there is a significant predilection for adult women compared with men with CD (3–8:1).[13–15] CD most often occurs in a young adult population (30s–40s).[8,15] Latency from lesion onset to symptom development is 2 to 3 years.[8,15]

### Normal Cortisol Physiology

A foundational understanding of normal cortisol physiology is instructive in conceptualizing the endocrinologic pathophysiology and associated clinical syndrome of CD. In the nonpathologic state, cortisol blood levels ebb and flow in a diurnal fashion. Cortisol levels are highest early in the morning on awakening, drop significantly in early afternoon, and reach a nadir at night (during sleep). Cortisol levels increase in times of physiologic stress and are profoundly affected by other external and internal factors. In the normal state, corticotropin-releasing hormone (CRH) is released from the paraventricular nuclei of the hypothalamus, enters the hypophyseal portal venous system, which in turn induces corticotroph cells in the anterior pituitary gland to secrete ACTH into the systemic vasculature.[8] Next, ACTH binds to specific receptors in the adrenal cortex, which results in adrenal output of cortisol (among other glucocorticoid steroids).[16] Cortisol participates in a self-regulatory, negative feedback loop to the hypothalamus, where it blunts CRH release.[17]

### Pathophysiology in Cushing Disease

In CD, the development of the clinical syndrome depends on hypersecretion of ACTH. Basophilic corticotroph cells in the anterior lobe of the pituitary gland can proliferate into a benign adenoma. The hypersecretion of ACTH results in constant excess production of glucocorticoid and cortisol hormones from the adrenal cortex.[18] A significant consequence of hypercortisolism in CD is the loss of the normal cyclical nature of cortisol secretion, leading to chronic suppression of CRH secretion from the hypothalamus.[8]

## Pathophysiologic State and Clinical Presentation of Patients with Cushing Disease

High circulating levels of cortisol and the loss of diurnal variation results in disastrous effects on normal body physiology in CS and CD.[7]

There is significant effect of CS on the cardiovascular system.[19] CS initially causes insulin resistance and dysregulation of glucose metabolism that leads to diabetes mellitus, obesity, dyslipidemia, and hypertension. CS is associated with increased low-density lipoprotein relative to high-density lipoprotein, even when compared with body mass index–matched control subjects.[20] This metabolic syndrome can lead to accelerated atherosclerosis, even in young adults.[5] Hypertension increases the risk of hemorrhagic and ischemic stroke.[21] Hypercortisolemia-associated hypercoagulability increases the risk of deep vein thrombosis, stroke, and pulmonary embolus, especially periprocedurally.[22,23] Cardiovascular pathology and risk factors caused by CD must be medically managed perioperatively and up to 5 years after cure.[20]

CS is associated with accelerated osteoporosis, with greater than one-half of patients with endogenous hypercortisolism exhibiting reduced x-ray absorptiometry scores compared with matched control subjects.[24] There is an increased risk of bone fracture (especially vertebral body fracture) in patients with CS, with almost 50% of patients experiencing a fracture during their disease.[25] Patients with CD require close endocrinologic follow-up for the treatment of osteoporosis, possibly with medications, such as bisphosphonates. CD can also cause growth hormone and bone marrow/immune suppression.[5,26]

There is often an underestimated effect of excess cortisol on cognitive function, mood, and health-related quality of life.[27] Patients with CD have increased risk of psychopathology, with major depression being the most common psychiatric affliction.[5] Rarely, fulminant psychosis can result. Additionally, patients with CD can experience cognitive and executive function decline, memory loss, and derangement in verbal/language processing.[28] These symptoms can persist even after treatment, because of irreversible brain matter loss, demonstrated in such regions as the hippocampus.[29]

CS and CD result in a characteristic phenotype that should prompt physicians to test for hypercortisolism. Hallmarks of CS include thinning hair, soft tissue plethora, acne, moon facies, central adiposity with muscle wasting, and an enlarged dorsocervical fat pad (termed "buffalo hump"). Patients with CS also exhibit various dermal changes including thin skin and abdominal striae. Additional findings on physical examination include purpura/easy bruising, lower extremity edema, and skin ulcers from poor wound healing. Women can experience amenorrhea and men can have decreased libido.[5,8] It is wise to view pictures of patients with CD from 5 to 10 years ago to best determine the effects of CS. This can also be a helpful tool to monitor for recovery and remission from CD after surgical treatment.

## Proving and Establishing the Cause of Hypercortisolism

If a patient is suspected to have CS, physicians must inspect the patient's daily medication list to ensure there is not a clear iatrogenic source of hypercortisolism. Confirming a diagnosis of CD is an arduous and complicated process. The goal of the work-up is to build enough data to support the case of CD (**Fig. 1**). Guidelines from the Endocrine Society state that the diagnosis of hypercortisolemia can be established with two positive screening tests.[30] A test with high diagnostic accuracy is first recommended: either a random urine cortisol, late night salivary cortisol, or 1 mg (overnight) or 2 mg (48 hour) dexamethasone suppression test (DST) is used. A positive test should be confirmed with a secondary, more specific assay, such as a midnight serum cortisol level or dexamethasone-CRH suppression test.[30]

# Cushing's Disease Diagnostic Workup

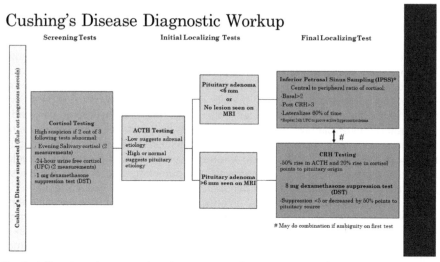

Fig. 1. A flowchart demonstrating the sequence of testing required for diagnosis of Cushing disease.

After hypercortisolism has been established, an endocrinologist should query the cause. Endogenous hypercortisolism is ACTH-dependent (ie, CD or ectopic ACTH-secreting tumor) or ACTH-independent (ie, cortical adrenal tumor).[8,31] Serum ACTH levels are obtained, and if high, establish the cause of hypercortisolism. Computed tomography of the abdomen and pelvis with intravenous contrast can confirm the presence of an adrenal mass.

Additional assays are required to further distinguish pituitary and ectopic ACTH-dependent causes of CS. Blood tests include CRH stimulation testing and high-dose DST. CRH stimulation testing relies on pituitary adenoma cells maintaining CRH receptors that continue to respond to bound CRH by releasing ACTH.[8] Therefore, exogenous CRH delivered during a stimulation test leads to elevated ACTH and cortisol in CD. In contrast, in an ectopic ACTH-secreting tumor that lacks CRH receptors, CRH administration does not lead to increased ACTH/cortisol levels.[17,32] Similarly, ACTH-producing adenoma cells in CD maintain their glucocorticoid negative feedback receptors, and their ACTH secretion is partially or fully suppressed by high-dose dexamethasone. In the high-dose, overnight DST, the patient is given 8 mg of dexamethasone and a morning plasma cortisol level is obtained; if the baseline level is suppressed greater than 68%, then CD is confirmed.[33]

There are many obstacles in this diagnostic process that create challenges for clinicians. Namely, the test results can be discordant or may not be replicable. Many laboratories have different reference values that make comparison of results less straightforward. Some testing, such as inferior petrosal sinus sampling (IPSS), is procedural or involves significant patient cooperation (eg, 24-hour urine testing). All of these factors can prolong the diagnostic process. Appropriate patient counseling of expectations for the steps of the process can build patient trust and provide reassurance.

## Imaging

Because of the high biochemical activity of CD pituitary adenomas, most are discovered as microadenomas (<1 cm in greatest diameter). These tumors consistently arise

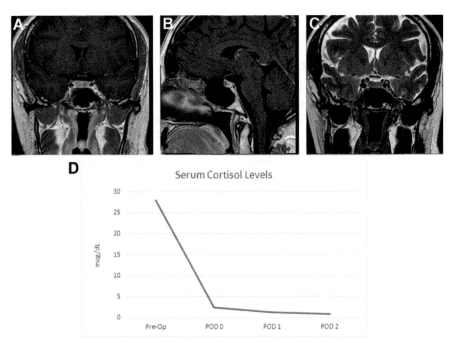

**Fig. 2.** Case of a 40-year-old woman with Cushing disease. (*A–C*) MRI of the brain, sella protocol showing a pituitary adenoma in the left anterior aspect of the pituitary gland within the sella. It is T1 nonenhancing (*A*, coronal; *B*, sagittal) with a small T2 hyperintense component (*C*, coronal). (*D*) There was a significant drop in morning cortisol following surgical resection from 28 μg/dL to 0.9 μg/dL by postoperative day 2.

from the anterior pituitary gland, but can also occur within the pituitary stalk and in the posterior lobe of the pituitary gland.[34] Following the diagnosis of ACTH-dependent hypercortisolism, an MRI of the pituitary and brain with and without gadolinium contrast is the next step for work-up. At a Pituitary Center of Excellence, there is often a specialized radiologic pituitary protocol created with input from the neuroradiology team to assist with visualizing microadenomas using high-resolution T2-weighted sequences (eg, constructive interference in steady state) obtained in thin cuts (1–1.5 mm) through the anterior skull base, with dynamic contrast enhancement. A focal lesion is detected in up to 60% of patients with CD. The microadenoma is commonly hypoenhancing in the early dynamic phase (**Fig. 2**). Addition of a spoiled gradient echo three-dimensional T1 sequence may increase the sensitivity of neuroimaging over conventional and dynamic sequences.[35–37]

With improved MRI protocols and MRI acquisition techniques, "radiologically silent" CD is rarer, but is still encountered in clinical practice.[37] In these cases, IPSS is used to further confirm a CD adenoma. In this procedure, a neurointerventional endovascular team accesses bilateral inferior petrosal sinuses with intravenous microcatheters. Intravenous CRH is administered and blood samplings of the inferior cavernous sinuses are taken at regular time intervals. In CD, ACTH levels following CRH stimulation are three times greater than baseline.[38–40] At high-volume centers, localization and/or lateralization of CD adenomas is achieved with IPSS with good sensitivity, where samples from one inferior petrosal sinus consistently exhibit higher ACTH levels than the contralateral side and correlate with a microadenoma.[41] For surgical planning, we often obtain a thin-cut computed tomography of the anterior skull base, which helps identify aberrant bony anatomy of the sphenoid sinus and the carotid arteries.

## SURGICAL TREATMENT OF CUSHING DISEASE

Complete surgical resection of a CD adenoma is the gold standard for treatment that can lead to cure. Most CD adenomas are amenable to the transsphenoidal (TS) surgical approach. Although the TS approach was first used with exterior magnification/illumination (loupes/headlight and operative microscope), most Pituitary Centers of Excellence now prefer the endonasal, endoscopic TS approach to the sella.[42–44] An experienced and skilled pituitary surgery team, comprised of a neurosurgeon and a skull base otolaryngology surgeon/rhinologist, can achieve excellent outcomes in the treatment of CD adenomas.

Because most CD adenomas are less than 1 cm in greatest dimension, localization is challenging, even with superior MRI acquisition techniques.[45] For this reason, we prefer the endoscope for visualization of the sellar area. The endoscopic endonasal approach to the sella has been well-described.[46] We emphasize a wide exposure of the pituitary sella, with removal of posterior sphenoid sinus wall and bone in the clival recess until both medial aspects of the cavernous sinus, the superior intercavernous sinus/sphenoid limbus, and the inferior sella above the clival recess are well-defined. Specific approaches to tumor resection depend on the presence of an identifiable adenoma on preoperative imaging.

### Exploiting the Histologic Pseudocapsule

A clear understanding of sellar surgical anatomy is critical for successful microadenoma resection. The layers of tissue encountered when resecting a pituitary adenoma include the dura, which has an outer (endosteal) layer and an inner (meningeal) layer with a potential space that expands laterally to house the cavernous sinus. Additional tissues encountered include the pituitary gland capsule, pituitary gland, adenoma pseudocapsule, and the pituitary adenoma.[47] It is important to study the preoperative MRI to identify the three-dimensional anatomy of the CD adenoma. Specifically, we like to note the side of the pituitary gland the adenoma resides, the location in the sagittal plane, and the relationship to the cavernous sinus wall. T2-weighted images can further indicate the consistency of the adenoma (eg, a T2-hyperintense adenoma may be more cystic).

Gross-total resection of a pituitary microadenoma depends on a reliable pseudocapsule that presents a boundary that is exploited for surgical success (Video 1). The histologic presence of the pseudocapsule was first identified by Costello in 1936, but further described by Hardy and then Oldfield in 2006.[47–49] The pseudocapsule develops as the benign adenoma grows slowly with the iterative division of a single cell. As the adenoma gains size, it progressively impinges on the normal pituitary gland around it. This pressure leads to a piling of several concentric layers of normal pituitary gland reticulin. Microadenomas 3 mm in size reliably demonstrate a robust reticulin pseudocapsule that differentiates the adenoma from the normal pituitary gland.[47] Recognition of the adenoma pseudocapsule and careful circumferential dissection of the pseudocapsule plane avoids tumor spillage and potential subtotal resection, leading to the greatest chance of CD remission.

### Surgical Technique

We start our intrasellar dissection by incising the meningeal layer of the dura with a Beaver blade. A small round disk dissector is used to develop the interdural plane, and angled microsciscors are used to sharply divide the meningeal dura to the medial cavernous sinus. It is common to encounter cavernous sinus bleeding in the interdural plane, which is easily controlled with thrombin powder and gentle pressure. The endosteal layer of the dura is then used to support further separation of the pituitary gland from the medial cavernous sinus, the inferior and posterior surfaces of the sella, and then superior surface. This circumferential dissection provides good all-around access to explore the gland. The endosteal dura is then sharply incised and swept away from the pituitary gland capsule with the round disk dissector.

If the adenoma is located in the anterior-most portion of the gland, the pseudocapsule may be encountered immediately following the dural opening. In most cases, there are a few millimeters of normal gland overlying the adenoma. If preoperative MRI assessment (in the coronal plane) indicated that the adenoma is in the center of the gland, the gland is incised with microscissors or the Beaver blade until the pseudocapsule is encountered, and the underlying adenoma is dissected and resected en bloc.

Often, the CD adenoma arise from the lateral aspect of the pituitary gland, abutting the cavernous sinus. In these cases, to ensure complete resection of the adenoma, we perform a partial transposition of the side of the pituitary gland with the adenoma. We bluntly dissect the plane between the pituitary gland and the cavernous sinus wall, gently coaxing the lobe of the pituitary gland into the sphenoid sinus. During this dissection, we carefully inspect for tumor invasion of the medial wall of the cavernous sinus. If there is clear contact of the adenoma with the medial wall of the cavernous sinus, we resect the medial wall with the tumor.[50,51] This step requires coagulation and sharp division of the inferior hypophyseal artery at the lateral and inferior aspect of the pituitary gland.

Only after the lateral wing of the pituitary gland has been transposed can we begin adenoma resection. The CD adenoma is classically paler than the surrounding gland and has a different consistency because of the pseudocapsule. We prefer to use gentle, blunt dissection with dull ring curettes and enucleators. Normal gland should be carefully maneuvered away from the adenoma, as it is coaxed from its pocket within the pituitary gland. It is imperative to preserve the integrity of the adenoma pseudocapsule, because intratumoral pressure is helpful for delivering the tumor from the gland. If the adenoma is greater than 1 cm, we prefer to transpose both lateral wings of the pituitary gland before adenoma dissection. After resection, the dura is reconstructed with synthetic collagen matrix and a nasoseptal flap if a cerebrospinal fluid leak is present.[52,53]

### Special Considerations for Radiographically Silent Cushing Disease

Without definite preoperative localization of the CD adenoma, there is a significantly lower chance of disease remission.[54] In these cases, we prefer to transpose the anterior lobe of the pituitary gland, such that both lateral wings are dissected free from the medial walls of the cavernous sinus. Using the data from prior IPSS for gross localization, we then make sequential sagittal incisions through the pituitary gland capsule and follow with blunt dissection within these cuts in search of a pseudocapsule. If no tumor is encountered, a selective hemihypophysectomy is performed, and pathologic analysis is undertaken in search of a microadenoma. Unfortunately, hypophysectomy may result in lifelong hypopituitarism.

### Risks of Surgery

With all TS approaches, there are present, but acceptable risks of surgery. These include sinonasal morbidity, bleeding, infection (meningitis), cerebrospinal fluid leak, hypopituitarism, and rarely, carotid injury. Certainly, disease recurrence in the presence of a subtotal resection is possible.

### Pathologic Analysis of Cushing Disease Adenoma

Histopathologic analysis of resected CD tumor reveals proliferation of basophilic cells in the typical appearance of an adenoma, with a thick reticulin wall. Immunohistochemistry staining for ACTH has made the pathologic diagnosis of CD more specific; however, false-positive errors are possible because nontumor corticotroph cells also stain for ACTH. In up to 80% of patients with hypercortisolism, ACTH-staining corticotrophs demonstrate replacement of normal cytoplasmic granules with hyaline material, called "Crooke hyaline changes."[8,55] This is an additional feature that confirms the diagnosis of CD, because Crooke changes do not occur outside of hypercortisolism.

### Postoperative Cushing Disease Management

The patient can recover from general anesthesia in the postanesthesia care unit. At high-volume centers, patients may be transferred to the general neurosurgical floor postoperatively. Serum sodium levels and urine output are followed to monitor for developing diabetes insipidus. Patients are followed by neurosurgical, otolaryngologic, and endocrinologic teams throughout their hospital stay. We emphasize nonnarcotic pain control, early mobilization, and initiation of low-molecular-weight heparin 24 hours postoperatively, because of the high risk of hypercoagulability in patients with CD.[56]

It is imperative to follow serum cortisol levels to confirm remission of CD in the immediate postoperative phase. The positive predictive value for CD remission if cortisol levels drop to less than 2 µg/dL during hospital admission approaches 100%.[57] Conversely, serum cortisol levels remaining greater than 10 µg/dL is highly predictive of a failed surgery.[57] If a patient achieves two serum cortisol levels less than 2 µg/dL or if they are symptomatically severely adrenally deficient (eg, hypotension, nausea, vomiting), we initiate physiologic cortisol-replacement therapy. If serum cortisol levels remain elevated and do not reach a nadir, we often reimage with MRI, and consider repeat surgery, as reported by others.[58,59] In these cases, a more thorough inspection of the resection cavity usually reveals residual tumor or invasion into the medial wall of the cavernous sinus. It is our preference to be more aggressive with early repeat surgery, because after healing and scarring has occurred, it is much more difficult to obtain a biochemical cure with delayed repeat surgery.[48,60]

## PERSISTENT OR RECURRENT CUSHING DISEASE

If hypocortisolism is not achieved following TS surgery, our preference is for early repeat surgery. At most Pituitary Centers of Excellence, outcomes for remission from CD should approach 90% or greater.[8,61] Certainly, auxiliary therapies may be needed to control refractory or recurrent CD.

### Medical Therapies

In general, there are three main classes of medical therapies that are used to normalize cortisol levels in the setting of persistent or recurrent CD. Each of the following medications are best deployed under the strict management of an experienced neuroendocrinologist. The first class are steroidogenesis inhibitors (eg, mitotane, ketoconazole, metyrapone, etomidate), which halt the production of cortisol at the level of the adrenal gland.[62] Possible side effects of these medications include hirsutism, gastrointestinal disturbance, and hepatic dysfunction. The second class includes glucocorticoid receptor antagonists (mifepristone), which are used to reduce the peripheral effect of hypercortisolism. Side effects include nausea and hypokalemia. Mifepristone is an abortifacient and should not be used in women who are pregnant or pursuing pregnancy.[8] A third class of agents is termed "corticotroph-directed agents," which bind somatostatin and dopamine receptors on CD adenomas (eg, pasireotide and cabergoline, respectively).[63] Osilodrostat is an inhibitor of a cytochrome P-450 enzyme that was recently tested on patients with CD in a multicenter, double-blind, phase III prospective trial. Results demonstrated rapid and effective reduction in hypercortisolism compared with placebo. Main side effects included nausea and hypocortisolism.[64]

### Radiation Therapy

Radiation therapy is used concomitantly with short-term medical therapy to achieve long-term control of recurrent or persistent CD. Various radiation modalities including fractionated radiotherapy, stereotactic radiosurgery, and proton radiotherapy have been used effectively in CD.[61,65–67] Long-term remission of CD is achieved with radiotherapy in 35% to 84% of cases.[61] Side effects of radiotherapy to the sellar region include hypopituitarism and optic neuropathy.

### Complete Adenectomy and Bilateral Adrenalectomy

Complete adenectomy and bilateral adrenalectomy were previously used as second-line therapies for refractory CD, but are now considered as last-resort because of advances in medical and radiation therapies. These procedures are reserved for patients with severe hypercortisolism, because they subject patients to lifelong dependence on exogenous steroid replacement.[61] A well-documented side effect of bilateral adrenalectomy is Nelson syndrome, occurring in up to 38% of patients, where loss of negative-feedback inhibition of residual corticotroph tumor results in surprising tumor growth and high ACTH serum levels.[68,69] Nelson syndrome may require surgical debulking to avoid irreversible optic nerve injury.

## CASE EXAMPLES
### Case 1

We evaluated a 40-year-old woman who featured phenotypic changes concerning for hypercortisolemia. These included long bone fractures, new anxiety, thinning of hair and hirsutism, weight gain, irregular menstrual cycles, prediabetic status, easy bruising, and fatigue. She was discovered to have an elevated 24-hour urine free cortisol, cortisol nonsuppression with low-dose dexamethasone testing, and elevated salivary cortisol. She exhibited elevated serum ACTH and cortisol on CRH testing. Her cortisol levels suppressed in response to high-dose dexamethasone. Neuroimaging revealed a 7-mm hypointense, nonenhancing adenoma on MRI (see **Fig. 2**). All test results were concordant and supported a diagnosis of CD. She underwent an endoscopic endonasal resection of her pituitary adenoma (Video 1). Postoperatively, her morning cortisol levels dropped from a preoperative level of 28 μg/dL to 0.9 μg/dL by postoperative day 2 (see **Fig. 2**). She was started on physiologic steroid replacement and has remained in remission.

### Case 2

A 49-year-old man was seen 4 years before presentation for work-up of hyperglycemia. Random ACTH was high at 119 pg/mL and morning cortisol at 19 μg/dL. Salivary cortisol was 0.15 without reference range, low-dose DST was unreliable. A 4- to 5-mm

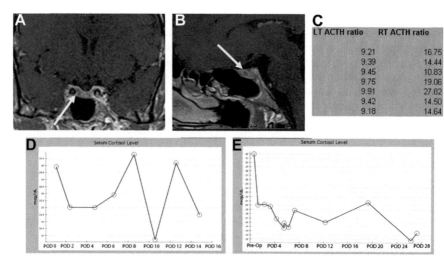

**Fig. 3.** Case of a 49-year-old man with Cushing disease and a "double adenoma." (*A, B*) MRI of the brain, sella protocol showing a pituitary adenoma (*arrow*) in the anterior right aspect of the pituitary gland abutting the cavernous sinus (*A*, coronal, *B*, sagittal). (*C*) Central/peripheral cortisol ratios from the right and left side of the pituitary gland during inferior petrosal sinus sampling, indicating higher relative ACTH levels from the right gland. (*D*) Preoperative and postoperative serum cortisol levels for first transsphenoidal resection of right pituitary adenoma, indicating persistently elevated levels. (*E*) Preoperative and postoperative serum cortisol levels for second transsphenoidal exploration, discovery, and resection of left pituitary adenoma, demonstrating cortisol nadir postoperatively to normal levels. POD, postoperative day.

pituitary adenoma was visualized on MRI, but because he was not overtly cushingoid in symptoms or appearance, this was believed to be a case of reactive hypercortisolemia (**Fig. 3**). He presented again in 2018 and underwent repeat endocrine testing, showing a high urinary free cortisol and nonsuppression with DST. ACTH increased by 50% after CRH stimulation testing. IPSS was performed, which revealed a higher central/peripheral ACTH ratio from the right pituitary compared with the left. He underwent an endoscopic endonasal TS approach to the sella. Pathologic specimen stained positive for follicle-stimulating hormone and luteinizing hormone but was negative for ACTH. The nadir morning cortisol postoperatively was 20 μg/dL (see **Fig. 3**). This was considered a failed intervention, and he was suspected of having a double adenoma. He underwent repeat surgery. The right gland was re-explored without another lesion discovered. A left side exploration, however, discovered a soft core of tissue consistent with adenoma. This was resected, and a small portion was consistent with adenoma, positive for ACTH and upregulated TBX19. Postoperative cortisol nadir was 11.7 μg/dL.

## SUMMARY

CD is a systemic, insidious, and profound disease that is difficult to diagnose and treat. It is characterized by ACTH-dependent, endogenous hypercortisolism secondary to a functional ACTH-secreting pituitary adenoma. Diagnostic work-up is critical but complicated and requires multidisciplinary evaluation that is best executed at a Pituitary Center of Excellence. Surgical resection can lead to biochemical cure and reversal of the deleterious effects of hypercortisolism for patients afflicted with CD. Biochemical assessments are the best way to assess for recurrence. For refractory cases, repeat surgery, medications, and radiation therapy are used to blunt the effects of CS.

## CLINICS CARE POINTS

- Physicians need a high index of suspicion for the diagnosis of CD.
- Surgical resection of CD can be curative.
- Patients with CD need close neuroradiological and endocrinological follow-up.

## DISCLOSURE OF FUNDING

Dr. David P. Bray is partly supported by the *Nell W. and William S. Elkin Research Fellowship in Oncology*, Winship Cancer Institute, Emory University Hospital, Atlanta, GA and supported in part by the National Center for Advancing Translational Sciences of the National Institutes of Health under Award Numbers UL1TR002378 and TL1TR002382.

## SUPPLEMENTARY DATA

Supplementary data related to this article can be found online at https://doi.org/10.1016/j.otc.2021.12.006.

## REFERENCES

1. Cushing H. The pituitary body and its disorders: clinical states produced by disorders of the hypophysis cerebri. Philadelphia: JB Lippincott; 1912.
2. Cushing H. The basophil adenomas of the pituitary body and their clinical manifestations (pituitary basophilism). J Neurosurg 1964;21(4):318–47.
3. McLaughlin N, Laws ER, Oyesiku NM, et al. Pituitary centers of excellence. Neurosurgery 2012;71(5):916–24.
4. Casanueva FF, Barkan AL, Buchfelder M, et al. Criteria for the definition of Pituitary Tumor Centers of Excellence (PTCOE): a Pituitary Society statement. Pituitary 2017;20(5):489–98.
5. Valassi E, Crespo I, Santos A, et al. Clinical consequences of Cushing's syndrome. Pituitary 2012;15(3):319–29.
6. Plotz CM, Knowlton AI, Ragan C. The natural history of Cushing's syndrome. Am J Med 1952;13(5):597–614.
7. Pivonello R, De Martino MC, De Leo M, et al. Cushing's syndrome. Endocrinol Metab Clin North Am 2008;37(1):135–49.
8. Lonser RR, Nieman L, Oldfield EH. Cushing's disease: pathobiology, diagnosis, and management. J Neurosurg 2017;126(2):404–17.
9. Lindholm J, Juul S, Jørgensen JOL, et al. Incidence and late prognosis of Cushing's syndrome: a population-based study. J Clin Endocrinol Metab 2001;86(1):117–23.
10. Etxabe J, Vazquez JA. Morbidity and mortality in Cushing's disease: an epidemiological approach. Clin Endocrinol (Oxf) 1994;40(4):479–84.
11. Ambrosi B, Faglia G. Epidemiology of pituitary tumors. Pituit Adenomas New Trends Basic Clin Res 1991;159–61.

12. Lamos EM, Munir KM. Cushing disease: highlighting the importance of early diagnosis for both de novo and recurrent disease in light of evolving treatment patterns. Endocr Pract 2014;20(9):945–55.

13. Boscaro M, Barzon L, Fallo F, et al. Cushing's syndrome. Lancet 2001;357(9258): 783–91.

14. Lonser RR, Wind JJ, Nieman LK, et al. Outcome of surgical treatment of 200 children with Cushing's disease. J Clin Endocrinol Metab 2013;98(3):892–901.

15. Zilio M, Barbot M, Ceccato F, et al. Diagnosis and complications of Cushing's disease: gender-related differences. Clin Endocrinol (Oxf) 2014;80(3):403–10.

16. Peytremann A, Nicholson WE, Brown RD, et al. Comparative effects of angiotensin and ACTH on cyclic AMP and steroidogenesis in isolated bovine adrenal cells. J Clin Invest 1973;52(4):835–42.

17. Vale W, Vaughan J, Smith M, et al. Effects of synthetic ovine corticotropin-releasing factor, glucocorticoids, catecholamines, neurohypophysial peptides, and other substances on cultured corticotropic cells. Endocrinology 1983; 113(3):1121–31.

18. Burch WM. Cushing's disease: a review. Arch Intern Med 1985;145(6):1106–11.

19. Pivonello R, Faggiano A, Lombardi G, et al. The metabolic syndrome and cardiovascular risk in Cushing's syndrome. Endocrinol Metab Clin 2005;34(2):327–39.

20. Colao A, Pivonello R, Spiezia S, et al. Persistence of increased cardiovascular risk in patients with Cushing's disease after five years of successful cure. J Clin Endocrinol Metab 1999;84(8):2664–72.

21. Toja PM, Branzi G, Ciambellotti F, et al. Clinical relevance of cardiac structure and function abnormalities in patients with Cushing's syndrome before and after cure. Clin Endocrinol (Oxf) 2012;76(3):332–8.

22. van der Pas R, Leebeek FWG, Hofland LJ, et al. Hypercoagulability in Cushing's syndrome: prevalence, pathogenesis and treatment. Clin Endocrinol (Oxf) 2013; 78(4):481–8.

23. Stuijver DJF, Van Zaane B, Feelders RA, et al. Incidence of venous thromboembolism in patients with Cushing's syndrome: a multicenter cohort study. J Clin Endocrinol Metab 2011;96(11):3525–32.

24. Mancini T, Doga M, Mazziotti G, et al. Cushing's syndrome and bone. Pituitary 2004;7(4):249–52.

25. Valassi E, Santos A, Yaneva M, et al. The European Registry on Cushing's syndrome: 2-year experience. Baseline demographic and clinical characteristics. Eur J Endocrinol 2011;165(3):383.

26. Britton S, Thoren M, Sjoberg HE. The immunological hazard of Cushing's syndrome. Br Med J 1975;4(5998):678–80.

27. Starkman MN, Giordani B, Berent S, et al. Elevated cortisol levels in Cushing's disease are associated with cognitive decrements. Psychosom Med 2001; 63(6):985–93.

28. Forget H, Lacroix A, Somma M, et al. Cognitive decline in patients with Cushing's syndrome. J Int Neuropsychol Soc 2000;6(1):20–9.

29. Starkman MN, Gebarski SS, Berent S, et al. Hippocampal formation volume, memory dysfunction, and cortisol levels in patients with Cushing's syndrome. Biol Psychiatry 1992;32(9):756–65.

30. Nieman LK, Biller BMK, Findling JW, et al. The diagnosis of Cushing's syndrome: an Endocrine Society clinical practice guideline. J Clin Endocrinol Metab 2008; 93(5):1526–40.

31. Newell-Price J, Trainer P, Besser M, et al. The diagnosis and differential diagnosis of Cushing's syndrome and pseudo-Cushing's states. Endocr Rev 1998;19(5): 647–72.
32. Nieman LK, Cutler GB Jr, Oldfield EH, et al. The ovine corticotropin-releasing hormone (CRH) stimulation test is superior to the human CRH stimulation test for the diagnosis of Cushing's disease. J Clin Endocrinol Metab 1989;69(1):165–9.
33. Tyrrell JB, Findling JW, Aron DC, et al. An overnight high-dose dexamethasone suppression test for rapid differential diagnosis of Cushing's syndrome. Ann Intern Med 1986;104(2):180–6.
34. Mason RB, Nieman LK, Doppman JL, et al. Selective excision of adenomas originating in or extending into the pituitary stalk with preservation of pituitary function. J Neurosurg 1997;87(3):343–51.
35. Arnaldi G, Angeli A, Atkinson AB, et al. Diagnosis and complications of Cushing's syndrome: a consensus statement. J Clin Endocrinol Metab 2003;88(12): 5593–602.
36. Wagner-Bartak NA, Baiomy A, Habra MA, et al. Cushing syndrome: diagnostic workup and imaging features, with clinical and pathologic correlation. Am J Roentgenol 2017;209(1):19–32.
37. Grober Y, Grober H, Wintermark M, et al. Comparison of MRI techniques for detecting microadenomas in Cushing's disease. J Neurosurg 2018;128(4):1051–7.
38. Flitsch J, Lüdecke DK, Knappe UJ, et al. Cavernous sinus sampling in selected cases of Cushing's disease. Exp Clin Endocrinol Diabetes 2002;110(7):329–35.
39. Graham KE, Samuels MH, Nesbit GM, et al. Cavernous sinus sampling is highly accurate in distinguishing Cushing's disease from the ectopic adrenocorticotropin syndrome and in predicting intrapituitary tumor location. J Clin Endocrinol Metab 1999;84(5):1602–10.
40. Oldfield EH, Chrousos GP, Schulte HM, et al. Preoperative lateralization of ACTH-secreting pituitary microadenomas by bilateral and simultaneous inferior petrosal venous sinus sampling. N Engl J Med 1985;312(2):100–3.
41. Wind JJ, Lonser RR, Nieman LK, et al. The lateralization accuracy of inferior petrosal sinus sampling in 501 patients with Cushing's disease. J Clin Endocrinol Metab 2013;98(6):2285–93.
42. Frank G, Pasquini E. Endoscopic endonasal cavernous sinus surgery, with special reference to pituitary adenomas. In: Frontiers of hormone research. Vol 34. ; 2006:64-82.
43. Prevedello DM, Doglietto F, Jane JA, et al. History of endoscopic skull base surgery: its evolution and current reality. J Neurosurg 2007;107(1):206–13.
44. Cavallo LM, Messina A, Esposito F, et al. Skull base reconstruction in the extended endoscopic transsphenoidal approach for suprasellar lesions. J Neurosurg 2007;107(4):713–20.
45. Dwyer AJ, Frank JA, Doppman JL, et al. Pituitary adenomas in patients with Cushing disease: initial experience with Gd-DTPA-enhanced MR imaging. Radiology 1987;163(2):421–6.
46. Starke RM, Reames DL, Chen C-J, et al. Endoscopic transsphenoidal surgery for Cushing disease: techniques, outcomes, and predictors of remission. Neurosurgery 2013;72(2):240–7.
47. Oldfield EH, Vortmeyer AO. Development of a histological pseudocapsule and its use as a surgical capsule in the excision of pituitary tumors. J Neurosurg 2006; 104(1):7–19.
48. Oldfield EH. Cushing's disease: lessons learned from 1500 cases. Clin Neurosurg 2017;64(CN):27–36.

49. Costello RT. Subclinical adenoma of the pituitary gland. Am J Pathol 1936; 12(2):205.

50. Truong HQ, Lieber S, Najera E, et al. The medial wall of the cavernous sinus. Part 1: surgical anatomy, ligaments, and surgical technique for its mobilization and/or resection. J Neurosurg 2018;1–9. https://doi.org/10.3171/2018.3.JNS18596.

51. Cohen-Cohen S, Gardner PA, Alves-Belo JT, et al. The medial wall of the cavernous sinus. Part 2: selective medial wall resection in 50 pituitary adenoma patients. J Neurosurg 2019;131(1):131–40.

52. Hadad G, Bassagasteguy L, Carrau RL, et al. A novel reconstructive technique after endoscopic expanded endonasal approaches: vascular pedicle nasoseptal flap. Laryngoscope 2006;116(10):1882–6.

53. Kassam AB, Thomas A, Carrau RL, et al. Endoscopic reconstruction of the cranial base using a pedicled nasoseptal flap. Neurosurgery 2008;63(1 SUPPL):44–53.

54. Sheehan JM, Beatriz Lopes M, Sheehan JP, et al. Results of transsphenoidal surgery for Cushing's disease in patients with no histologically confirmed tumor. Neurosurgery 2000;47(1):33–9.

55. Oldfield EH, Vance ML, Louis RG, et al. Crooke's changes In Cushing's syndrome depends on degree of hypercortisolism and individual susceptibility. J Clin Endocrinol Metab 2015;100(8):3165–71.

56. Shepherd DM, Jahnke H, White WL, et al. Randomized, double-blinded, placebo-controlled trial comparing two multimodal opioid-minimizing pain management regimens following transsphenoidal surgery. J Neurosurg 2017;128(2):444–51.

57. Hameed N, Yedinak CG, Brzana J, et al. Remission rate after transsphenoidal surgery in patients with pathologically confirmed Cushing's disease, the role of cortisol, ACTH assessment and immediate reoperation: a large single center experience. Pituitary 2013;16(4):452–8.

58. Dickerman RD, Oldfield EH. Basis of persistent and recurrent Cushing disease: an analysis of findings at repeated pituitary surgery. J Neurosurg 2002;97(6): 1343–9.

59. Ram Z, Nieman LK, Cutler GB, et al. Early repeat surgery for persistent Cushing's disease. J Neurosurg 1994;80(1):37–45.

60. Friedman RB, Oldfield EH, Nieman LK, et al. Repeat transsphenoidal surgery for Cushing's disease. J Neurosurg 1989;71(4):520–7.

61. Tritos NA, Biller BMK, Swearingen B. Management of Cushing disease. Nat Rev Endocrinol 2011;7(5):279–89.

62. Nieman LK, Biller BMK, Findling JW, et al. Treatment of Cushing's syndrome: an Endocrine Society clinical practice guideline. J Clin Endocrinol Metab 2015; 100(8):2807–31.

63. Lacroix A, Gu F, Gallardo W, et al. Efficacy and safety of once-monthly pasireotide in Cushing's disease: a 12 month clinical trial. Lancet Diabetes Endocrinol 2018; 6(1):17–26.

64. Pivonello R, Fleseriu M, Newell-Price J, et al. Efficacy and safety of osilodrostat in patients with Cushing's disease (LINC 3): a multicentre phase III study with a double-blind, randomised withdrawal phase. Lancet Diabetes Endocrinol 2020; 8(9):748–61.

65. Sheehan JM, Vance ML, Sheehan JP, et al. Radiosurgery for Cushing's disease after failed transsphenoidal surgery. J Neurosurg 2000;93(5):738–42.

66. Littley MD, Shalet SM, Beardwell CG, et al. Long-term follow-up of low-dose external pituitary irradiation for Cushing's disease. Clin Endocrinol (Oxf) 1990; 33(4):445–55.

67. Jagannathan J, Sheehan JP, Pouratian N, et al. Gamma knife surgery for Cushing's disease. J Neurosurg 2007;106(6):980–7.
68. Assié G, Bahurel H, Coste J, et al. Corticotroph tumor progression after adrenalectomy in Cushing's disease: a reappraisal of Nelson's syndrome. J Clin Endocrinol Metab 2007;92(1):172–9.
69. Nelson DH, Meakin JW, Dealy JB Jr, et al. ACTH-producing tumor of the pituitary gland. N Engl J Med 1958;259(4):161–4.

# Acromegaly
## Medical and Surgical Considerations

Alexandra M. Giantini-Larsen, MD[1],
Rafael Uribe-Cardenas, MD, MHS[1], Rupa Gopalan Juthani, MD*

KEYWORDS

- Acromegaly • Insulinlike growth factor-1 • Growth hormone • Somatotrophinoma
- Remission rates • Transsphenoidal resection • Stereotactic radiosurgery

KEY POINTS

- Acromegaly results from excessive secretion of growth hormone (GH) and insulinlike growth factor (IGF-1), most commonly of pituitary origin, and recognized clinically by dysmorphic features, such as jaw prognathism, acral overgrowth, arthritis, and soft tissue swelling.
- Transsphenoidal resection of GH-secreting adenomas is the primary therapy for individuals with acromegaly.
- Serum GH level should be measured during the postoperative hospitalization. A GH level of less than 1.0 ng/mL is a predictor of remission and decreased mortality. Persistent secretion is seen even in cases with apparent gross total resection, because of microscopic disease.
- Surgical debulking is recommended for tumors with parasellar and cavernous sinus invasion in which gross total resection is not possible.
- Stereotactic radiosurgery and systemic medications are used in cases of residual or recurrent tumor. Three classes of medications used are somatostatin analogues, dopamine agonists, and a genetically engineered human GH analogue.

## INTRODUCTION

Acromegaly is a complex clinical syndrome characterized by diffuse somatic and endocrinologic changes that results from excessive secretion of growth hormone (GH) and insulinlike growth factor 1 (IGF-1). Hypersecretion of GH is most commonly of pituitary origin, but cases of extrapituitary excessive release of GH have been reported. Acromegaly is not a common condition; a recent study by Crisafulli and colleagues[1] estimated the global prevalence to be 5.9 cases per 100,000 persons and

Department of Neurological Surgery, Weill Cornell Medicine, 525 East 68th Street, Box 99, New York, NY 10065, USA
[1] These authors contributed equally to the preparation of this article
* Corresponding author.
*E-mail address:* rgj9002@med.cornell.edu

Otolaryngol Clin N Am 55 (2022) 331–341
https://doi.org/10.1016/j.otc.2021.12.007
0030-6665/22/© 2022 Elsevier Inc. All rights reserved.

oto.theclinics.com

an incidence ratio of 0.38 per 100,000 person-years. There are regional variations in the epidemiology of the disease, which may be secondary to underdiagnosis or lack of adequate reporting. A study using claims-based data concluded that incidence and prevalence in the United States may be higher than previously reported in European studies. Based on data collected in that study, the authors concluded that there are approximately 3000 new cases of acromegaly each year in the United States, with a total prevalence of approximately 25,000 cases.[2] Disease awareness coupled with improved diagnostic tools may account for this apparent increased incidence of the disease.[3]

The manifestations of acromegaly are wide-ranging and can have a profound impact on the individuals who suffer from it, with a significant impact on life expectancy. A study measuring mortality in those with acromegaly from 1987 to 2013, broken into three time cohorts (1987–1995, 1996–2004, and 2005–2013), found a decrease in standardized morality ratio with standardized morality ratio of 3.45 during the first time period to standardized morality ratio of 1.86 during the last time period.[4] This corresponded with a significant increase in surgical resection from 58% to 72% and a significant decrease in the prevalence of hypopituitarism from 41% to 23% during the same time periods. A prompt diagnosis is essential to establish adequate treatment as early as possible to prevent long-term metabolic complications and to decrease the possibility of irreversible structural abnormalities. Adequate biochemical control of the disease is associated with decreased costs, improvement in quality of life, and decreased mortality.[5] Factors that determine the overall morbidity and mortality in patients with acromegaly include age, levels of GH and IGF-1 before and after treatment, tumor size, extent of resection, and the duration of symptoms before diagnosis and treatment.[6]

## EVALUATION OF ACROMEGALY

Acromegaly is most commonly recognized clinically by the characteristic dysmorphic features present in affected individuals. Because these changes occur over a long period of time, they are often recognized late in the course of the disease and include jaw prognathism, acral overgrowth, arthritis, and soft tissue swelling.[7] Patients are typically referred by ancillary specialties, such as optometry or dentistry, after presenting with complaints of decreased vision or bite disturbances. The history and physical examination are critical in identifying acromegaly. In addition to the characteristic dysmorphisms discussed previously, common complaints include noticeable change in ring size, shoe size, and height depending on age of onset. The most common visual finding in patients with acromegaly is a characteristic visual field deficit consisting of bitemporal hemianopsia, resulting from mass effect on the optic chiasm.[8]

Patients suspected of having acromegaly secondary to a pituitary tumor require a multidisciplinary approach to diagnosis and treatment (**Fig. 1**). The first step toward making a diagnosis is to confirm the elevation of GH and IGF-1. Because of significant variation in GH levels throughout the day, random GH levels are not recommended for the diagnosis of acromegaly, and IGF-1 is favored for baseline diagnosis and subsequent monitoring. If IGF-1 levels are equivocal or elevated, patients typically undergo an oral glucose tolerance test. Lack of GH suppression to less than 1 μg/L after documented hyperglycemia induced by an oral glucose load is confirmatory of the disease.[9] As with any patient with a pituitary tumor, patients with acromegaly require a complete endocrine panel to assess the functioning of the anterior and posterior gland. Up to 25% of GH-secreting adenomas have a mixed-cell population with a

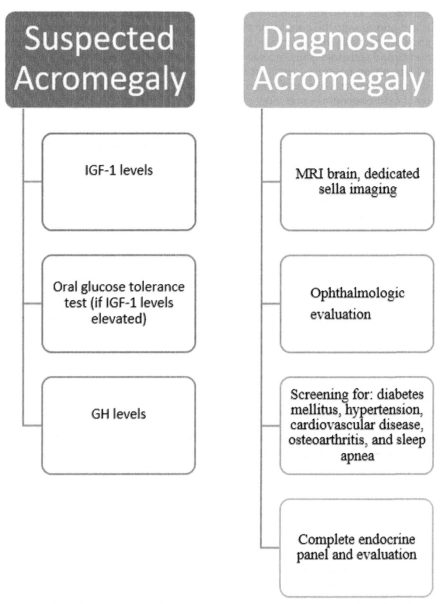

**Fig. 1.** Work-up for suspected and diagnosed acromegaly. Representative algorithms for the work-up of acromegaly, including laboratory testing, examination, and imaging.

proportion of cells causing hyperprolactinemia (ie, somatomammotroph tumors).[6] Elevations in prolactin may also be seen with macroadenomas because of compression of the pituitary infundibulum with resultant decrease in the negative feedback of prolactin, resulting in a "stalk-effect" elevation.[7]

Given that most cases of acromegaly arise from a pituitary adenoma, imaging of the brain is paramount in the diagnosis of the disease. Most pituitary adenomas in acromegaly are macroadenomas (ie, tumors with a maximum diameter >1 cm);

therefore MRI of the brain with and without contrast is often sufficient to diagnose the tumors and assess their anatomic relationships with important surrounding neurovascular structures including the cavernous sinuses, internal carotid arteries, optic chiasm, and sphenoid sinus. However, dedicated MRI "pituitary protocol" with early and late phase contrast-enhanced imaging of the sella is recommended in cases where the diagnosis of acromegaly is strongly suspected. This allows for identification of macroadenomas and most microadenomas (tumors with a maximum diameter <1 cm). Dynamic imaging of the sella is performed by injecting intravenous gadolinium and obtaining coronal cuts through the pituitary at variable time intervals to assess the distribution of contrast medium in the hypophyseal tissue. The normal gland enhances early, whereas adenomas tend to be observed as hypointense lesions in the first sequences, only to enhance in a delayed fashion in comparison with the surrounding normal parenchyma. This technique further allows for identification of the normal gland relative to the tumor, which is critical during surgical planning and performance.[10] Additional imaging may be obtained for surgical planning only as needed, including high-resolution imaging for stereotaxis. Maxillofacial computed tomography scans are helpful for the transsphenoidal approach to better identify the bony anatomy. Vascular imaging is only obtained for very large tumors with encasement or severe displacement of vessels, which may be encountered during surgery.

A complete ophthalmologic evaluation is necessary in all patients including formal visual field testing in cases where the optic apparatus is compressed by the adjacent tumor. Patients with acromegaly should also be screened for commonly associated comorbidities including diabetes mellitus, hypertension, cardiovascular disease, osteoarthritis, and sleep apnea. If any of these conditions is present, it should be treated rigorously and followed longitudinally.[9]

## DISCUSSION: THERAPEUTIC OPTIONS

The primary mode of treatment of patients with acromegaly secondary to a pituitary adenoma is surgery (**Fig. 2**). In most cases, the recommended approach is endoscopic endonasal, which should be performed at a high-volume center by surgeons with experience treating these cases. Some tumors require a combined approach with a craniotomy, although an initial attempted endonasal resection is often favored. A maximal safe resection is recommended in all cases. Current guidelines advise against the use of preoperative medical treatment to achieve biochemical response after surgery. The exception is made in cases of severe sleep apnea with thick pharyngeal tissues or high-output cardiac failure, in which somatostatin receptor ligands are recommended preoperatively to reduce surgical risk from associated comorbidities.[9] Once surgery is performed, a random level of GH is measured on the first postoperative day (**Fig. 3**). A GH of less than 1 μg/L has been associated with statistically decreased observed to expected mortality ratio, and that reduction of GH to less than 1 μg/L or normalization of serum IGF-1 levels reduces mortality associated with acromegaly.[11] Starke and colleagues[12] found the best predictor of remission after surgical resection was in-hospital GH level of less than 1.15 ng/mL. Therefore, the target serum GH should be less than 1 ng/mL. If the level is greater than 1 μg/L, then a second level should be measured after a glucose load. IGF-1 levels are slower to normalize and are therefore measured 12 weeks after surgery, and under the direction of an endocrinologist. Levels may continue to decrease during this period, and persistent elevation within the first 3 months is not indicative of treatment failure. In cases in which biochemical remission is achieved and there is no evidence of residual

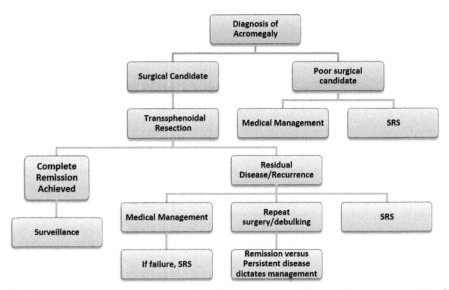

**Fig. 2.** Management of acromegaly. Algorithmic representation of the management of acromegaly, with surgery as a first-line treatment. SRS, stereotactic radiosurgery.

tumor on MRI, no additional medical management is recommended. Patients with residual disease (biochemical or anatomic) require additional treatment.[13] If there is residual tumor that is surgically resectable, repeat surgery should be the first line of

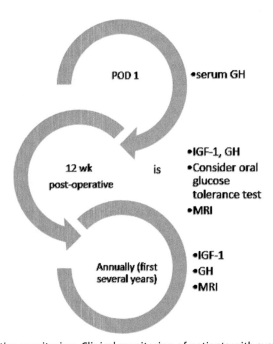

**Fig. 3.** Postoperative monitoring. Clinical monitoring of patients with suspected gross total resection on initial postoperative MRI. POD, postoperative day.

treatment. If the tumor is not resectable or the patient is not an operative candidate for other medical reasons, medical management should be considered.

## INDICATIONS FOR SURGERY

Patients with GH-secreting pituitary adenomas are recommended to undergo surgical resection if medically able. The primary goal of surgery for somatotrophinomas is to decrease IGF-1 levels to a normal range controlled for the patient's gender and age, in addition to achieving relief of mass effect in cases of macroadenoma. Normalization of pituitary function, including resolution or improvement in hypopituitarism, can often be achieved as a result of surgical resection.[14] Treatment paradigms are aimed to control the myriad of medical complications that result from excessive GH secretion, and effects from tumor mass effect. In 2014, the Endocrine Society Clinical Guidelines Subcommittee published a Clinical Practice Guideline for the treatment of acromegaly.[9] The Endocrine Society commissioned a systematic review that included 35 studies that compared surgical and medical treatment in patients with acromegaly that were treatment-naive and found that surgical resection provided a significantly higher remission rate when compared with medical therapy (67% vs 45%; $P = .02$).[15] Remission rates after surgery were significantly higher at longer follow-up times (>24 months) compared with medical treatment (66% vs 44%; $P = .04$), but not statistically higher at shorter follow-up times (<6 months) (37% vs 26%; $P = .22$). Therefore, surgical resection is recommended as first-line therapy for individuals with acromegaly from pituitary adenoma.

## SURGICAL TECHNIQUES: ENDOSCOPIC VERSUS MICROSURGICAL TRANSSPHENOIDAL SURGERY

The Endocrine Society group recommends transsphenoidal surgery as the primary therapy for most patients diagnosed with acromegaly.[9] Multiple single institutional studies have assessed endoscopic versus microsurgical transsphenoidal surgery for the resection of somatotrophinomas. Starke and colleagues[12] did not find a statistical difference between the endoscopic and microsurgical transsphenoidal surgery approaches in achieving remission, but did report that remission was associated with lower preoperative GH levels (<45 ng/mL) and Knosp score of 0 to 2. Chen and coworkers[16] published a comprehensive literature review with findings that both approaches produced similar rates of remission. The overall long-term remission rates were 69.2% versus 70.2% for the microsurgical versus endoscopic groups, respectively. Phan and colleagues[17] found patients with noninvasive macroadenomas were significantly more likely to achieve remission with an endoscopic resection. Fathalla and colleagues[18] found no significant difference in remission rates, but found a significantly higher rate of gross total resection in the endoscopic group. In cases of cavernous sinus involvement, there was a higher rate of gross total resection that did not reach significance in the endoscopic versus microsurgical group. Juthani and colleagues[19] found that adjuvant use of the intraoperative MRI significantly increased the rate of gross total resection for endoscopic and microscopic approaches. This study found a significantly higher rate of remission in tumors resected endoscopically versus microscopically, and progression-free survival was significantly correlated with the extent of resection on postoperative MRI.

The endoscopic approach has largely supplanted the use of microscopic technique because of improvements in visualization that are widely accepted to achieve superior results for resection of pituitary macroadenomas and secretory adenomas, particularly in cases of extrasellar tumor involvement. Advances in endoscopic technique and robust cerebrospinal fluid leak repair using vascularized nasoseptal flaps have

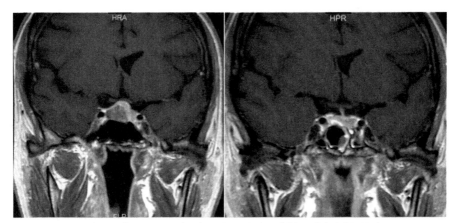

**Fig. 4.** Preoperative and postoperative imaging. Coronal T1-weighted MRI shows representative GH-secreting adenoma preoperatively (*left*) with mass effect on optic chiasm and displacement of the enhancing pituitary gland to the left, and postoperatively (*right*) following endoscopic transsphenoidal approach resulting in gross total resection and resolution of mass effect.

allowed for more aggressive resection, even in cases of cavernous sinus involvement. **Fig. 4** demonstrates a typical GH-staining pituitary adenoma resected via an endoscopic transsphenoidal approach, with resultant gross total resection.

Differences in remission rates are most pronounced in macroadenomas. Remission rates are affected by preoperative hormone levels, tumor size, and extent. In a study evaluating remission rates based on size, Chen and coworkers[16] reported long-term remission rates in microadenomas of 76.9% versus 73.5% and in macroadenomas rates of 40.2% versus 61.5%, when comparing microsurgical and endoscopic approaches, respectively. Statistical comparison analysis was unable to be performed because of limitations in the literature. However, a potential benefit of endoscopic resection for pituitary macroadenomas has been noted. For macroadenomas, the advantage is likely caused by increased field of view with the panoramic scope, improved lighting, and direct visualization of the tumor.[20] Complications that could arise from surgical resection include cerebrospinal fluid leak, meningitis, diabetes insipidus, panhypopituitarism, and rarely injury to the internal carotid artery and visual field deficit not present preoperatively.[21]

### *Other Considerations: Subtotal Resection/Debulking*

For individuals who have extensive parasellar disease and Knosp grade 3+ cavernous sinus involvement precluding gross total resection, debulking surgery as an initial treatment option is still recommended to improve response to medical therapy.[9] Surgical debulking without gross total resection is associated with increased response to somatostatin analogues (SSA) postoperatively and decrease in GH levels and tumor size.[22,23] In these cases, reduction in medication doses and decreased dependency on polypharmacy is the primary goal. After debulking surgery is performed, individuals are initiated on systemic medications as outlined previously. IGF-1 and GH levels are monitored for response to therapy. If a lack of response occurs, or the individual is unable to tolerate medications because of side effect profile, stereotactic radiosurgery (SRS) is considered.

## THERAPEUTIC OPTIONS: MEDICAL THERAPY

Medical treatment is recommended alone or in combination with further therapy in cases of persistent GH secretion refractory to surgical therapy.[9,13] There are three classes of medications used for the treatment of patients with acromegaly with persistent disease after surgical resection. The first class, SSAs include octreotide and lanreotide. Pasireotide, a second-generation SSA, has higher affinity for subtypes 1 to 3 and 5 of the somatostatin receptor. Dopamine agonists, such as cabergoline, also decrease GH production in addition to having an inhibitory effect on prolactin release, making them useful in patients with somatomammotroph tumors. Pegvisomant is a newer pharmacologic agent that acts by antagonizing the GH receptor in peripheral tissues.[24] Newer medications and new formulations of existing drugs are currently being developed or tested in an effort to improve adherence to treatment and biochemical control of the disease.[25]

SSAs mimic the inhibitory effects of somatostatin on the anterior pituitary. Octreotide was the first SSA to be introduced, but because of its short half-life of approximately 2 hours, longer acting compounds were developed. These include octreotide long-acting release and lanreotide. The second-generation SSA, pasireotide showed better biochemical control in a randomized clinical trial compared with octreotide; however, the reported biochemical efficacy of all SSAs varies greatly across the literature. Common side effects of SSAs include gastrointestinal symptoms, such as nausea, diarrhea, and abdominal pain, with potential to cause biliary sludge and cholelithiasis. Most importantly, SSAs can impair insulin secretion, which is particularly concerning in this patient population because of their heightened risk for developing diabetes mellitus.

Dopamine agonists, such as bromocriptine, and the more selective drug cabergoline, may be used in patients with tumors that cosecrete prolactin. Current guidelines suggest the use of cabergoline in cases with only modest elevations of IGF-1. Dopamine agonists are used in conjunction with SSAs, but are inferior to SSAs when used alone for the biochemical management of disease. Common side effects include constipation, nausea, and postural hypotension. Pegvisomant, a genetically engineered human GH analogue, competes with physiologic GH for binding to the somatostatin receptor. Because of its potential to cause transaminitis, liver function tests must be performed regularly during treatment.[26] SSAs or pegvisomant are recommended in cases with significant biochemical disease. The overall goal of treatment is to achieve an age-normalized IGF-1 level or a random GH level less than 1.0 µg/L.[9] The cost of these agents can become prohibitively high in patients with refractory GH secretion, emphasizing the importance of surgical resection in disease control.[27]

## THERAPEUTIC OPTIONS: RADIOSURGERY

For individuals who have undergone surgical resection with persistent residual tumor that is not easily accessible, most often because of cavernous sinus invasion, and have failed medical therapy, radiosurgery is used for tumor control. Ability to successfully perform radiosurgery depends on extent of disease involvement and proximity to the optic chiasm, which is dose limiting. The Endocrine Society commissioned a systematic review of 31 studies to compare conventional fractioned radiation therapy with SRS and found that SRS was associated with a higher remission rate and lower rate of endocrinologic complications, although the data lacked statistical significance.[28] A recent large international multicenter retrospective cohort study looking at SRS for persistent or recurrent acromegaly after surgical resection found a durable endocrine remission at 10 years in 59% of individuals who received SRS.[29] The only independent predictor of durable remission was the discontinuation of IGF-1-lowering mediations before SRS. Relapse after post-SRS remission occurred in 9% of cases with mean time to recurrence of 17 months. After radiosurgery, annual GH/IGF-1 levels should be checked following medical withdrawal, and complete hormone panel to screen for hypopituitarism as a delayed side effect of radiation therapy. The rate of endocrine remission and endocrine control increased between the 5-year and 10-year post-SRS analysis.[30] The 10-year estimated endocrine control rate was 56.9%, and the estimated 10-year radiographic local control rate was 92.8%. The rates of visual field deficit and hypopituitarism after SRS were estimated at 2.7% and 26.8% after SRS in a systemic review and meta-analysis.

## SUMMARY

Acromegaly is a challenging and often devastating disease with impact on nearly all organ systems. Aggressive management with early surgical resection and prompt treatment is critical for controlling the manifestations of this disease. Gross total resection and hormone remission is the primary goal of surgery; however, there is significant benefit from debulking surgery even in cases of tumors that are not amenable to gross total resection. The use of medical therapies and radiosurgery is recommended for surgically refractive disease. Long-term, multidisciplinary follow-up is critical to management.

## CLINICS CARE POINTS

- The primary treatment of acromegaly from pituitary somatotrophinoma is transsphenoidal resection.
- A postoperative GH level of less than 1.0 ng/mL is a predictor of remission and decreased mortality.
- Surgical debulking is recommended when gross total resection is not possible because of parasellar spread and invasion into the cavernous sinus.
- Systemic medication and stereotactic radiosurgery are used for recurrent or persistent disease after resection.

## DISCLOSURE

The authors have nothing to disclose.

## REFERENCES

1. Crisafulli S, Luxi N, Sultana J, et al. Global epidemiology of acromegaly: a systematic review and meta-analysis. Eur J Endocrinol 2021;185(2):251–63.
2. Broder MS, Chang E, Cherepanov D, et al. Incidence and prevalence of acromegaly in the United States: a claims-based analysis. Endocr Pract 2016; 22(11):1327–35.
3. Colao A, Grasso LFS, Giustina A, et al. Acromegaly. Nat Rev Dis Primers 2019; 5(1):20.
4. Esposito D, Ragnarsson O, Granfeldt D, et al. Decreasing mortality and changes in treatment patterns in patients with acromegaly from a nationwide study. Eur J Endocrinol 2018;178(5):459–69.

5. Whittington MD, Munoz KA, Whalen JD, et al. Economic and clinical burden of comorbidities among patients with acromegaly. Growth Horm IGF Res 2021;59: 101389.
6. Melmed S. Medical progress: acromegaly. N Engl J Med 2006;355(24):2558–73.
7. Ioachimescu AG. Acromegaly: achieving timely diagnosis and improving outcomes by personalized care. Curr Opin Endocrinol Diabetes Obes 2021;28(4): 419–26.
8. Chanson P, Salenave S. Acromegaly. Orphanet J Rare Dis 2008;3:17.
9. Katznelson L, Laws ER Jr, Melmed S, et al. Acromegaly: an endocrine society clinical practice guideline. J Clin Endocrinol Metab 2014;99(11):3933–51.
10. Marro B, Zouaoui A, Sahel M, et al. MRI of pituitary adenomas in acromegaly. Neuroradiology 1997;39(6):394–9.
11. Holdaway IM, Rajasoorya RC, Gamble GD. Factors influencing mortality in acromegaly. J Clin Endocrinol Metab 2004;89(2):667–74.
12. Starke RM, Raper DM, Payne SC, et al. Endoscopic vs microsurgical transsphenoidal surgery for acromegaly: outcomes in a concurrent series of patients using modern criteria for remission. J Clin Endocrinol Metab 2013;98(8):3190–8.
13. Katznelson L. Approach to the patient with persistent acromegaly after pituitary surgery. J Clin Endocrinol Metab 2010;95(9):4114–23.
14. Ribeiro-Oliveira A Jr, Barkan A. The changing face of acromegaly: advances in diagnosis and treatment. Nat Rev Endocrinol 2012;8(10):605–11.
15. Abu Dabrh AM, Mohammed K, Asi N, et al. Surgical interventions and medical treatments in treatment-naïve patients with acromegaly: systematic review and meta-analysis. J Clin Endocrinol Metab 2014;99(11):4003–14.
16. Chen CJ, Ironside N, Pomeraniec IJ, et al. Microsurgical versus endoscopic transsphenoidal resection for acromegaly: a systematic review of outcomes and complications. Acta Neurochir (Wien) 2017;159(11):2193–207.
17. Phan K, Xu J, Reddy R, et al. Endoscopic Endonasal versus microsurgical transsphenoidal approach for growth hormone-secreting pituitary adenomas-systematic review and meta-analysis. World Neurosurg 2017;97:398–406.
18. Fathalla H, Cusimano MD, Di Ieva A, et al. Endoscopic versus microscopic approach for surgical treatment of acromegaly. Neurosurg Rev 2015;38(3): 541–8 [discussion: 548-549].
19. Juthani RG, Reiner AS, Patel AR, et al. Radiographic and clinical outcomes using intraoperative magnetic resonance imaging for transsphenoidal resection of pituitary adenomas. J Neurosurg 2020;134(6):1824–35.
20. Dallapiazza RF, Jane JA Jr. Outcomes of endoscopic transsphenoidal pituitary surgery. Endocrinol Metab Clin North Am 2015;44(1):105–15.
21. Jane JA Jr, Starke RM, Elzoghby MA, et al. Endoscopic transsphenoidal surgery for acromegaly: remission using modern criteria, complications, and predictors of outcome. J Clin Endocrinol Metab 2011;96(9):2732–40.
22. Karavitaki N, Turner HE, Adams CB, et al. Surgical debulking of pituitary macroadenomas causing acromegaly improves control by lanreotide. Clin Endocrinol (Oxf) 2008;68(6):970–5.
23. Petrossians P, Borges-Martins L, Espinoza C, et al. Gross total resection or debulking of pituitary adenomas improves hormonal control of acromegaly by somatostatin analogs. Eur J Endocrinol 2005;152(1):61–6.
24. Ezzat S, Caspar-Bell GM, Chik CL, et al. Predictive markers for postsurgical medical management of acromegaly: a systematic review and consensus treatment guideline. Endocr Pract 2019;25(4):379–93.

25. Antunes X, Kasuki L, Gadelha MR. New and emerging pharmacological treatment options for acromegaly. Expert Opin Pharmacother 2021;1–9.
26. Manjila S, Wu OC, Khan FR, et al. Pharmacological management of acromegaly: a current perspective. Neurosurg Focus 2010;29(4):E14.
27. Leonart LP, Borba HHL, Ferreira VL, et al. Cost-effectiveness of acromegaly treatments: a systematic review. Pituitary 2018;21(6):642–52.
28. Abu Dabrh AM, Asi N, Farah WH, et al. Radiotherapy versus radiosurgery in treating patients with acromegaly: a systematic review and meta-analysis. Endocr Pract 2015;21(8):943–56.
29. Ding D, Mehta GU, Patibandla MR, et al. Stereotactic radiosurgery for acromegaly: an international multicenter retrospective cohort study. Neurosurgery 2019;84(3):717–25.
30. Singh R, Didwania P, Lehrer EJ, et al. Stereotactic radiosurgery for acromegaly: an international systematic review and meta-analysis of clinical outcomes. J Neurooncol 2020;148(3):401–18.

# Nonfunctioning Pituitary Lesions

Benjamin P. Brownlee, MD[a], Daljit Mann, MD[a], Chad Glenn, MD[b,1],
Kibwei A. McKinney, MD[a],*

## KEYWORDS

- Nonfunctioning pituitary adenoma • Silent pituitary adenoma
- Silent lactotroph adenoma • Silent corticotroph adenoma
- Silent gonadotroph adenoma • Silent thyrotroph adenoma
- Silent somatotroph adenoma • Null-cell adenoma

## KEY POINTS

- This article provides an in-depth review of the salient clinical and pathologic features of nonfunctioning pituitary adenomas.
- The article discusses the spectrum of features of nonfunctioning adenomas, based on their clinical, biochemical, hormonal, and molecular patterns of expression.
- The various subtypes of nonfunctioning adenomas are reviewed, thus providing a differential diagnosis according to their histopathologic features, including factors related to their overall prognosis.
- The diagnostic evaluation and management options for nonfunctioning adenomas are detailed, including the indications for expectant management, medical therapy, and surgical intervention.

## INTRODUCTION

Pituitary adenomas are a common pathology seen by neurosurgeons and otolaryngologists. The overall prevalence of pituitary adenoma in the general population ranges from 1 in 865 to 1 in 2688 adults. Of these tumors, between 15% and 54% are nonfunctioning pituitary adenomas (NFPAs).[1] Most NFPAs are macroadenomas, defined as an adenoma greater than 10 mm in diameter. Because of their size, they typically present with mass effect, manifested by clinical symptoms including headache, hypopituitarism, cranial nerve deficits, and visual field defects, rather than pituitary hypersecretion. Silent pituitary adenoma (SPA) is a rare subset of NFPA defined as pituitary neuroendocrine tumors that express transcription factors (TFs) for

[a] Department of Otolaryngology – Head and Neck Surgery, University of Oklahoma Health Sciences Center, 800 Stanton L. Young Boulevard, Suite 1400, Oklahoma City, OK 73104, USA;
[b] Department of Neurological Surgery, University of Oklahoma Health Sciences Center, Oklahoma City, OK, USA
[1] Present address: 6468 Valley Ridge Drive, Edmond, OK 73034.
* Corresponding author.
*E-mail address:* kibwei-mckinney@ouhsc.edu

Otolaryngol Clin N Am 55 (2022) 343–350
https://doi.org/10.1016/j.otc.2021.12.015
0030-6665/22/© 2022 Elsevier Inc. All rights reserved.

hormone synthesis, but do not present with signs or symptoms of hormone hyperse-cretion. Each type of active adenoma may also have a silent equivalent. These nonfunctioning lesions tend to be more aggressive than their hypersecreting counter-parts and have a higher rate of recurrence.[2–4]

SPA represents a clinical spectrum (totally silent, clinically silent, and whispering) that can change during the course of disease (**Table 1**).[2] On either side of this spec-trum lies null-cell adenoma, which is clinically and biochemically silent, and func-tioning adenoma, which, as the name suggests, is a clinically significant pituitary adenoma hypersecreting hormones and is no longer considered to be an SPA.

Pathologically, SPA is divided into seven distinct subtypes according to the 2017 World Health Organization classification of pituitary adenomas: silent lactotroph, silent somatotroph, silent thyrotroph, silent corticotroph, silent gonadotroph, PIT1-positive plurihormonal adenoma, and null-cell.[2,3] Each of these seven subtypes is unique in its biochemical profile and its pattern of staining on immunohistochemistry (IHC), as shown in **Table 2**. In the following sections, the unique characteristics of each type are discussed.

## SILENT LACTOTROPH

Silent lactotrophs are differentiated from other subtypes by their positive staining for prolactin. However, it is exceedingly rare for a silent lactotroph to present clinically. A large retrospective cohort study from the United Kingdom revealed a prevalence of silent lactotrophs in surgical patients of only 0.6%,[5] whereas other studies have suggested that the prevalence is somewhat higher, at around 1.65%.[2] This subtype stains positive for prolactin 1 on IHC and expresses the TFs PIT1 and estrogen recep-tor-$\alpha$ (ER$\alpha$).[2] Despite its rare clinical presentation, approximately one-half of inciden-tally discovered pituitary masses stain positive for prolactin on autopsy.[6]

## SILENT SOMATOTROPH

A silent somatotroph is a growth hormone (GH)-secreting tumor that does not present with signs or symptoms of acromegaly. It is uncommon, representing approximately 2% to 4% of all pituitary adenomas.[7] This subtype is classified into two separate groups: densely granulated somatotroph adenoma and sparsely granulated somato-troph adenoma. This classification schema, which is also used for secreting somato-troph adenomas, is further subdivided by three characteristics: GH expression, the presence of $\alpha$-subunit, and positive staining for low-molecular-weight keratin. Silent somatotrophs are more frequently sparsely granulated somatotroph adenoma, with weak GH expression, no $\alpha$-subunit expression, and low-molecular-weight keratin stains in a predominantly juxtanuclear globular pattern.[8] This contrasts with densely

| Table 1 Spectrum of silent pituitary adenoma | | | | |
|---|---|---|---|---|
| | Clinical | Biochemical | Hormone (IHC) | Transcription Factor |
| Null-cell | Silent | Silent | Negative | Negative |
| Totally silent | Silent | Silent | Positive | Positive |
| Clinically silent | Silent | Mild | Positive | Positive |
| Whispering | Borderline | Positive | Positive | Positive |
| Functioning | Positive | Positive | Positive | Positive |

*Abbreviation:* IHC, immunohistochemistry.

| Table 2 | | |
| --- | --- | --- |
| Silent pituitary adenomas and identification markers | | |
| SPA Subtype | Transcription Factor | IHC: Hormone |
| Null cell | None | Silent |
| Lactotroph | PIT-1, Erα | Prolactin |
| Somatotroph | PIT-1 | GH |
| Thyrotroph | PIT-1, GATA-2 | TSHβ |
| Corticotroph | TPIT | ACTH |
| Gonadotroph | SF-1, Erα | LH:FSH <1 |
| Plurihormonal | PIT-1 | GH, PRL, TSHβ |

*Abbreviations:* ACTH, adrenocorticotropic hormone; ERα, estrogen receptor-α; FSH, follicle-stimulating hormone; GH, growth hormone; LH, luteinizing hormone; PRL, prolactin; SF-1, steroidogenic factor-1; TPIT, T-box transcription factor; TSH, thyroid-stimulating hormone.

granulated somatotroph adenoma, which has strong GH expression with an α-subunit, in addition to a perinuclear pattern of staining.

These tumors typically present in young females during the work-up of headaches that are refractory to routine medical management. This subtype of nonfunctioning tumors carries the TF PIT1, similarly to silent lactotrophs, but IHC differentiates between these diagnoses based on positive staining for GH. Typically, patients have normal insulin growth factor 1 and GH levels; however, up to one-third of patients may have elevated GH levels that eventually progress to acromegaly.[1,7] Additionally, when compared with their hypersecreting counterpart, they tend to occur at a younger age, with a more invasive clinical course and a higher propensity toward tumor recurrence.[9] A link between silent somatotroph and familial isolated pituitary adenoma, an autosomal-dominant disease with incomplete penetrance, has been made because of a mutation in the tumor suppressor gene *aryl hydrocarbon receptor-interacting protein*.[10]

## SILENT THYROTROPH

Silent thyrotroph adenomas represent another rare type of SPA, with an overall prevalence of about 3.5%.[11] These tumors express thyroid hormone and are differentiated from thyroid-stimulating hormone (TSH)-secreting pituitary adenomas by the absence of hyperthyroidism. There is no evidence to date that the silent and active forms have different natural progressions.[11] Patients most commonly present with headache and visual disturbance caused by extrasellar extension, which is seen in more than half of cases.[2]

Like silent lactotroph and silent somatotroph, silent thyrotrophs show nuclear expression of PIT1. In contrast to the other types, these tumors also express GATA-binding protein-2. On IHC, these tumors typically show variable TSHβ and α-subunit expression, ranging from 1% to 90%.[2] There is evidence to suggest that there is a direct correlation between TSHβ expression and clinical hyperthyroidism, with higher expression being associated with clinical hyperthyroidism.[11] Like their active counterpart, silent thyrotroph tumors express somatostatin receptor 2 (SSTR2) and somatostatin receptor 5 (SSTR5), and there are early indications that they may also respond well to somatostatin analogues, such as octreotide.[12]

## SILENT CORTICOTROPH

Silent corticotroph adenoma (SCA) can be totally silent with absent clinical features of Cushing syndrome and normal cortisol levels or clinically silent with absent clinical features but elevated adrenocorticotropic hormone (ACTH) levels. SCAs comprise 3% to 6% of all pituitary adenomas and account for 40% of all corticotroph cell-line tumors.[2] SCAs usually present as macroadenomas with mass-related symptoms, are more common in younger age, and have a predilection for females. When compared with silent gonadotroph adenomas (SGAs), SCAs behave more aggressively and involve the cavernous sinus more frequently.[13]

Diagnostically, a heterogeneous appearance on MRI comprised of cystic and hemorrhagic components suggests SCA. The presence of multiple microcysts in a clinically silent pituitary macroadenoma has a sensitivity of 76% and a specificity of 95% for predicting an SCA.[14] SCAs are divided into two subtypes on histopathology. Type 1 SCA has densely granulated, strong ACTH immunoreactivity and is indistinguishable from a functional adenoma. In contrast, type 2 SCA is sparsely granulated with weak and focal ACTH immunoreactivity. IHC staining for T-box transcription factor has been shown to be a reliable marker for corticotroph cell lineage.[15] SCAs have increased rate of tumor recurrence when compared with SGAs (36% vs 10%), and retrospective studies have demonstrated that tumors with fewer cystic compartments and greater preoperative ACTH levels are risk factors for recurrence.[16]

## SILENT GONADOTROPH

SGAs are the most common form of SPA tumor, comprising up to 73% of all SPAs.[13] Functioning gonadotroph adenomas and SGAs preferentially secrete follicle-stimulating hormone (FSH), and usually have a luteinizing hormone/FSH ratio less than 1.[17] These hormonal levels are helpful for preoperative identification of the tumor and postoperative monitoring. IHC staining for the TF steroidogenic factor-1 in gonadotroph adenomas is helpful in classifying hormone-negative tumors and is exclusive to SGAs. Other TFs identified with SGA include DAX1 and ERα, although ERα is also expressed by lactotroph tumors. Some SGAs show expression of dopamine receptor type 2 and somatostatin receptor with evidence of tumor shrinkage with the use of dopamine agonists[18] and tumor stabilization following the initiation of somatostatin analogues.[19]

## PIT1-POSITIVE PLURIHORMONAL ADENOMA

PIT1-positive plurihormonal adenoma, which was previously named silent adenoma type III, is an uncommon monomorphous (single cell origin) tumor with a prevalence of 0.9%, which uniformly expresses PIT1 and more than one adenohypophyseal hormone from the PIT1 lineage.[1,20] These tumors are known to be clinically and biologically aggressive, often present at a much younger age than other SPA, and may actually present with clinical symptoms, such as hyperthyroidism, amenorrhea, or acromegaly. Furthermore, there is reported association between PIT1-positive plurihormonal adenoma and multiple endocrine neoplasia type 1 syndrome.[2] In addition to the expression of PIT1, the histopathologic hallmark is nuclear inclusions, known as nuclear spheridia, which may also be seen on hematoxylin-eosin stain, and focal or scattered positivity to GH, prolactin, and TSHβ.[20] Despite being aggressive, they are sensitive to radiation.

## NULL-CELL ADENOMA

Null-cell adenoma is a diagnosis of exclusion that requires immunonegativity for all adenohypophyseal hormones and a lack of cell-specific TFs. When SPA are appropriately tested for TFs and pituitary hormones, the prevalence of null-cell adenoma decreases to approximately 1% of all NFPAs.[13] Null-cell adenomas generally have unfavorable outcomes when compared with other SPAs because of a higher risk of early recurrence and cavernous sinus invasion. When compared specifically with SGAs, null-cell adenomas tend to be larger macroadenomas with more extensive cavernous sinus invasion. Decreased p27 expression on IHC is a negative prognostic indicator and is associated with shorter tumor volume doubling times and accelerated growth of residual tumor postoperatively.[21]

## CLINICAL EVALUATION

Patients with NFPAs typically present with an incidentally found sellar mass on imaging, or more commonly, symptoms related to mass effect from a macroadenoma. Presenting symptoms may include headache, vision changes from compression of the optic chiasm, and hypopituitarism.

The appropriate work-up of a patient with a newly found macroadenoma includes endocrinologic assessment of hormone secretion to identify hypersecreting or nonfunctioning tumors. Preoperative levels of luteinizing hormone, FSH, TSH/free T4, GH/insulin growth factor 1, prolactin, and ACTH should be assessed. In SPAs, there is an absence of preoperative clinical signs of hypersecretion, typically with normal laboratory values. Only SCAs are detected preoperatively, with an increase in ACTH levels in the presence of normal morning cortisol levels. It may also be identified with normal corticotroph levels while all other pituitary hormones are deficient. If adrenal insufficiency or central hypothyroidism is identified, it is recommended to begin glucocorticoid or thyroid hormone supplementation. If identified, treatment of preoperative hypogonadism or GH deficiency is not recommended. Preoperative detection of hormone deficiency also allows for the opportunity to monitor hormone status, which helps to guide therapeutic decision-making. Hyperprolactinemia may be seen with NFPAs because of pituitary stalk compression. It is imperative to accurately make the diagnosis because the management of prolactinomas differs from NFPAs. Patients with NFPA were usually found to have prolactin levels less than 100 ng/mL, whereas a prolactin level greater than 250 ng/mL was seen only in patients with prolactinomas.[22]

A thorough clinical examination includes the evaluation of all cranial nerves and is not complete without an ophthalmologic evaluation, particularly if the patient has any preoperative visual complaints. Preoperative ophthalmology consultation is also necessary if tumor abuts the optic nerve, to establish a baseline examination.

The gold standard for radiologic evaluation of a pituitary mass is MRI with and without gadolinium contrast. On postcontrast T1-weighted images, NFPAs typically appear hypointense relative to the native pituitary gland, secondary to delayed enhancement. MRI evaluation allows for surgical planning with identification of the relationship of the tumor to nearby structures, including the optic nerves, internal carotid arteries, and cavernous sinuses. A preoperative, noncontrast computed tomography scan with thin cross-sections through the sinuses and skull base allows for superior identification of sinonasal bony landmarks and are used for intraoperative navigation in conjunction with MRI.

## NONOPERATIVE MANAGEMENT

Surgery is generally recommended as first-line treatment of NFPAs. However, active surveillance, medical therapies, or radiation therapy may be indicated for some patients. For asymptomatic microadenomas that are incidentally found, active surveillance of endocrine function and repeat MRI at intervals of 6 to 12 months may be considered on an individualized basis. If there is evidence of rapid tumor growth or development of new symptoms during the surveillance period, transsphenoidal pituitary surgery is recommended. Initial treatment with radiation therapy is typically only considered for patients with significant comorbidities, deeming them poor surgical candidates. Some SPAs, including SGA and silent thyrotroph adenomas, have been shown to respond to dopamine agonists and somatostatin analogues. However, these treatments are usually reserved for the treatment of residual tumor postoperatively.

## OPERATIVE MANAGEMENT

Surgical intervention is indicated for symptomatic nonfunctioning pituitary macroadenomas. Absolute indications for surgery include macroadenoma with visual field disturbances or other visual abnormalities with adenoma abutting the optic nerves, or in patients with pituitary apoplexy. Relative indications for surgery include patients with headache or pituitary dysfunction alone, because surgical intervention does not guarantee improvement in these symptoms.[23] The current technique used for the approach to pituitary adenomas is transsphenoidal surgery via an endoscopic or microscopic approach. Gross total resection of tumor may not be possible in cases with extensive cavernous sinus invasion. SCAs and null-cell adenomas are associated with these high-risk features. Postoperative complications include cerebrospinal fluid leak, meningitis, vascular injury, diabetes insipidus, and new visual field deficits.

## POSTOPERATIVE CONSIDERATIONS

Postoperative imaging and endocrine and ophthalmology evaluations should be considered for patients, although there is a lack of evidence for a standardized approach to the timing and frequency of the evaluations. MRI is usually completed 3 to 6 months after surgery to allow for resolution of blood products and packing materials and accurate assessment for residual tumor. The timing for further repeat imaging is decided on an individualized basis depending on residual tumor size or location of residual tumor.

SCA and null-cell adenomas are associated with more aggressive features, such as cavernous sinus invasion, and have a high recurrence rate. In patients with recurrent or residual tumors, postoperative radiation therapy should be considered as adjuvant treatment to stop tumor growth. However, because of concerns of complications of radiotherapy and permanent side effect profile, medical management with dopamine agonists or somatostatin analogues has been investigated with successful results. Temozolomide is a chemotherapeutic oral alkylating agent that has been used in tumors showing aggressive behavior, with progression of disease after surgery and/or irradiation.[24,25]

## SUMMARY

SPAs represent a spectrum of hormone-secreting tumors without the clinical manifestations of their functioning counterparts. Silent tumors can have variable expression of hormone and cell-line-specific TFs that can help make the correct diagnosis. Correct identification of the subtype of SPA has a significant impact on prognosis, clinical course, and management of the tumor.

## CLINICS CARE POINTS

- 15% to 54% of pituitary tumors are nonfunctioning pituitary adenomas (NFPA), a clinical diagnosis based on patient signs and symptoms.

- Because of their indolent clinical course, these lesions often present at advanced stages, only after their size results in clinically evident cranial neuropathies or compressive symptoms.
- Silent pituitary adenomas (SPA) describe a spectrum of disease based on the pathologic characteristics, including the biochemical, hormonal, and molecular patterns of expression of each tumor. Clinical work-up of these tumors includes early assessment of hormone levels to identify the presence or absence of hypersecretion.
- Null-cell adenoma is a diagnosis of exclusion that lacks any expression of biochemical or hormonal markers, representing less than 1% of pituitary adenomas overall.
- The other SPA subtypes are distinguished from one another based on their cell line of origin. The subtype is determined pathologically based on positive immunohistochemistry staining for the hormone produced by the predominant cell line.
- Other transcription factors have been elucidated that may help in differentiating between these tumors and, in some cases, provide prognostic information.
- Silent lactotroph adenomas constitute one-half of incidentally discovered tumors and have an increased expression of transcription factors PIT1 and ERα.
- Silent somatotroph adenomas are subdivided into densely or sparsely granulated tumors. They show weaker growth hormone and no α-subunit expression, and stain poorly for low-molecular-weight keratin.
- Silent thyrotroph adenomas demonstrate positive staining for PIT1 and GATA-binding protein-2, with variable α-subunit expression. Similar to secreting thyrotroph adenomas, these tumors may respond to medical management with somatostatin analogues.
- Silent corticotroph adenomas stain positively for T-box transcription factor and have a more aggressive clinical presentation, including a greater likelihood of cavernous sinus invasion and clinical recurrence following surgical extirpation.
- Silent gonadotroph adenomas express dopamine receptor type 2 (D2R) and somatostatin receptor (SSTR) and may respond to treatment with somatostatin analogues.
- Early neuro-ophthalmologic evaluation should also be considered to identify any subtle, subclinical changes that may provide the indication for surgical intervention.

## DISCLOSURE

The authors have nothing to disclose.

## REFERENCES

1. Molitch ME. Diagnosis and treatment of pituitary adenomas: a review. JAMA 2017;317(5):516–24.
2. Drummond J, Roncaroli F, Grossman AB, et al. Clinical and pathological aspects of silent pituitary adenomas. J Clin Endocrinol Metab 2019;104(7):2473–89.
3. Trouillas J, Jaffrain-Rea ML, Vasiljevic A, et al. How to classify the pituitary neuro-endocrine tumors (PitNET)s in 2020. Cancers (Basel) 2020;12(2):514.
4. Ezzat S, Asa SL, Couldwell WT, et al. The prevalence of pituitary adenomas: a systematic review. Cancer 2004;101(3):613–9.
5. Tampourlou M, Ntali G, Ahmed S, et al. Outcome of nonfunctioning pituitary adenomas that regrow after primary treatment: a study from two large UK centers. J Clin Endocrinol Metab 2017;102(6):1889–97.
6. Mavrakis AN, Tritos NA. Diagnostic and therapeutic approach to pituitary incidentalomas. Endocr Pract 2004;10(5):438–44.
7. Langlois F, Woltjer R, Cetas JS, et al. Silent somatotroph pituitary adenomas: an update. Pituitary 2018;21(2):194–202.

8. Asa SL, Ezzat S. An update on pituitary neuroendocrine tumors leading to acromegaly and gigantism. J Clin Med 2021;10(11):2254.

9. Naritaka H, Kameya T, Sato Y, et al. Morphological characterization and subtyping of silent somatotroph adenomas. Pituitary 1999;1(3–4):233–41.

10. Hernández-Ramírez LC, Gabrovska P, Dénes J, et al, International FIPA Consortium. Landscape of familial isolated and young-onset pituitary adenomas: prospective diagnosis in AIP mutation carriers. J Clin Endocrinol Metab 2015;100(9): E1242–54.

11. Kirkman MA, Jaunmuktane Z, Brandner S, et al. Active and silent thyroid-stimulating hormone-expressing pituitary adenomas: presenting symptoms, treatment, outcomes, and recurrence. World Neurosurg 2014;82(6):1224–31.

12. Kuzu F, Bayraktaroğlu T, Zor F, et al. A thyrotropin-secreting macroadenoma with positive growth hormone and prolactin immunostaining: a case report and literature review. Niger J Clin Pract 2015;18(5):693–7.

13. Nishioka H, Inoshita N, Mete O, et al. The complementary role of transcription factors in the accurate diagnosis of clinically nonfunctioning pituitary adenomas. Endocr Pathol 2015;26(4):349–55.

14. Cazabat L, Dupuy M, Boulin A, et al. Silent, but not unseen: multimicrocystic aspect on T2-weighted MRI in silent corticotroph adenomas. Clin Endocrinol (Oxf) 2014;81(4):566–72.

15. Vallette-Kasic S, Figarella-Branger D, Grino M, et al. Differential regulation of proopiomelanocortin and pituitary-restricted transcription factor (TPIT), a new marker of normal and adenomatous human corticotrophs. J Clin Endocrinol Metab 2003;88(7):3050–6.

16. Langlois F, Lim DST, Varlamov E, et al. Clinical profile of silent growth hormone pituitary adenomas; higher recurrence rate compared to silent gonadotroph pituitary tumors, a large single center experience. Endocrine 2017;58(3):528–34.

17. Hanson PL, Aylwin SJ, Monson JP, et al. FSH secretion predominates in vivo and in vitro in patients with non-functioning pituitary adenomas. Eur J Endocrinol 2005;152(3):363–70.

18. Vieira Neto L, Wildemberg LE, Moraes AB, et al. Dopamine receptor subtype 2 expression profile in nonfunctioning pituitary adenomas and in vivo response to cabergoline therapy. Clin Endocrinol (Oxf) 2015;82(5):739–46.

19. Fusco A, Giampietro A, Bianchi A, et al. Treatment with octreotide LAR in clinically non-functioning pituitary adenoma: results from a case-control study. Pituitary 2012;15(4):571–8.

20. Mete O, Lopes MB. Overview of the 2017 WHO classification of pituitary tumors. Endocr Pathol 2017;28(3):228–43.

21. Balogun JA, Monsalves E, Juraschka K, et al. Null cell adenomas of the pituitary gland: an institutional review of their clinical imaging and behavioral characteristics. Endocr Pathol 2015;26(1):63–70.

22. Hong JW, Lee MK, Kim SH, et al. Discrimination of prolactinoma from hyperprolactinemic non-functioning adenoma. Endocrine 2010;37(1):140–7.

23. Esposito D, Olsson DS, Ragnarsson O, et al. Non-functioning pituitary adenomas: indications for pituitary surgery and post-surgical management. Pituitary 2019; 22(4):422–34.

24. Even-Zohar N, Greenman Y. Management of NFAs: medical treatment. Pituitary 2018;21(2):168–75.

25. Greenman Y, Stern N. Optimal management of non-functioning pituitary adenomas. Endocrine 2015;50(1):51–5.

# Giant Pituitary Adenoma – Special Considerations

Oliver Y. Tang, BS[a], Wayne D. Hsueh, MD[b,c], Jean Anderson Eloy, MD[b,c,d], James K. Liu, MD[b,c,d],*

## KEYWORDS

- Pituitary adenoma • Tumor • Skull base • Transsphenoidal surgery
- Endoscopic endonasal surgery • Neurosurgery • Microsurgery • Tumor outcomes

## KEY POINTS

- Giant pituitary adenomas (GPAs) encompass 5% to 15% of pituitary adenomas and primarily present with mass effect symptoms, such as visual impairment and visual field defects.
- With the possible exception of prolactinomas, first-line treatment is maximal safe resection to relieve parasellar decompression.
- The endoscopic endonasal transsphenoidal (EET) approach has served as the predominant surgical approach for treating GPAs since its development.
- While the EET, microsurgical transsphenoidal, and transcranial approach achieve gross total resection rates greater than 40% and recurrence rates less than 15%, the EET has the lowest perioperative mortality (0.6%) and highest visual improvement rates (82.1%).
- The selection of surgical approaches should be done on a case-by-case basis. Selected cases may benefit from a combined above and below approach.

## INTRODUCTION

Giant pituitary adenomas (GPAs) have posed a formidable challenge in the management of pituitary tumors since their original description by Jefferson in the 1940s, who documented a 35% postoperative mortality in patients with tumors exhibiting significant suprasellar extension.[1] GPAs are estimated to compose 5% to 15% of all pituitary adenomas[1–4] and are most commonly defined in the literature as pituitary adenomas with a maximum diameter in any dimension of greater than 4 cm.[2–5] However, other definitions

---

[a] Department of Neurosurgery, Warren Alpert Medical School of Brown University, 222 Richmond Street, Providence, RI 02903, USA; [b] Department of Otolaryngology–Head and Neck Surgery, Rutgers New Jersey Medical School, 90 Bergen Street Room, Suite 8100, Newark, NJ 07101, USA; [c] Department of Neurological Surgery, Rutgers New Jersey Medical School, 90 Bergen Street Room, Suite 8100, Newark, NJ 07101, USA; [d] Saint Barnabas Medical Center, RWJ Barnabas Health, Livingston, NJ, USA
* Corresponding author.
*E-mail address:* james.liu.md@rutgers.edu
Twitter: @oliverytang (O.Y.T.); @SkullBaseMD (J.K.L.)

Otolaryngol Clin N Am 55 (2022) 351–379
https://doi.org/10.1016/j.otc.2021.12.008
0030-6665/22/© 2022 Elsevier Inc. All rights reserved.

for this clinical entity include a maximum diameter of greater than 3 cm,[6–10] presence of suprasellar extension greater than 2 cm,[11–13] or tumor volume of greater than 10 cm$^3$.[14] Like pituitary adenomas overall, most GPAs are nonfunctioning, and the most common functioning subtype is prolactinoma.[2,8,9,12,15–25] Several case series have demonstrated that GPAs have a slight male predominance and are more common with higher age.[2,3,26–30] Although nearly all GPAs have cytologically benign features on histology,[4,31–34] these lesions invariably necessitate medical management or surgical decompression because of their invasive nature and compression of parasellar neurovascular structures.

Three surgical approaches have primarily been used for GPA resection: the microsurgical transsphenoidal (MT) approach, endoscopic endonasal transsphenoidal (EET) approach, and the transcranial (TC) approach. Recent studies have also used a combined transsphenoidal-TC approach to resect the tumor in an above and below manner. Regardless of modality, surgical outcomes of GPAs are significantly poorer than those of their nongiant counterparts, with lower rates of gross total resection (GTR) and increased treatment morbidity and recurrence rates consistently documented.[5,21,35–45] The goal of this article is to summarize the management of GPAs, including indications, special considerations, and existing evidence for each of the surgical modalities.

## Overview of Giant Pituitary Adenoma

### Clinical presentation

Because most GPAs are nonfunctional, their presenting symptoms are most commonly caused by compression of local structures from multidimensional extension beyond the sella.[46] In accordance with several studies documenting that the most common direction of GPA extension is into the suprasellar region,[6,33,36,47] the predominant presenting symptom for GPA is visual impairment and visual field defects, caused by compression of the optic chiasm and nerves.[2,4,13,14,19,40,48–53] Suprasellar extension into the ventricular system and mass effect may also cause headache or hydrocephalus. Lateral extension into the cavernous sinus and medial temporal lobe may result in epilepsy and cranial nerve palsies, such as ophthalmoplegia.[54] With significant anterior extension into the nasopharynx, GPAs may be mistaken as a sinonasal tumor because of symptoms like nasal obstruction, epistaxis, or rhinorrhea.[55–57] Inferior and infrasellar extension to the occipital condyles may cause craniocervical joint instability.[58] Finally, posterior extension into the posterior fossa may result in signs of brainstem compression.[58]

In the realm of endocrine function, partial hypopituitarism is present in most GPA patients, and panhypopituitarism has been described in 17% to 33% of patients.[2,41] Zhang and colleagues determined that rates of hypopituitarism are higher for GPAs, compared with their large (3–4 cm) counterparts.[59] The most common endocrine symptom is hypogonadism, caused by either mass effect or hyperprolactinemia.[2] For functional tumors with hormonal hypersecretion, patients may present with galactorrhea, amenorrhea, and hypogonadism (prolactinoma), acromegaly (somatotropinoma), or hyperthyroidism (thyrotropinoma).[2]

### Anatomic Classification Systems

Several classification systems are useful in staging the local invasion of GPAs. The modified Wilson-Hardy system classifies tumors based on degree of sellar destruction (grade of I-V based on involvement and destruction of sellar floor) and extrasellar extension (stage of 0 or A-E depending on suprasellar or parasellar invasion).[60] In a series of 118 GPAs, Goel and colleagues proposed a classification system designed to inform surgical approach, probability of GTR, and need for adjuvant radiotherapy: grade I (confinement within the sellar dura and underneath the sellar diaphragm with no evidence of cavernous sinus [CS] invasion), grade II (CS invasion), grade III (elevation of the dura of superior CS), and grade IV (supradiaphragmatic-subarachnoid extension and vascular encasement).[4] The most frequently used classification scheme for modern case series was proposed by Knosp and colleagues, based on the degree of cavernous sinus invasion seen on magnetic resonance imaging (MRI): 0 (within the medial aspect of the supra- and intracavernous internal carotid arteries [ICAs]), 1 (within the cross-sectional centers of the ICAs), 2 (within the lateral aspects of the ICAs), 3 (beyond the lateral aspects of the ICAs), and 4 (total vascular encasement).[61] A 2015 modification divided grade 3 into 3A (superior CS invasion) and 3B (inferior CS invasion), after determining that rates of surgical invasion were significantly higher for 3B.[62]

### Medical management and adjunct treatment

Giant prolactinomas present a notable exception to the rule that surgical management is necessitated for GPAs, because dopamine receptor agonists, such as bromocriptine or cabergoline, serve as the treatment of choice for giant prolactinomas (**Fig. 1**).[23,28,63–68] Several studies have documented that medical management of prolactinoma reduces mass effect and levels of serum hyperprolactinemia in 70% to 98.8% of cases.[23,28,63–65,68] Nevertheless, rare complications of treatment that have been documented because of the rapid decrease of tumor size and warrant attention include cerebral or optic chiasmal herniation, seizures and cerebrospinal fluid (CSF) leakage.[57,69–71] Despite the success of hormonal treatment for prolactinomas, minimal efficacy has been demonstrated for the hormonal treatment of nonfunctional or nonprolactinoma functional adenomas via agents like somatostatin, but medical management may be used as a neoadjuvant or adjuvant treatment for tumor remnant stabilization.[2,72,73]

Radiotherapy for GPAs does not serve as a first-line therapy, but fractionated stereotactic or gamma knife radiosurgery has been established as effective adjuvant treatment for recurrent or residual tumor.[17,18,36,74–78] The most common complication documented after radiotherapy for GPA is hypopituitarism.[2,17,18,74,79] Previously irradiated GPAs undergoing surgical resection have also been shown to have increased difficulty of subsequent surgery and skull base reconstruction, which is a notable consideration for tumors that may require reoperation.[14,52,80,81] In addition, visual loss is a reported complication following radiotherapy for GPA. In summary, the multifaceted treatment approach necessitated for GPAs emphasizes the multidisciplinary approach required for treating these challenging clinical entities.

### Surgical indications, approaches, and complications

Most GPAs require surgical management to relieve mass effect and decompress key neural structures in order to restore visual function and preserve residual pituitary function. In the instance of giant prolactinomas, which may undergo medical therapy as first-line treatment, surgical indications include continued mass effect despite dopamine therapy, dopamine intolerance, or pituitary apoplexy.[2,48] Visual improvement is among the most common aims of GPA surgery, and a 43% to 99% improvement rate has been documented in case series across all surgical modalities.[8–11,13,14,16–21,24,25,34,43,46,53,80,82–86] Although the MT and TC approaches served as the 2 primary approaches for resecting lesions through the 20th century until the adoption of the EET approach in the 1990s,[2] the EET approach has grown to become the first-line approach for most GPAs at many

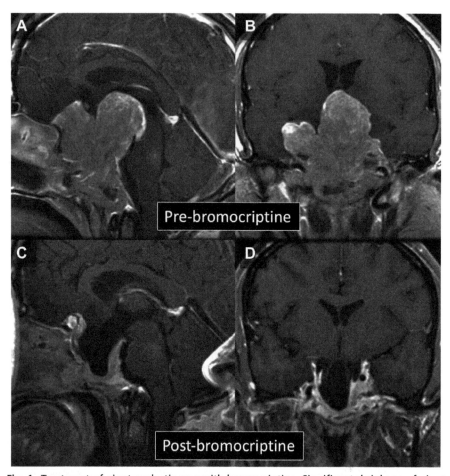

**Fig. 1.** Treatment of giant prolactinoma with bromocriptine. Significant shrinkage of giant invasive prolactinoma after 6 months of treatment with bromocriptine. (*A*) Sagittal and (*B*) coronal MRI before treatment. (*C*) Sagittal and (*D*) coronal MRI after treatment.

institutions,[6,14,19,40,44,45,52,53,84,87–90] including the authors' practice. In the authors' review of all published case series on GPA surgery, although only 94 total GPA patients undergoing EET were in the literature in 2011, the number of EET patients with reported outcomes as of 2021 (n = 1060) greatly outnumbers MT (n = 699) and TC (n = 513) patients (**Fig. 2**).

When considering the extent of maximal safe resection, several factors have been shown to be predictive of extent of resection. Two distinct tumor morphologies have been associated with poorer extent of resection: dumbbell-shaped (suprasellar extension connected to a constricted neck in a hiatus through the sellar diaphragm) and multilobular (lack of wide connections between tumor components) GPAs.[9,17,24,34,38,40,43,53,91] In contrast, round GPAs and the presence of a major cystic component are associated with higher rates of GTR.[38,48,92] Tumors with a fibrous consistency, which are estimated to make up 5% to 7.5% of cases, pose a significant challenge in transsphenoidal removal because of poor descent of the suprasellar tumor component following sellar debulking.[7,13,38,93] Retrosellar extension has been

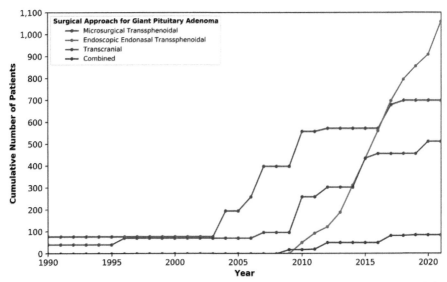

**Fig. 2.** Cumulative patient total for case series on GPA surgery. Cumulative patient totals for all published case series on GPA from 1990-2021, stratified by surgical approach.

consistently documented as a prognosticator of lower extent of resection.[6,9,38,40] Additionally, several case series have validated that CS invasion greatly hinders GTR,[3,9,17,34,43,46,51,52,94] especially in the presence of significant lateral extension because of the need to respect the natural boundary of the cranial nerves in the lateral wall of the CS. For example, Koutourousiou and colleagues reported a 0% GTR rate for Knosp grade 4 GPAs.[17] GPAs that have been previously treated via surgery or radiotherapy have been established as more challenging lesions to resect, because of post-treatment scarring and obliteration of anatomic landmarks.[14,52,80,81] Finally, although tumor maximum diameter is most commonly used to define GPAs, several studies have argued that cubic volume may play a more reliable role than maximum diameter in predicting resectability.[14,38,46,95]

Beyond limited GTR rates, perioperative complications are another notable challenge for GPA patients. In 1 series of 1240 pituitary adenoma patients, giant status (>4 cm) was the only characteristic predictive of surgical morbidity on multivariable analysis.[37] Postoperative hypopituitarism and diabetes insipidus are common complications, with permanent endocrine dysfunction documented in over 20% of patients in 1 review of 431 patients.[5,50,79] Current guidelines recommend postoperative endocrinologic follow-up for up to 1 year for patients with normal pituitary function, as compared to lifetime follow-up for patients with abnormal pituitary function or who undergo radiation therapy.[96] Other common complications include CSF leak, meningitis, cranial nerve palsy, and vascular sequelae like perioperative hemorrhage, or vasospasm.[37,97] One of the most feared and fatal complications following GPA resection is postoperative pituitary apoplexy, which is posited to be caused by release of tumor vasculature or venous congestion in residual tumor, resulting in hemorrhagic conversion.[98,99] Patients primarily present with excruciating headache, visual symptoms, ophthalmoplegia, nausea, and vomiting within the first 24 hours,[98,100] but rarer cases after several days have been reported.[101] Kurwale and colleagues documented a mortality rate of 92% in their 13-patient GPA series.[100] Postoperative pituitary apoplexy requires emergent treatment with intravenous corticosteroids and transsphenoidal decompression. Although Omodaka and colleagues proposed preoperative emboli-zation as a method to decrease surgical morbidity for GPA,[102] this strategy has yet to be validated by other studies.

## Surgical Approaches for Giant Pituitary Adenoma

### Microsurgical transsphenoidal approach

Although Harvey Cushing played a monumental role in pioneering the removal of pitu-itary tumors via the transsphenoidal approach, operating on 231 tumors from 1910 to 1935 with a mortality rate of only 5.6%, it has been documented that large pituitary tumors specifically motivated Cushing's transition toward the transfrontal approach, which he believed achieved improved radical tumor resection and decompres-sion.[103–105] Cushing's influence and reduction of TC mortality rates to 4.6% caused the TC approach to dominate from the 1930s to 1950s. Nevertheless, the transsphe-noidal approach was resurrected over the subsequent 3 decades because of the work of surgeons like Dott, Guiot, and Hardy.[103] Hardy's landmark 1971 paper discussed the integration of an operating microscope into the transsphenoidal approach for accessing the sella turcica.[106]

MT surgery may be performed through either an endonasal or sublabial approach. In contrast to the TC approach, it confers the advantages of accessing pathology before critical neurovascular structures and avoiding retraction of the brain or optic apparatus.[14,21,76,91,107] Compared with the endoscopic 2-dimensional view in the EET approach, the MT approach also offers a stereoscopic view. Nevertheless, because of its narrow surgical corridor and straight surgical view, the MT approach is limited in removing GPAs with significant suprasellar extension or complete supra-sellar location.[6,52,80,89] Several studies have studied intraoperative MRI as a potential adjunct to address these visualization concerns, but this area warrants further research.[81,108,109] Although earlier studies have documented surgical maneuvers to promote descent of the suprasellar tumor component including the Valsalva maneu-ver, jugular compression, or air or saline injection into the lumbar cistern, the utility of these techniques is limited in certain GPAs, such as fibrous tumors.[13,19]

Eleven case series encompassing 699 GPA patients have been published on using the MT approach for GPA resection (**Table 1**).[3,4,6,12,14,21,34,37,93,108,110] GTR was accomplished in 44.7% of patients (239/535); improvement of visual symptoms was documented in 64.2% of patients (194/302), and tumor recurrence or progression was observed in 8.9% of patients (24/269).

### Endoscopic endonasal transsphenoidal approach

The EET approach is a more recent development, and the use of an endoscope for pi-tuitary surgery was only first reported by Bushe and Halves in 1978.[111] The universal adoption of the endoscope by otolaryngologists for surgical treatment of inflammatory sinonasal disorders prompted further exploration of endoscopic applications for pitu-itary surgery, including a landmark 50-patient series in 1997 by Jho and Carrau.[112] As described earlier, the EET has since evolved into the first-line approach for most GPAs.

Advantages offered by the EET approach, compared with the older MT approach, include panoramic visualization, illumination, and wider access of the sellar and para-sellar regions.[46,85,91] This may be supplemented with further modalities like intraoper-ative navigation and micro-Doppler.[86] The typical EET approach begins with middle and inferior turbinate lateralization and wide sphenoidotomy, with parasellar exposure from 1 lateral optic carotid recess to the other and from the tuberculum sellae to the clivus.[5,89,113,114] The tumor is subsequently debulked using microsurgical techniques

**Table 1**
**Giant pituitary adenoma case series for the microsurgical transsphenoidal approach (n = 11)**

| Author (Year) | Number of Patients | Mean Follow-Up in Months | Mean Diameter in Centimeters | Extent of Resection | | | Improvement of Visual Symptoms (%) | Complications | Recurrence or Progression |
|---|---|---|---|---|---|---|---|---|---|
| | | | | GTR (%) | STR (%) | PR (%) | | | |
| Akbari et al,[6] 2018[a] | 19 | NR | 3.2 | 3 (16%) | 16 (84%) | 0 (0%) | NR | Mortality: 2 (11%)<br>CSF leak: 2 (11%)<br>New HP: 11 (58%)<br>New DI: 4 (21%)<br>Meningitis: 1 (5%) | NR |
| Barzaghi et al,[37] 2007 | 54 | NR | NR | NR | NR | NR | NR | Mortality: 2 (4%)<br>CSF leak: 1 (2%) | NR |
| Baumann et al,[108] 2010 | 6 | 25 | NR | 4 (67%) | 2 (33%) | NR | 6/6 (100%) | CSF leak: 1 (17%)<br>New DI: 2 (33%) | 0 (0%) |
| Cusimano et al,[14] 2012[c] | 14 | 73.9 | 3.7 | 2 (14%) | NR | NR | 12/14 (86%) | New HP: 5 (36%)<br>New DI: 2 (17%) | 3 (21%) |
| Goel et al,[4] 2004 | 118 | 31 | NR | 35 (30%) | 48 (41%) | 35 (30%) | 39/118 (33%) | Mortality: 2 (2%)<br>CSF leak: 5 (4%)<br>Meningitis: 4 (3%)<br>ICH: 2 (2%) | NR |
| Karki et al,[21] 2017 | 59 (48% NF) | 40.6 | NR | 44 (75%) | 11 (19%) | 4 (7%) | 42/59 (71%) | CSF leak: 14 (24%)<br>New HP: 15 (25%)<br>New DI: 11 (19%) | 2 (3%) |
| Mohr et al,[12] 1990[b] | 77 (69% NF) | NR | NR | 49 (64%) | 26 (34%) | NR | 58/63 (92%) | Mortality: 4 (5%)<br>New DI: 5 (7%)<br>ICH: 4 (5%) | 19 (25%) |
| Mortini et al,[3] 2007 | 85 | 56.9 | 4.7 | 13 (15%) | 54 (64%) | 0 (0%) | NR | Mortality: 2 (11%)<br>CSF leak: 1 (1%)<br>New HP: 9 (11%)<br>New DI: 7 (8%)<br>Apoplexy: 8 (8%) | NR |

(continued on next page)

**Table 1**
*(continued)*

| Author (Year) | Number of Patients | Mean Follow-Up in Months | Mean Diameter in Centimeters | Extent of Resection | | | Improvement of Visual Symptoms (%) | Complications | Recurrence or Progression |
|---|---|---|---|---|---|---|---|---|---|
| | | | | GTR (%) | STR (%) | PR (%) | | | |
| Nishioka et al,[34] 2017 | 49 | 62.2 | 4.8 | 15 (31%) | 19 (49%) | 15 (31%) | 37/42 (88%) | New HP or DI: 6 (12%)<br>New ND: 1 (2%) | 0 (0%) |
| Sinha et al,[48] 2010 | 110 | 29.6 | 5.4 | NR | NR | NR | NR | CSF leak: 11 (7%)<br>New DI: 15 (9%)<br>Meningitis: 8 (5%)<br>ICH: 7 (4%)<br>Vascular injury: 6 (4%) | NR |
| Wang et al,[110] 2006 | 64 | 37.5 | NR | 51 (80%) | 13 (20%) | 0 (0%) | NR | CSF leak: 5 (8%)<br>New HP: 1 (2%)<br>New DI: 26 (41%) | 0 (0%) |
| Zhao et al,[93] 2010 | 44 | NR | NR | 27 (61%) | 14 (32%) | 3 (7%) | NR | NR | NR |

*Abbreviations:* CSF, cerebrospinal fluid; GTR, gross total resection; HCP, hydrocephalus; HP, hypopituitarism; ICH, intracranial hemorrhage; ND, neurologic deficit; NF, nonfunctional; NR, not reported; PR, partial resection; STR, subtotal resection.

[a] GPAs were defined by this study as having a maximum diameter of greater than 3 cm, rather than greater than 4 cm.
[b] GPAs were defined by this study as having suprasellar extension of greater than 2 cm.
[c] GPAs were defined by this study as greater than 10 cm[3] in volume.

(**Figs. 3** and **4**). Several extended EET approaches have been extensively described, with the most common entailing removal of the tuberculum and planum sphenoidale for lesions with significant anterior or suprasellar extension (**Figs. 5** and **6**). This transplanum-transtuberculum approach not only improves suprasellar access, but also creates simultaneous intracapsular and extracapsular corridors for tumor dissection.[5,80,89,93,114,115] The transethmoid-transpterygoid route allows exposure of the medial and lateral CS compartments bilaterally, unlike the TC approach, which only confers unilateral CS access.[14,88] The transclival approach allows improved access to the posterior fossa.[40,43] Several case reports have documented the success of these extended techniques even for GPAs traditionally considered more challenging for a transsphenoidal route, such as fibrous and dumbbell-shaped tumors.[13,19,116] Beyond the innovation of these extended approaches, other variations of the EET have been developed to reduce surgical morbidity. For example, Pezzutti and colleagues recently outlined a second floor strategy to reduce postoperative apoplexy

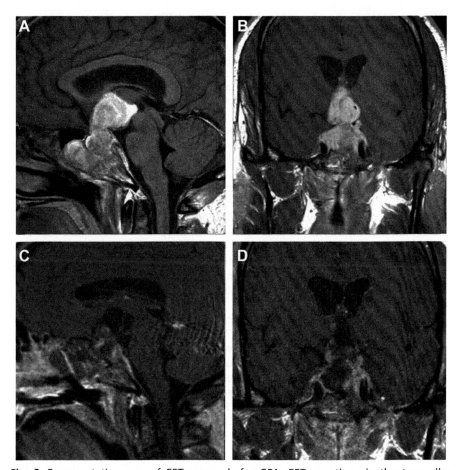

**Fig. 3.** Representative case of EET approach for GPA. EET resection via the transsellar corridor of GPA with significant suprasellar extension into the retrochiasmatic space and third ventricle. A near-total resection was achieved with residual microscopic tumor in the left cavernous sinus that was treated with radiosurgery. (*A*) Sagittal and (*B*) coronal preoperative MRI. (*C*) Sagittal and (*D*) coronal postoperative MRI.

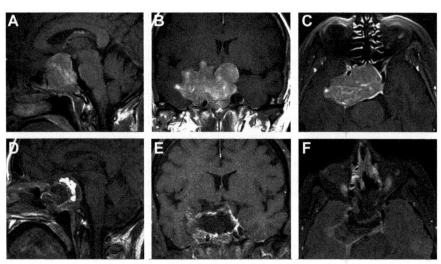

**Fig. 4.** EET resection of GPA with significant lateral resection. EET resection via the transsellar corridor of GPA with significant right lateral extension from cavernous sinus invasion. A gross total resection was achieved through the transsellar corridor using angled endoscopy and angled curved suctions. (*A*) Sagittal, (*B*) coronal, and (*C*) axial preoperative MRI. (*D*) Sagittal, (*E*) coronal, and (*F*) axial postoperative MRI.

risk, which involves resecting a GPA's suprasellar portion before its sellar portion.[99] An EET procedure ends with skull base repair, which is accomplished by multilayer reconstruction involving a combination of fascia lata grafts, dural substitutes, and pedicled nasoseptal flap (see **Fig. 6**).[5,117] Although a CSF leak has traditionally been considered one of the most prevalent and worrisome complications of the EET approach,[85] this complication has decreased markedly since the introduction of the pedicled nasoseptal flap by Hadad and colleagues,[117] with 1 case series documenting a CSF leak reduction from 16.7% to 7.4% after its adoption.[40] An alternate flap, such as turbinate or pericranial, may be utilized if the nasoseptal flap is nonviable because of previous radiotherapy or surgery.[115] Because of these advances, 1 review of 431 patients determined that permanent diabetes insipidus (DI) or hypopituitarism is now the most common postoperative complication (20.8%), compared with CSF leak (8.8%).[5]

In a 2012 review by Komotar and colleagues comparing all 3 surgical modalities for GPA, EET achieved higher rates of GTR (47.2%) and visual improvement (91.1%) and lower rates of hypopituitarism (1.1%) and recurrence (2.1%), with no documented CSF leaks.[107] Nevertheless, because of the nascency of this technique, this article only assessed 106 patients across 3 case series. Two more recent reviews of exclusively endoscopic procedures have documented GTR rates of 20% to 61.9% of cases and visual improvement in 61.8% to 97.4% of cases.[5,89] Despite these advantages, other studies have asserted that the EET approach faces limitations in resecting certain GPAs, particularly tumors with significant subfrontal, temporal, or lateral CS extension.[51,85]

Twenty-five case series encompassing 1060 GPA patients have been published on using the EET approach for GPA resection (**Table 2**).[6,8,9,13,14,16,17,19,24,34,40,43,45,46,51–53,80,84–86,90,91,115,118] GTR was accomplished in 42.0% of patients (445/1060); improvement of visual symptoms was documented in 82.1% of patients (600/731); and tumor recurrence or progression was observed in 12.7% of patients (95/747).

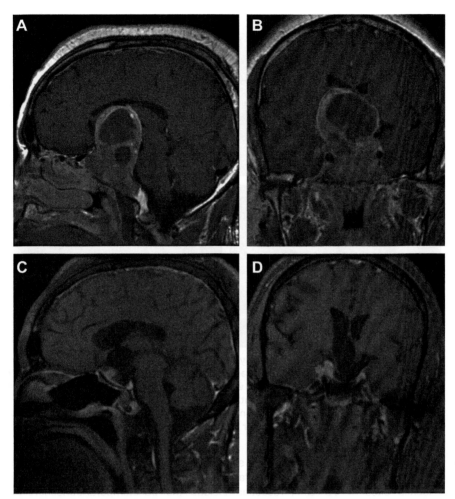

**Fig. 5.** Extended EET Resection with transplanum-transtuberculum approach of GPA with significant suprasellar extension. GPA with significant suprasellar extension into the third ventricle resected via endoscopic transplanum-transtuberculum approach. The residual tumor invading both cavernous sinuses was controlled with intensity-modulated radiation therapy. Postoperative MRI confirmed near-total resection. (*A*) Sagittal and (*B*) coronal preoperative MRI. (*C*) Sagittal and (*D*) coronal postoperative MRI.

## Transcranial approach

Although the TC approach is estimated to play a role in treating only 1% to 10% of all GPAs,[10,20,83,119,120] it serves a notable niche for tumors that may be challenging to address via either transsphenoidal approach. Indications for the TC approach include tumors with a dumbbell morphology or minimal communication between intra- and suprasellar components, encasement of the optic apparatus or cerebral arteries, or irregular or asymmetric extension into subfrontal, temporal lobes, posterior fossa, or retrochiasmatic region (**Fig. 7**).[3,15,19,40,83,84,88,99,100,107,119,121–123] The TC approach may also be beneficial for patients with anatomic variations or comorbid pathology, such as a shallow sella, narrow intercarotid space, ectatic carotid arteries, or concurrent aneurysms.[10,15,124] Finally, the TC approach may be used in patients with previous

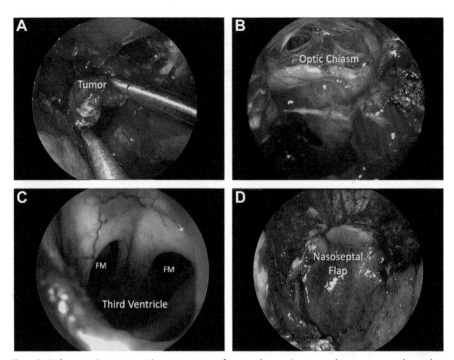

**Fig. 6.** Relevant intraoperative anatomy for endoscopic transplanum-transtuberculum approach. Intraoperative photos of case presented in **Fig. 5** via the endoscopic transplanum-transtuberculum approach, with relevant surgical anatomy and landmarks. (*A*) Debulking of the tumor. (*B*) Visualization of the optic chiasm. (*C*) Visualization of the third ventricle and both foramina of Monro (FM). (*D*) Use of pedicled nasoseptal flap for skull base reconstruction following tumor resection.

transsphenoidal surgery or concurrent sinusitis.[10,124] The most common surgical approaches include the pterional, subfrontal, and fronto-orbitozygomatic,[103] but other approaches cited in TC GPA resection include the transtemporal-transchoroidal, transcallosal-transventricular, and basal interhemispheric.[10] Although the TC approach holds utility for GPAs with specific indications and is an important component of a pituitary surgeon's armamentarium, it is notable that these procedures carry the well-known risks that come with a craniotomy, with certain case series documenting minor and major surgical morbidity rates of up to 75% and 35%, respectively.[3,119]

Eleven case series encompassing 513 GPA patients have been published on using a TC approach for GPA resection (**Table 3**).[3,10,11,14,18,20,25,41,48,82,83] GTR was accomplished in 41.9% of patients (138/329); improvement of visual symptoms was documented in 71.1% of patients (205/288), and tumor recurrence or progression was observed in 11.9% of patients (27/226).

### Combined approach

An above and below angle of attack for resecting GPAs, involving the simultaneous performance of supra- and infrasellar surgical approaches, was first proposed by Loyo and colleagues in 1984.[125] Several case series characterizing these combined approaches have emphasized their utility for dumbbell-shaped GPAs, fibrous GPAs, and GPAs with asymmetric extension in the sagittal or coronal plane.[7,126] The aforementioned indications for a TC approach, such as the necessity for dissecting the

**Table 2**
Giant pituitary adenoma case series for the endoscopic endonasal transsphenoidal approach (n = 25)

| Author (Year) | Number of Patients | Mean Follow-Up in Months | Mean Diameter in Centimeters | Extent of Resection | | | Improvement of Visual Symptoms (%) | Complications | Recurrence or Progression |
| --- | --- | --- | --- | --- | --- | --- | --- | --- | --- |
| | | | | GTR (%) | STR (%) | PR (%) | | | |
| Akbari et al,[6] 2018[a] | 16 | NR | 3.5 | 13 (81%) | 3 (20%) | NR | NR | Mortality: 2 (13%)<br>New HP: 12 (75%)<br>New DI: 5 (31%)<br>CSF leak: 3 (19%)<br>Meningitis: 2 (13%) | NR |
| Chabot et al,[52] 2015 | 6 | 12 | NR | 3 (50%) | 3 (50%) | NR | 3/5 (60%) | NR | NR |
| Chibbaro et al,[53] 2021 | 96 (100% NF) | 52.4 | 4.7 | 34 (35%) | 62 (65%) | NR | 77/78 (99%) | CSF leak: 7 (7%)<br>New DI: 37 (38%)<br>HCP: 1 (1%)<br>Meningitis: 7 (7%)<br>Apoplexy: 2 (2%) | 16 (17%) |
| Chohan et al,[46] 2016 | 62 | 22 | NR | 29 (47%) | NR | NR | 39/52 (63%) | CSF leak: 1 (2%)<br>ICH: 1 (2%) | 0 (0%) |
| Constantino et al,[8] 2016[a] | 28 (82% NF) | 30 | 4.6 | 4 (14%) | 14 (51%) | 10 (36%) | 9/12 (75%) | Mortality: 2 (7%)<br>CSF leak: 5 (18%)<br>New DI: 16 (57%)<br>Meningitis: 2 (7%)<br>Sinusitis: 2 (7%)<br>ICH: 1 (4%)<br>Vascular injury: 1 (4%)<br>Synechiae: 6 (21%) | 9 (32%) |
| Cusimano et al,[14] 2012[c] | 29 | 73.9 | 4.0 | 6 (21%) | NR | NR | 25/29 (96%) | New HP: 9 (31%)<br>New DI: 2 (7%) | 7 (24%) |

*(continued on next page)*

**Table 2**
*(continued)*

| Author (Year) | Number of Patients | Mean Follow-Up in Months | Mean Diameter in Centimeters | Extent of Resection | | | Improvement of Visual Symptoms (%) | Complications | Recurrence or Progression |
|---|---|---|---|---|---|---|---|---|---|
| | | | | GTR (%) | STR (%) | PR (%) | | | |
| de Paiva Neto et al,[16] 2010 | 51 (76% NF) | 12 | 4.5 | 21 (41%) | 30 (59%) | NR | 31/38 (82%) | CSF leak: 1 (2%)<br>Meningitis: 0 (0%)<br>Sinusitis: 3 (6%)<br>ICH: 2 (4%)<br>Vascular injury: 0 (0%) | 10 (20%) |
| Elshazly et al,[17] 2018 | 55 (93% NF) | 41 | 5.1 | 24 (44%) | 31 (56%) | NR | 32/48 (67%) | CSF leak: 1 (2%)<br>New HP: 8 (15%)<br>New DI: 13 (24%)<br>Apoplexy: 1 (2%) | 6 (11%) |
| Fallah et al,[91] 2020 | 35 | 12 | NR | 26 (74%) | 5 (14%) | 4 (11%) | NR | NR | NR |
| Gondim et al,[19] 2014 | 50 (84% NF) | | 5.4 | 19 (38%) | 9 (18%) | 22 (44%) | 38/48 (76%) | CSF leak: 4 (8%)<br>New HP: 18 (36%)<br>New DI: 23 (46%)<br>Meningitis: 1 (2%) | 10 (20%) |
| Han et al,[84] 2017 | 43 | 46.9 | 4.7 | 11 (26%) | 22 (51%) | 10 (23%) | 35/43 (81%) | CSF leak: 2 (5%)<br>New HP: 4 (9%)<br>New DI: 1 (3%)<br>Meningitis: 1 (2%) | 3 (7%) |
| Jamaluddin et al,[118] 2021 | 10 | 24.6 | NR | 3 (38%) | 5 (63%) | NR | 6/6 (100%) | CSF leak: 0 (0%)<br>New DI: 2 (25%)<br>Meningitis: 0 (0%) | 0 (0%) |
| Juraschka et al,[9] 2014[a] | 73 (89% NF) | 8.0 | 4.1 | 16 (24%) | 35 (53%) | 15 (23%) | 46/53 (87%) | CSF leak: 7 (10%)<br>New HP: 3 (4%)<br>HCP: 2 (3%)<br>Meningitis: 2 (3%)<br>Sinusitis: 10 (14%) | NR |

| Study | N | | | | | | | Complications | |
|---|---|---|---|---|---|---|---|---|---|
| Koutourousiou et al,[40] 2013 | 54 | 37.9 | 5.0 | 11 (20%) | 25 (46%) | 18 (33%) | 36/45 (80%) | CSF leak: 9 (17%)<br>New HP: 9 (17%)<br>New DI: 5 (10%)<br>CN palsy: 7 (13%)<br>Meningitis: 3 (6%)<br>Apoplexy: 2 (4%) | 8 (15%) |
| Kuo et al,[85] 2016 | 38 | 72.9 | NR | 8 (21%) | 30 (79%) | NR | 27/38 (71%) | CSF leak: 0 (0%)<br>New HP: 10 (26%)<br>New DI: 1 (3%)<br>ICH: 3 (8%)<br>Vascular injury: 1 (3%) | 1 (3%) |
| Kutlay et al,[115] 2018 | 27 | 28 | NR | 21 (78%) | 6 (22%) | NR | NR | CSF leak: 3 (11%)<br>New DI: 3 (11%)<br>CN palsy: 1 (4%) | NR |
| Nakao et al,[13] 2011[b] | 43 | 63.6 | 4.8 | 20 (47%) | 23 (53%) | NR | 42/43 (98%) | CSF leak: 0 (0%)<br>New HP: 2 (5%)<br>New DI: 11 (26%) | 0 (0%) |
| Nishioka et al,[34] 2017 | 60 | 62.2 | 4.8 | 19 (32%) | 26 (43%) | 15 (25%) | 44/53 (83%) | New HP or DI: 7 (12%)<br>New ND: 4 (7%) | 0 (0%) |
| Peto et al,[51] 2020 | 10 | 5.9 | NR | 4 (40%) | 5 (50%) | NR | 5/9 (56%) | CSF leak: 7 (70%) | NR |
| Rahimli et al,[43] 2021 | 44 | 38.5 | NR | 28 (64%) | 10 (23%) | 6 (14%) | 27/33 (82%) | Mortality: 2 (5%)<br>CSF leak: 5 (11%)<br>New DI: 20 (46%)<br>Vascular injury: 3 (7%) | 4 (9%) |
| Sankhla et al,[80] 2013 | 13 | NR | NR | 8 (62%) | 4 (31%) | 1 (8%) | 11/13 (85%) | NR | NR |
| Wang et al,[90] 2015 | 115 | 28.8 | NR | 87 (76%) | NR | NR | NR | Mortality: 0 (0%)<br>Coma: 1 (1%) | NR |
| Yang et al,[86] 2019 | 60 (88% NF) | 42.5 | 5.2 | 28 (47%) | 32 (53%) | NR | 44/60 (73%) | CSF leak: 1 (2%)<br>New HP: 8 (13%)<br>New DI: 10 (17%) | 13 (22%) |

(continued on next page)

**Table 2**
*(continued)*

| Author (Year) | Number of Patients | Mean Follow-Up in Months | Mean Diameter in Centimeters | Extent of Resection | | | Improvement of Visual Symptoms (%) | Complications | Recurrence or Progression |
|---|---|---|---|---|---|---|---|---|---|
| | | | | GTR (%) | STR (%) | PR (%) | | | |
| Yano et al,[24] 2017 | 34 (82% NF) | 76 | 4.6 | 0 (0%) | 16 (47%) | 18 (53%) | 23/25 (92%) | CSF leak: 2 (6%)<br>New HP: 4 (12%)<br>New DI: 7 (21%)<br>HCP: 1 (3%)<br>Vascular injury: 2 (6%) | 8 (24%) |
| Zheng et al,[45] 2020 | 8 | NR | NR | 2 (25%) | 6 (75%) | NR | NR | NR | NR |

*Abbreviations:* CSF, cerebrospinal fluid; GTR, gross total resection; HCP, hydrocephalus; HP, hypopituitarism; ICH, intracranial hemorrhage; ND, neurologic deficit; NF, nonfunctional; NR, not reported; PR, partial resection; STR, subtotal resection.

a GPAs were defined by this study as having a maximum diameter of greater than 3 cm, rather than greater than 4 cm.

b GPAs were defined by this study as having suprasellar extension of greater than 2 cm

c GPAs were defined by this study as greater than 10 cm$^3$ in volume.

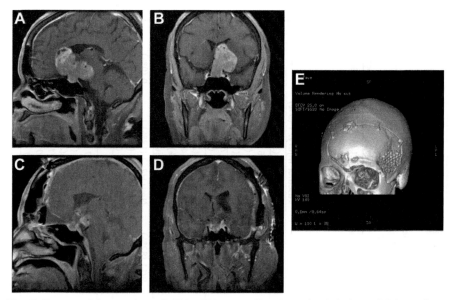

**Fig. 7.** Transcranial resection of GPA. GPA extending into the left frontal lobe, sylvian fissure, and retrochiasmatic space resected transcranially via a left modified 1-piece orbito-zymatic approach. A transcranial approach was chosen over either transsphenoidal approaches because of the GPA's significant asymmetric anterior and lateral extension. Postoperative MRI confirmed a near-total resection. (*A*) Sagittal and (*B*) coronal preoperative MRI. (*C*) Sagittal and (*D*) coronal postoperative MRI. (*E*) 3-dimensional computed tomography reconstruction showing the extended modified 1-piece orbitozygomatic approach used for the transcranial resection.

GPA from neurovascular structures, also serve as indications for a combined approach,[84] and D'Ambriosio and colleagues have advocated for consideration of a combined approach in any patient who is a TC candidate.[126] In the combined transsphenoidal-TC approach, the TC surgeon primarily focuses on playing a protective role for intradural structures and delivering the tumor bulk toward the sella as it is manipulated by the transsphenoidal surgeon,[127] enabling minimal violation of the tumor capsule.[126] The combined approach may also be preferred to a staged operation due to removal of residual tumor to minimize the risk of postoperative apoplexy or edema.[119] Nevertheless, it is important to note that the combined approach is logistically challenging and requires 2 surgical teams, operative fields, sets of operating instruments, and potentially operating microscopes.[128]

Eight case series encompassing 96 GPA patients have been published on using a combined surgical approach for GPA resection (**Table 4**).[7,22,34,84,120,126,127,129] These case series have combined a TC procedure with the MT approach,[7,120] the EET approach,[22,84,126,129] or both transsphenoidal modalities.[34,127] Other case reports have documented endeavors to make the TC portion of the procedure more minimally invasive via an endoscopic transventricular approach[130–132] or keyhole craniotomy.[133] Although studies have raised the concern about infection risks due to open communication between nasal flora and the intradural space,[126] no intracranial infections or meningitis cases were documented across the 8 articles.

### Comparison of surgical approaches

There were no significant differences across the 3 surgical approaches in pooled rates for GTR (MT: 44.7%, EET: 42.0%, TC: 41.9%) or tumor recurrence or progression (MT: 8.9%,

**Table 3**
Giant pituitary adenoma case series for the transcranial approach (n = 11)

| Author (Year) | Number of Patients | Mean Follow-Up in Months | Mean Diameter in Centimeters | Extent of Resection | | | Improvement of Visual Symptoms (%) | Complications | Recurrence or Progression |
|---|---|---|---|---|---|---|---|---|---|
| | | | | GTR (%) | STR (%) | PR (%) | | | |
| Cusimano et al,[14] 2012c | 29 | 73.9 | 4.0 | 0 (0%) | NR | NR | 21/29 (72%) | Mortality: 1 (3%)<br>New HP: 12 (41%)<br>New DI: 3 (10%)<br>HCP: 1 (3%)<br>ICH: 4 (14%)<br>Vascular injury: 1 (3%) | 9 (31%) |
| Fu et al,[18] 2016 | 21 (71% NF) | 54.3 | NR | NR | NR | NR | 6/17 (35%) | New HP: 7 (33%) | 8 (38%) |
| Goel etal,[82] 1996 | 30 | 13 | NR | 0 (0%) | NR | NR | 11/22 (50%) | Mortality: 6 (20%)<br>CSF leak: 2 (7%)<br>New HP: 4 (13%)<br>New DI: 2 (7%)<br>CN palsy: 5 (17%) | 2 (7%) |
| Graillon et al,[20] 2020 | 19 (79% NF) | 57 | 5.2 | 4 (21%) | 13 (69%) | 2 (11%) | 10/19 (53%) | New HP: 5 (27%)<br>New DI: 8 (42%)<br>ICH: 2 (11%)<br>Vascular injury: 3 (16%) | 0 (0%) |
| Guo et al,[83] 2012 | 15 | 40 | NR | 10 (67%) | 5 (33%) | NR | 9/11 (82%) | New HP: 2 (13%)<br>New DI: 12 (80%)<br>CN palsy: 1 (7%) | 0 (0%) |
| Jeffreys et al,[11] 1989b | 41 | NR | NR | 31 (76%) | 10 (24%) | NR | 34/41 (82%) | NR | NR |
| Mortini et al,[3] 2007 | 26 | 56.9 | 4.7 | 1 (4%) | 11 (42%) | NR | NR | Mortality: 1 (4%)<br>CSF leak: 2 (8%)<br>New HP: 6 (23%)<br>New DI: 4 (15%)<br>Apoplexy: 0 (0%)<br>ICH: 1 (4%) | NR |

| Shen et al,[10] 2020[a] | 37 | 12 | 4.8 | 21 (57%) | 15 (40%) | 1 (3%) | 16/37 (43%) | CSF leak: 0 (0%)<br>New HP: 18 (49%)<br>New DI: 20 (54%)<br>CN palsy: 3 (8%)<br>HCP: 1 (3%)<br>Meningitis: 10 (27%)<br>ICH: 2 (5%) | NR |
|---|---|---|---|---|---|---|---|---|---|
| Sinha et al,[48] 2010 | 163 | 29.6 | 5.4 | NR | NR | NR | NR | CSF leak: 2 (2%)<br>New DI: 7 (6%)<br>Meningitis: 3 (3%)<br>ICH: 6 (5%)<br>Vascular injury: 0 (0%) | NR |
| Yildirim et al,[41] 2015 | 20 | NR | NR | 14 (70%) | 6 (30%) | NR | NR | New HP: 3 (15%)<br>New DI: 2 (10%) | NR |
| Zhang et al,[25] 2015 | 112 (81% NF) | 19.5 | 4.8 | 57 (51%) | 26 (23%) | 29 (26%) | 98/112 (88%) | Mortality: 3 (3%) | 8 (7%) |

*Abbreviations:* CSF, cerebrospinal fluid; GTR, gross total resection; HCP, hydrocephalus; HP, hypopituitarism; ICH, intracranial hemorrhage; ND, neurologic deficit; NF, nonfunctional; NR, not reported; PR, partial resection; STR, subtotal resection.

[a] GPAs were defined by this study as having a maximum diameter of greater than 3 cm, rather than greater than 4 cm.
[b] GPAs were defined by this study as having suprasellar extension of greater than 2 cm.
[c] GPAs were defined by this study as greater than 10 cm$^3$ in volume.

**Table 4**
Giant pituitary adenoma case series for the combined approach (n = 8)

| Author (Year) | Number of Patients | Mean Follow-Up in Months | Mean Diameter in Centimeters | Extent of Resection GTR (%) | Extent of Resection STR (%) | Extent of Resection PR (%) | Improvement of Visual Symptoms (%) | Complications | Recurrence or Progression |
|---|---|---|---|---|---|---|---|---|---|
| Alleyne et al,[7] 2002[a] | 10 | 31 | NR | 4 (40%) | 6 (60%) | NR | 9/9 (100%) | New HP: 1 (10%)<br>New DI: 2 (20%)<br>HCP: 1 (10%)<br>Vascular injury: 1 (10%) | 0 (0%) |
| D'Ambrosio et al,[126] 2009 | 9 | 51.6 | NR | 4 (44%) | 5 (55%) | NR | 7/9 (78%) | CSF leak: 1 (11%)<br>New HP: 1 (11%)<br>New DI: 3 (33%)<br>CN palsy: 1 (11%) | 4 (44%) |
| Han et al,[84] 2017 | 13 | 46.9 | 4.7 | 6 (46%) | 3 (23%) | 4 (31%) | 11/13 (85%) | CSF leak: 0 (0%)<br>New HP: 4 (31%)<br>New DI: 1 (8%)<br>Meningitis: 0 (0%) | 1 (17%) |
| Kuga et al,[22] 2019 | 3 (67% NF) | 32 | 4.4 | 0 (0%) | 3 (100%) | 0 (0%) | 2/3 (67%) | New HP: 2 (67%)<br>New DI: 1 (33%) | 1 (33%) |
| Leung et al,[127] 2011 | 7 | 53 | 4.9 | 3 (43%) | 4 (57%) | NR | 0/1 (0%) | CSF leak: 1 (14%) | 0 (0%) |
| Leung et al,[129] 2012 | 2 | NR | 4.5 | 1 (50%) | NR | NR | 2/2 (100%) | New DI: 2 (100%) | NR |
| Nishioka et al,[120] 2012 | 23 | 32.7 | 4.7 | 5 (22%) | 17 (74%) | 1 (4%) | NR | CSF leak: 1 (4%)<br>CN palsy: 5 (22%)<br>HCP: 1 (4%) | 0 (0%) |
| Nishioka et al,[34] 2017 | 19 | 62.2 | 4.8 | 4 (21%) | 10 (53%) | 5 (26%) | 6/15 (40%) | New HP or DI: 5 (28%)<br>New ND: 5 (28%) | 0 (0%) |

*Abbreviations:* CSF, cerebrospinal fluid; GTR, gross total resection; HCP, hydrocephalus; HP, hypopituitarism; ICH, intracranial hemorrhage; ND, neurologic deficit; NF, nonfunctional; NR, not reported; PR, partial resection; STR, subtotal resection.
[a] GPAs were defined by this study as having a maximum diameter of greater than 3 cm, rather than greater than 4 cm.

EET: 12.7%, TC: 11.9%). However, perioperative mortality rates for EET (0.6%) were significantly lower than those for MT (1.8%, $P=.047$) and TC (2.3%, $P=.009$). Moreover, EET exhibited higher rates of visual improvement (82.1%) compared with MT (64.2% $P<.001$) and TC (71.1%, $P<.001$).

## DISCUSSION

GPAs are a challenging clinical entity, in that, apart from dopamine treatment for prolactinomas, they invariably require surgical decompression to ameliorate visual and endocrine function. Rates of GTR for GPAs are significantly lower compared with their nongiant counterparts, and factors associated with lower extent of maximal safe resection include dumbbell or multilobular morphology, retrosellar and CS extension, and previous surgery or irradiation. Nevertheless, GTR rates of 40% have been documented across all 3 primary surgical modalities (MT, EET, and TC), and visual improvement has been observed for 43% to 99% of patients.

In the authors' updated review comparing surgical approaches for GPAs, the EET approach—the most commonly used procedure for GPA resection in modern practice—had comparable rates of GTR and tumor recurrence or progression but achieved lower perioperative mortality rates and superior restoration of visual function compared with MT and TC. Extended EET approaches also enable resection of tumors previously thought unfavorable for a transsphenoidal route.[115] With the addition of articles from the past decade, the rates of GTR and visual improvement for EET have slightly worsened in comparison to the 2012 review by Komotar and colleagues,[107] potentially because of a regression toward the mean, as the inclusion of more recent studies has resulted in pooled results that may be reflective of the well-documented and challenging learning curve of the EET procedure.[14,41,53,115,127] Improved rates of GTR and visual improvement have also been observed for the MT and TC approaches with the inclusion of more recent case series, which may reflect an improved quality of surgical management for GPA across all modalities. In interpreting these results, it is also important to note that the case reports from which these outcomes were drawn may be subject to publication bias. Moreover, because this article aimed to provide the most thorough review of GPA literature, there may be heterogeneity in GPA and extent of resection definitions, primary or recurrent status, and concurrent use of medical management or radiosurgery for the patients included. Finally, there may be selection bias between approaches, such as TC cases potentially encompassing especially challenging tumors.[22,84] Nevertheless, the authors' results corroborate earlier findings of EET as a safe and effective approach for most GPAs.

However, there is no single surgical approach that is advisable for all GPAs. The optimal surgical modality for any individual patient should be selected by the anatomic considerations of his or her GPA, and all 3 approaches complementary components of a pituitary surgeon's armamentarium. Moreover, the utilization of combined transsphenoidal-TC approaches, reported for over 100 GPA patients, has been demonstrated to enable safer tumor debulking for more challenging lesions and reduces the risk of postoperative sequelae from residual tumor, such as pituitary apoplexy, that may occur in between staged procedures.[119] Continued research in reducing the invasiveness of the TC component of these combined procedures is important in improving surgical outcomes for GPA patients.

## SUMMARY

GPAs make up 5% to 15% of pituitary adenomas, but have significantly higher rates of extrasellar invasion, subtotal resection, surgical morbidity, and recurrence. With the possible exception of giant prolactinomas, GPAs invariably require surgical decompression. On review of 3 decades of case series encompassing 699 MT, 1060 EET, and 513 TC patients, gross total resection and recurrence rates were comparable across modalities, but the EET approach had lower perioperative mortality and superior restoration of visual function, making it the preferred technique for resection of most GPAs. Nevertheless, each approach has a unique set of indications and choice of modality should be informed on a case-by-case basis based on a GPA's anatomic considerations. Combined transsphenoidal-TC approaches for minimizing residual tumor represent another potential strategy.

## CLINICS CARE POINTS

- Giant pituitary adenomas (GPAs) encompass 5% to 15% of pituitary adenomas and are predominantly nonfunctional tumors that present with mass effect symptoms. With the possible exception of prolactinomas, first-line treatment is maximal safe resection to relieve parasellar decompression.

- The endoscopic endonasal transsphenoidal (EET) approach is the predominant surgical approach for treating GPAs. While the EET, microsurgical transsphenoidal, and transcranial approach achieve gross total resection rates greater than 40% and recurrence rates less than 15%, the EET has the lowest perioperative mortality (0.6%) and highest rates of visual improvement (82.1%).

- The selection of surgical approaches should be done on a case-by-case basis. Selected cases may benefit from a combined above and below approach.

## DISCLOSURE

The authors have nothing to disclose.

## REFERENCES

1. Jefferson G. Extrasellar extensions of pituitary adenomas: (section of neurology). Proc R Soc Med 1940;33(7):433–58.
2. Iglesias P, Rodriguez Berrocal V, Diez JJ. Giant pituitary adenoma: histological types, clinical features and therapeutic approaches. Endocrine 2018;61(3): 407–21.
3. Mortini P, Barzaghi R, Losa M, et al. Surgical treatment of giant pituitary adenomas: strategies and results in a series of 95 consecutive patients. Neurosurgery 2007;60(6):993–1002.
4. Goel A, Nadkarni T, Muzumdar D, et al. Giant pituitary tumors: a study based on surgical treatment of 118 cases. Surg Neurol 2004;61(5):436–45.
5. Marigil Sanchez M, Karekezi C, Almeida JP, et al. Management of giant pituitary adenomas: role and outcome of the endoscopic endonasal surgical approach. Neurosurg Clin N Am 2019;30(4):433–44.
6. Akbari H, Malek M, Ghorbani M, et al. Clinical outcomes of endoscopic versus microscopic transsphenoidal surgery for large pituitary adenoma. Br J Neurosurg 2018;32(2):206–9.
7. Alleyne CH Jr, Barrow DL, Oyesiku NM. Combined transsphenoidal and pterional craniotomy approach to giant pituitary tumors. Surg Neurol 2002;57(6): 380–90.
8. Constantino ER, Leal R, Ferreira CC, et al. Surgical outcomes of the endoscopic endonasal transsphenoidal approach for large and giant pituitary adenomas:

institutional experience with special attention to approach-related complications. Arq Neuropsiquiatr 2016;74(5):388–95.

9. Juraschka K, Khan OH, Godoy BL, et al. Endoscopic endonasal transsphenoidal approach to large and giant pituitary adenomas: institutional experience and predictors of extent of resection. J Neurosurg 2014;121(1):75–83.

10. Shen M, Chen Z, Shou X, et al. Surgical outcomes and predictors of visual function alterations after transcranial surgery for large-to-giant pituitary adenomas. World Neurosurg 2020;141:e60–9.

11. Jeffreys RV. The surgical treatment of large pituitary adenomas. Br J Neurosurg 1989;3(2):147–52.

12. Mohr G, Hardy J, Comtois R, et al. Surgical management of giant pituitary adenomas. Can J Neurol Sci 1990;17(1):62–6.

13. Nakao N, Itakura T. Surgical outcome of the endoscopic endonasal approach for non-functioning giant pituitary adenoma. J Clin Neurosci 2011;18(1):71–5.

14. Cusimano MD, Kan P, Nassiri F, et al. Outcomes of surgically treated giant pituitary tumours. Can J Neurol Sci 2012;39(4):446–57.

15. Chibbaro S, Ganau M, Gubian A, et al. The role of endoscopic endonasal approach in the multimodal management of giant pituitary adenoma: case report and literature review. Asian J Neurosurg 2018;13(3):888–92.

16. de Paiva Neto MA, Vandergrift A, Fatemi N, et al. Endonasal transsphenoidal surgery and multimodality treatment for giant pituitary adenomas. Clin Endocrinol (Oxf) 2010;72(4):512–9.

17. Elshazly K, Kshettry VR, Farrell CJ, et al. Clinical outcomes after endoscopic endonasal resection of giant pituitary adenomas. World Neurosurg 2018;114: e447–56.

18. Fu P, He YS, Cen YC, et al. Microneurosurgery and subsequent gamma knife radiosurgery for functioning pituitary macroadenomas or giant adenomas: One institution's experience. Clin Neurol Neurosurg 2016;145:8–13.

19. Gondim JA, Almeida JP, Albuquerque LA, et al. Giant pituitary adenomas: surgical outcomes of 50 cases operated on by the endonasal endoscopic approach. World Neurosurg 2014;82(1–2):e281–90.

20. Graillon T, Castinetti F, Fuentes S, et al. Transcranial approach in giant pituitary adenomas: results and outcome in a modern series. J Neurosurg Sci 2020; 64(1):25–36.

21. Karki M, Sun J, Yadav CP, et al. Large and giant pituitary adenoma resection by microscopic transsphenoidal surgery: Surgical outcomes and complications in 123 consecutive patients. J Clin Neurosci 2017;44:310–4.

22. Kuga D, Toda M, Ozawa H, et al. Endoscopic endonasal approach combined with a simultaneous transcranial approach for giant pituitary tumors. World Neurosurg 2019;121:173–9.

23. Yang MS, Hong JW, Lee SK, et al. Clinical management and outcome of 36 invasive prolactinomas treated with dopamine agonist. J Neurooncol 2011;104(1): 195–204.

24. Yano S, Hide T, Shinojima N. Efficacy and complications of endoscopic skull base surgery for giant pituitary adenomas. World Neurosurg 2017;99:533–42.

25. Zhang Y, Xu B, Jiang J, et al. [Treatment for giant pituitary adenomas through transcranial approach in a series of 112 consecutive patients]. Zhonghua Wai Ke Za Zhi 2015;53(3):197–201.

26. Sinha S, Sarkari A, Mahapatra AK, et al. Pediatric giant pituitary adenomas: are they different from adults? A clinical analysis of a series of 12 patients. Childs Nerv Syst 2014;30(8):1405–11.

27. Liu J, Li C, Xiao Q, et al. Comparison of pituitary adenomas in elderly and younger adults: clinical characteristics, surgical outcomes, and prognosis. J Am Geriatr Soc 2015;63(9):1924–30.
28. Maiter D, Delgrange E. Therapy of endocrine disease: the challenges in managing giant prolactinomas. Eur J Endocrinol 2014;170(6):R213–27.
29. Delgrange E, Trouillas J, Maiter D, et al. Sex-related difference in the growth of prolactinomas: a clinical and proliferation marker study. J Clin Endocrinol Metab 1997;82(7):2102–7.
30. Iglesias P, Arcano K, Trivino V, et al. Giant non-functioning pituitary adenoma: clinical characteristics and therapeutic outcomes. Exp Clin Endocrinol Diabetes 2021;129(4):309–13.
31. Chacko G, Chacko AG, Lombardero M, et al. Clinicopathologic correlates of giant pituitary adenomas. J Clin Neurosci 2009;16(5):660–5.
32. Madsen H, Borges TM, Knox AJ, et al. Giant pituitary adenomas: pathologic-radiographic correlations and lack of role for p53 and MIB-1 labeling. Am J Surg Pathol 2011;35(8):1204–13.
33. Chang CY, Luo CB, Teng MM, et al. Computed tomography and magnetic resonance imaging characteristics of giant pituitary adenomas. J Formos Med Assoc 2000;99(11):833–8.
34. Nishioka H, Hara T, Nagata Y, et al. Inherent tumor characteristics that limit effective and safe resection of giant nonfunctioning pituitary adenomas. World Neurosurg 2017;106:645–52.
35. Gokalp HZ, Deda H, Attar A, et al. The neurosurgical management of prolactinomas. J Neurosurg Sci 2000;44(3):128–32.
36. Garibi J, Pomposo I, Villar G, et al. Giant pituitary adenomas: clinical characteristics and surgical results. Br J Neurosurg 2002;16(2):133–9.
37. Barzaghi LR, Losa M, Giovanelli M, et al. Complications of transsphenoidal surgery in patients with pituitary adenoma: experience at a single centre. Acta Neurochir (Wien) 2007;149(9):877–85.
38. Azab WA, Nasim K, Abdelnabi EA, et al. Endoscopic endonasal excision of large and giant pituitary adenomas: radiological and intraoperative correlates of the extent of resection. World Neurosurg 2019;126:e793–802.
39. Batista RL, Trarbach EB, Marques MD, et al. Nonfunctioning pituitary adenoma recurrence and its relationship with sex, size, and hormonal immunohistochemical profile. World Neurosurg 2018;120:e241–6.
40. Koutourousiou M, Gardner PA, Fernandez-Miranda JC, et al. Endoscopic endonasal surgery for giant pituitary adenomas: advantages and limitations. J Neurosurg 2013;118(3):621–31.
41. Yildirim AE, Sahinoglu M, Ekici I, et al. Nonfunctioning pituitary adenomas are really clinically nonfunctioning? clinical and endocrinological symptoms and outcomes with endoscopic endonasal treatment. World Neurosurg 2016;85:185–92.
42. Ogawa Y, Ikeda H, Tominaga T. Clinicopathological study of prognostic factors in patients with pituitary adenomas and Ki-67 labeling index of more than 3. J Endocrinol Invest 2009;32(7):581–4.
43. Rahimli T, Hidayetov T, Yusifli Z, et al. Endoscopic endonasal approach to giant pituitary adenomas: surgical outcomes and review of the literature. World Neurosurg 2021;149:e1043–55.
44. Han YL, Chen DM, Zhang C, et al. Retrospective analysis of 52 patients with prolactinomas following endoscopic endonasal transsphenoidal surgery. Medicine (Baltimore) 2018;97(45):e13198.

45. Zheng Y, Chen DM, Wang Y, et al. Surgical management of growth hormone-secreting pituitary adenomas: a retrospective analysis of 33 patients. Medicine (Baltimore) 2020;99(19):e19855.

46. Chohan MO, Levin AM, Singh R, et al. Three-dimensional volumetric measurements in defining endoscope-guided giant adenoma surgery outcomes. Pituitary 2016;19(3):311–21.

47. Black PM, Zervas NT, Candia G. Management of large pituitary adenomas by transsphenoidal surgery. Surg Neurol 1988;29(6):443–7.

48. Sinha S, Sharma BS. Giant pituitary adenomas–an enigma revisited. Microsurgical treatment strategies and outcome in a series of 250 patients. Br J Neurosurg 2010;24(1):31–9.

49. Ilovayskaya IA, Dreval AV, Krivosheeva YG, et al. [Clinical and functional characteristics of giant pituitary adenomas in the population of patients in the Moscow region]. Zh Vopr Neirokhir Im N N Burdenko 2018;82(6):76–81.

50. Landeiro JA, Fonseca EO, Monnerat AL, et al. Nonfunctioning giant pituitary adenomas: Invasiveness and recurrence. Surg Neurol Int 2015;6:179.

51. Peto I, Abou-Al-Shaar H, White TG, et al. Sources of residuals after endoscopic transsphenoidal surgery for large and giant pituitary adenomas. Acta Neurochir (Wien) 2020;162(10):2341–51.

52. Chabot JD, Chakraborty S, Imbarrato G, et al. Evaluation of outcomes after endoscopic endonasal surgery for large and giant pituitary macroadenoma: a retrospective review of 39 consecutive patients. World Neurosurg 2015;84(4):978–88.

53. Chibbaro S, Signorelli F, Milani D, et al. Primary Endoscopic Endonasal Management of Giant Pituitary Adenomas: Outcome and Pitfalls from a Large Prospective Multicenter Experience. Cancers (Basel) 2021;13(14):3603.

54. Joshi SM, Chopra IS, Powell M. Hydrocephalus caused by giant pituitary tumors: case series and guidelines for management. Br J Neurosurg 2009;23(1):30–2.

55. Beriat GK, Dogan C, Akmansu SH, et al. A rare cause of nasal obstruction: giant invasive nonfunctioning pituitary adenoma. Kulak Burun Bogaz Ihtis Derg 2010;20(6):309–13.

56. Prawira A, Lazinski D, Siu LL, et al. Giant prolactinoma presenting as a base of skull tumor with nasopharyngeal extension: a potential diagnostic pitfall in neuroendocrine lesions of the base of skull. Head Neck Pathol 2017;11(4):537–40.

57. Abe D, Ogiwara T, Nakamura T, et al. Treatment strategy for giant invasive macroprolactinoma with spontaneous cerebrospinal fluid rhinorrhea: a case report and literature review. World Neurosurg 2020;144:19–23.

58. Zaben MJ, Harrisson SE, Mathad NV. Giant prolactinoma causing craniocervical junction instability: a case report. Br J Neurosurg 2011;25(6):754–6.

59. Zhang R, Wang Z, Gao L, et al. Clinical characteristics and postoperative recovery of hypopituitarism in patients with nonfunctional pituitary adenoma. World Neurosurg 2019;126:e1183–9.

60. Wilson CB. A decade of pituitary microsurgery. The Herbert Olivecrona lecture. J Neurosurg 1984;61(5):814–33.

61. Knosp E, Steiner E, Kitz K, et al. Pituitary adenomas with invasion of the cavernous sinus space: a magnetic resonance imaging classification compared with surgical findings. Neurosurgery 1993;33(4):610–7.

62. Micko AS, Wohrer A, Wolfsberger S, et al. Invasion of the cavernous sinus space in pituitary adenomas: endoscopic verification and its correlation with an MRI-based classification. J Neurosurg 2015;122(4):803–11.

63. Lv L, Hu Y, Yin S, et al. Giant prolactinomas: outcomes of multimodal treatments for 42 cases with long-term follow-up. Exp Clin Endocrinol Diabetes 2019; 127(5):295–302.

64. Shimon I, Sosa E, Mendoza V, et al. Giant prolactinomas larger than 60 mm in size: a cohort of massive and aggressive prolactin-secreting pituitary adenomas. Pituitary 2016;19(4):429–36.

65. Moraes AB, Silva CM, Vieira Neto L, et al. Giant prolactinomas: the therapeutic approach. Clin Endocrinol (Oxf) 2013;79(4):447–56.

66. Andujar-Plata P, Villar-Taibo R, Ballesteros-Pomar MD, et al. Long-term outcome of multimodal therapy for giant prolactinomas. Endocrine 2017;55(1):231–8.

67. Yu C, Wu Z, Gong J. Combined treatment of invasive giant prolactinomas. Pituitary 2005;8(1):61–5.

68. Shrivastava RK, Arginteanu MS, King WA, et al. Giant prolactinomas: clinical management and long-term follow up. J Neurosurg 2002;97(2):299–306.

69. Koguchi M, Nakahara Y, Ebashi R, et al. Status epilepticus induced by treatment with dopamine agonist therapy for giant prolactinoma: a case report. J Med Case Rep 2019;13(1):18.

70. Dhanwal DK, Sharma AK. Brain and optic chiasmal herniations into sella after cabergoline therapy of giant prolactinoma. Pituitary 2011;14(4):384–7.

71. Kalinin PL, Shkarubo AN, Astafieva LI, et al. [Cerebrospinal fluid rhinorrhea in primary treatment of large and giant prolactinomas with dopamine agonists]. Zh Vopr Neirokhir Im N N Burdenko 2017;81(6):32–9.

72. Lv L, Hu Y, Zhou P, et al. Presurgical treatment with somatostatin analogues in growth hormone-secreting pituitary adenomas: a long-term single-center experience. Clin Neurol Neurosurg 2018;167:24–30.

73. Shimon I, Jallad RS, Fleseriu M, et al. Giant GH-secreting pituitary adenomas: management of rare and aggressive pituitary tumors. Eur J Endocrinol 2015; 172(6):707–13.

74. Minniti G, Scaringi C, Poggi M, et al. Fractionated stereotactic radiotherapy for large and invasive non-functioning pituitary adenomas: long-term clinical outcomes and volumetric MRI assessment of tumor response. Eur J Endocrinol 2015;172(4):433–41.

75. Zhao K, Liu X, Liu D, et al. Fractionated gamma knife surgery for giant pituitary adenomas. Clin Neurol Neurosurg 2016;150:139–42.

76. Agrawal A, Cincu R, Goel A. Current concepts and controversies in the management of non-functioning giant pituitary macroadenomas. Clin Neurol Neurosurg 2007;109(8):645–50.

77. Fisher BJ, Gaspar LE, Noone B. Giant pituitary adenomas: role of radiotherapy. Int J Radiat Oncol Biol Phys 1993;25(4):677–81.

78. Yildiz F, Zorlu F, Erbas T, et al. Radiotherapy in the management of giant pituitary adenomas. Radiother Oncol 1999;52(3):233–7.

79. Nelson PB, Goodman ML, Flickenger JC, et al. Endocrine function in patients with large pituitary tumors treated with operative decompression and radiation therapy. Neurosurgery 1989;24(3):398–400.

80. Sankhla SK, Jayashankar N, Khan GM. Surgical management of selected pituitary macroadenomas using extended endoscopic endonasal transsphenoidal approach: early experience. Neurol India 2013;61(2):122–30.

81. Berkmann S, Schlaffer S, Nimsky C, et al. Intraoperative high-field MRI for trans-sphenoidal reoperations of nonfunctioning pituitary adenoma. J Neurosurg 2014;121(5):1166–75.
82. Goel A, Nadkarni T. Surgical management of giant pituitary tumours–a review of 30 cases. Acta Neurochir (Wien) 1996;138(9):1042–9.
83. Guo F, Song L, Bai J, et al. Successful treatment for giant pituitary adenomas through diverse transcranial approaches in a series of 15 consecutive patients. Clin Neurol Neurosurg 2012;114(7):885–90.
84. Han S, Gao W, Jing Z, et al. How to deal with giant pituitary adenomas: trans-sphenoidal or transcranial, simultaneous or two-staged? J Neurooncol 2017; 132(2):313–21.
85. Kuo CH, Yen YS, Wu JC, et al. Primary endoscopic transnasal transsphenoidal surgery for giant pituitary adenoma. World Neurosurg 2016;91:121–8.
86. Yang C, Zhang J, Li J, et al. The role of multimodal navigation in endoscopic en-donasal surgery for giant pituitary adenomas. Gland Surg 2019;8(6):663–73.
87. Cappabianca P, Cavallo LM, Solari D, et al. Size does not matter. The intrigue of giant adenomas: a true surgical challenge. Acta Neurochir (Wien) 2014;156(12): 2217–20.
88. de Divitiis E, de Divitiis O. Surgery for large pituitary adenomas: what is the best way? World Neurosurg 2012;77(3–4):448–50.
89. Cappabianca P, Cavallo LM, de Divitiis O, et al. Endoscopic endonasal extended approaches for the management of large pituitary adenomas. Neuro-surg Clin N Am 2015;26(3):323–31.
90. Wang F, Zhou T, Wei S, et al. Endoscopic endonasal transsphenoidal surgery of 1,166 pituitary adenomas. Surg Endosc 2015;29(6):1270–80.
91. Fallah N, Taghvaei M, Sadaghiani S, et al. Surgical outcome of endoscopic en-donasal surgery of large and giant pituitary adenomas: an institutional experi-ence from the Middle East. World Neurosurg 2019;132:e802–11.
92. Goel A, Shah A, Jhawar SS, et al. Fluid-fluid level in pituitary tumors: analysis of management of 106 cases. J Neurosurg 2010;112(6):1341–6.
93. Zhao B, Wei YK, Li GL, et al. Extended transsphenoidal approach for pituitary adenomas invading the anterior cranial base, cavernous sinus, and clivus: a single-center experience with 126 consecutive cases. J Neurosurg 2010; 112(1):108–17.
94. Woodworth GF, Patel KS, Shin B, et al. Surgical outcomes using a medial-to-lateral endonasal endoscopic approach to pituitary adenomas invading the cavernous sinus. J Neurosurg 2014;120(5):1086–94.
95. Hofstetter CP, Nanaszko MJ, Mubita LL, et al. Volumetric classification of pitui-tary macroadenomas predicts outcome and morbidity following endoscopic en-donasal transsphenoidal surgery. Pituitary 2012;15(3):450–63.
96. Ziu M, Dunn IF, Hess C, et al. Congress of neurological surgeons systematic re-view and evidence-based guideline on posttreatment follow-up evaluation of pa-tients with nonfunctioning pituitary adenomas. Neurosurgery 2016;79(4): E541–3.
97. Billings M, Dahlin R, Zampella B, et al. Conditions associated with giant pituitary tumors at the time of surgery effecting outcome morbidity and mortality. Surg Neurol Int 2019;10:92.
98. Goel A, Deogaonkar M, Desai K. Fatal postoperative 'pituitary apoplexy': its cause and management. Br J Neurosurg 1995;9(1):37–40.
99. Pezzutti DL, Magill ST, Albonette-Felicio T, et al. Endoscopic Endonasal Trans-tubercular Approach for Resection of Giant Pituitary Adenomas With

Subarachnoid Extension: The "Second Floor" Strategy to Avoid Postoperative Apoplexy. World Neurosurg 2021;153:e464–72.

100. Kurwale NS, Ahmad F, Suri A, et al. Post operative pituitary apoplexy: preoperative considerations toward preventing nightmare. Br J Neurosurg 2012;26(1):59–63.

101. Patel SK, Christiano LD, Eloy JA, et al. Delayed postoperative pituitary apoplexy after endoscopic transsphenoidal resection of a giant pituitary macroadenoma. J Clin Neurosci 2012;19(9):1296–8.

102. Omodaka S, Ogawa Y, Sato K, et al. Preoperative embolization and immediate removal of a giant pituitary adenoma: a case report. BMC Res Notes 2017;10(1):63.

103. Couldwell WT. Transsphenoidal and transcranial surgery for pituitary adenomas. J Neurooncol 2004;69(1–3):237–56.

104. Cohen-Gadol AA, Laws ER, Spencer DD, et al. The evolution of Harvey Cushing's surgical approach to pituitary tumors from transsphenoidal to transfrontal. J Neurosurg 2005;103(2):372–7.

105. Liu JK, Das K, Weiss MH, et al. The history and evolution of transsphenoidal surgery. J Neurosurg 2001;95(6):1083–96.

106. Hardy J. Transsphenoidal hypophysectomy. J Neurosurg 1971;34(4):582–94.

107. Komotar RJ, Starke RM, Raper DM, et al. Endoscopic endonasal compared with microscopic transsphenoidal and open transcranial resection of giant pituitary adenomas. Pituitary 2012;15(2):150–9.

108. Baumann F, Schmid C, Bernays RL. Intraoperative magnetic resonance imaging-guided transsphenoidal surgery for giant pituitary adenomas. Neurosurg Rev 2010;33(1):83–90.

109. Li J, Cong Z, Ji X, et al. Application of intraoperative magnetic resonance imaging in large invasive pituitary adenoma surgery. Asian J Surg 2015;38(3):168–73.

110. Wang RZ, Yin J, Su CB, et al. [Extended transsphenoidal operation for giant and invasive pituitary adenomas]. Zhonghua Wai Ke Za Zhi 2006;44(22):1548–50.

111. Bushe KA, Halves E. [Modified technique in transsphenoidal operations of pituitary adenomas. Technical note (author's transl)]. Acta Neurochir (Wien) 1978;41(1–3):163–75.

112. Jho HD, Carrau RL. Endoscopic endonasal transsphenoidal surgery: experience with 50 patients. J Neurosurg 1997;87(1):44–51.

113. Kalyvas A, Millesi M, Gentili F. Endoscopic extra-capsular resection of a giant pituitary adenoma: how I do it. Acta Neurochir (Wien) 2021;163(6):1711–5.

114. de Divitiis E, Cavallo LM, Cappabianca P, et al. Extended endoscopic endonasal transsphenoidal approach for the removal of suprasellar tumors: Part 2. Neurosurgery 2007;60(1):46–58.

115. Kutlay M, Durmaz A, Ozer I, et al. Extended endoscopic endonasal approach to the ventral skull base lesions. Clin Neurol Neurosurg 2018;167:129–40.

116. Kato T, Sawamura Y, Abe H. [Transsphenoidal-transtuberculum Sellae approach for supradiaphragmatic tumors]. No Shinkei Geka 1998;26(7):583–8.

117. Hadad G, Bassagasteguy L, Carrau RL, et al. A novel reconstructive technique after endoscopic expanded endonasal approaches: vascular pedicle nasoseptal flap. Laryngoscope 2006;116(10):1882–6.

118. Jamaluddin MA, Patel BK, George T, et al. Endoscopic Endonasal Approach for Giant Pituitary Adenoma Occupying the Entire Third Ventricle: Surgical Results and a Review of the Literature. World Neurosurg 2021;154:e254–63.

119. Pratheesh R, Rajaratnam S, Prabhu K, et al. The current role of transcranial surgery in the management of pituitary adenomas. Pituitary 2013;16(4):419–34.
120. Nishioka H, Hara T, Usui M, et al. Simultaneous combined supra-infrasellar approach for giant/large multilobulated pituitary adenomas. World Neurosurg 2012;77(3–4):533–9.
121. Musluman AM, Cansever T, Yilmaz A, et al. Surgical results of large and giant pituitary adenomas with special consideration of ophthalmologic outcomes. World Neurosurg 2011;76(1–2):141–8.
122. King WA, Rodts GE, Becker DP, et al. Microsurgical management of giant pituitary tumors. Skull Base Surg 1996;6(1):17–26.
123. Honegger J, Ernemann U, Psaras T, et al. Objective criteria for successful transsphenoidal removal of suprasellar nonfunctioning pituitary adenomas. A prospective study. Acta Neurochir (Wien) 2007;149(1):21–9.
124. Musleh W, Sonabend AM, Lesniak MS. Role of craniotomy in the management of pituitary adenomas and sellar/parasellar tumors. Expert Rev Anticancer Ther 2006;6(Suppl 9):S79–83.
125. Loyo M, Kleriga E, Mateos H, et al. Combined supra-infrasellar approach for large pituitary tumors. Neurosurgery 1984;14(4):485–8.
126. D'Ambrosio AL, Syed ON, Grobelny BT, et al. Simultaneous above and below approach to giant pituitary adenomas: surgical strategies and long-term follow-up. Pituitary 2009;12(3):217–25.
127. Leung GK, Law HY, Hung KN, et al. Combined simultaneous transcranial and transsphenoidal resection of large-to-giant pituitary adenomas. Acta Neurochir (Wien) 2011;153(7):1401–8.
128. Couldwell WT. Giant pituitary tumor combined approach. World Neurosurg 2012;77(3–4):451–2.
129. Leung GK, Yuen MM, Chow WS, et al. An endoscopic modification of the simultaneous 'above and below' approach to large pituitary adenomas. Pituitary 2012;15(2):237–41.
130. Greenfield JP, Leng LZ, Chaudhry U, et al. Combined simultaneous endoscopic transsphenoidal and endoscopic transventricular resection of a giant pituitary macroadenoma. Minim Invasive Neurosurg 2008;51(5):306–9.
131. Romano A, Chibbaro S, Marsella M, et al. Combined endoscopic transsphenoidal-transventricular approach for resection of a giant pituitary macroadenoma. World Neurosurg 2010;74(1):161–4.
132. Ojha BK, Husain M, Rastogi M, et al. Combined transsphenoidal and simultaneous trans-ventricular-endoscopic decompression of a giant pituitary adenoma: case report. Acta Neurochir (Wien) 2009;151(7):843–7.
133. Takeuchi K, Nagatani T, Watanabe T, et al. A purely endoscopic and simultaneous transsphenoidal and transcranial keyhole approach for giant pituitary adenoma resection: a technical case report. NMC Case Rep J 2015;2(3):101–5.

# Surgical Considerations in Endoscopic Pituitary Approaches for the Otolaryngologist

Timothy Fan, BS, Alan D. Workman, MD, MTR, Stacey T. Gray, MD*

## KEYWORDS

- Endoscopic • Transnasal • Transsphenoidal • Pituitary tumors • Pituitary surgery

## KEY POINTS

- Endoscopic endonasal surgery is the preferred approach to pituitary lesions, and it holds unique advantages over both microscopic surgeries and open techniques.
- Gain of functional space and adequate visualization are critical aspects of the endoscopic surgical approach.
- Transnasal transsphenoidal endoscopic surgery progresses through nasal, sphenoidal, and sellar stages, with important principles and nuances at each step.

## INTRODUCTION

### History

With immediate decompression and no systemic adverse effects, surgical resection is the first-line therapy for pituitary adenomas, besides prolactinomas.[1] Pituitary adenomas share intricate anatomic relationships with nearby neurovascular structures, rendering surgical resection challenging in inexperienced hands. In the past century, advances in surgical knowledge and technology propelled major changes in approaches to resection, skull base reconstruction, and instrumentation, progressively decreasing morbidity and mortality while increasing curative rates. The first transsphenoidal pituitary surgery was performed by Schloffer via a superior nasal route in 1907.[2] Two years later, Kanavel introduced an inferior nasal approach to reduce facial tissue resection and improve suprasellar visualization.[3] In 1910, Cushing standardized and popularized the sublabial transseptal transsphenoidal approach as well as the transfrontal transcranial approach for challenging operations.[4] Guiot incorporated

The authors have no conflicts of interest or any funding sources to declare.
Department of Otolaryngology – Head and Neck Surgery, Harvard Medical School, Massachusetts Eye and Ear Infirmary, 243 Charles Street, Boston, MA 02114, USA
* Corresponding author.
E-mail address: Stacey_Gray@meei.harvard.edu

radiofluoroscopy and the microscope in pituitary surgeries in 1971, refining the resection accuracy without sacrificing normal pituitary tissue.[5] In 1992, Jankowski performed the first transsphenoidal pituitary surgery with an endoscope to improve peripheral and superior field visualization, further optimizing the operative safety profile.[6]

The introduction of the endoscopic approach transformed pituitary surgery. In contrast to the microscope, the endoscope offers a panoramic view, eliminating traditional operative blind spots in the suprasellar and parasellar compartments.[7] The use of angled endoscopes, distal tip illumination, and lens irrigation systems provides ideal visualization and functional space for pituitary surgery.[7,8] The micro-Doppler can also be used to further ensure safety and accuracy.[9] Compared with traditional approaches, endoscopic transnasal transsphenoidal pituitary surgery minimizes tissue trauma and has been reported to improve postoperative outcomes, while minimizing operative risks and perioperative morbidity. Endoscopic pituitary surgery has been reported to result in decreased blood loss, increased gross tumor resection, faster visual improvement, better endocrine outcomes, quicker recovery, shorter hospitalization, lower health care costs, and lower rates of postoperative cerebrospinal fluid (CSF) leak, septal perforation, and epistaxis.[8,10–12] Previous experience with endoscopic sinonasal surgeries uniquely prepare otolaryngologists to excel at an endoscopic approach to assist neurosurgical colleagues with pituitary surgery.[13] It is this collaboration between Neurosurgery and Otolaryngology that is critical for successful outcomes, using the expertise of both specialties.

## Preoperative Preparation

Creation of a safe dissection field relies on hemostasis and accurate presurgical planning. Before the operation, the surgeon should inquire about potential bleeding disorders, abnormal coagulation studies, and hypertension. When possible, the patient should stop medications that interfere with normal platelet function, including aspirin, nonsteroidal antiinflammatory drugs, antiplatelet medications, anticoagulant medications, and herbal supplements.[14–16] Total intravascular anesthesia has been reported to prevent intranasal vasodilation and to lower mean arterial pressure and heart rate, both of which are contributors to increased intraoperative hemorrhage.[17] The application of topical intranasal vasoconstrictors, such as oxymetazoline and epinephrine, at the start of the case is also frequently used to decrease bleeding.

Careful presurgical preparation enhances intraoperative decision-making and optimizes surgical outcomes. Careful review of computed tomography (CT) and magnetic resonance imaging (MRI) images is essential for otolaryngologists and neurosurgeons to evaluate relevant anatomy, assess tumor size and location, and preemptively identify foreseeable complications. A plan for skull base reconstruction should also be reviewed preoperatively. For patients with a history of previous sinonasal and/or pituitary surgery, an in-office nasal examination may assist with identification of landmarks and detection of distorted anatomy. The choanal arch is an easily identifiable and consistent landmark, which can help with identification of the face of the sphenoid sinus.[18] The use of intraoperative neuronavigation (image guidance) is beneficial for maintaining midline orientation within the sphenoid sinus, which is crucial for safe and complete resection; however, understanding and recognition of anatomic surgical landmarks is absolutely necessary for successful surgery. Preoperative preparation is especially important in the setting of reoperation, where septal and intrasellar scarring, tumor spillage, and higher morbidity are anticipated.[19] When significant supra- and/or parasellar extension is discovered on imaging, extended approaches may be warranted.[20–22] Options for skull base reconstruction, including the availability of nasal tissue, should be assessed before surgery. As with any surgery, otolaryngologists should be well versed with the patient's medical history, anatomy, and have contingency plans in place for complications before each pituitary surgery. It is especially important to have a preoperative plan in place for an intraoperative vascular injury, and this should be discussed with the team ahead of time. Should a vascular injury occur, it is critical to have the necessary supplies available to address the injury immediately and to have each team member understand their role during such a complication.

*Application*

Endoscopic pituitary surgeries may be performed with a 2-, 3-, or 4-handed approach via uninostril or binostril approaches. Uninostril entry is less invasive and can be appropriate for smaller and noncomplicated pituitary adenomas. In addition, for patients with significant unilateral nasal pathology (such as significant septal deviation), a uninostril approach may be suitable to minimize disrupting the existing structures. Large pituitary adenomas with supra- or parasellar extension, fibrous consistency, or revision surgery often prompt the need for binostril access. In general, a binostril approach offers maneuverability for 2-surgeon 4-handed surgery, but specific choices depend on patient characteristics and surgeon preferences. Although brief operative considerations are described in this article, the specific techniques and equipment used vary among otolaryngologists. Endoscopic transnasal transsphenoidal pituitary surgeries proceed through nasal, sphenoidal, and sellar stages, with special considerations for each step (**Box 1**). In addition to considering the extent of surgery necessary, care should be taken to avoid secondary injury to nasal tissue in order to preserve normal sinonasal function. Plans for skull base reconstruction, including the need for a nasoseptal flap, should also be determined before any surgical dissection.

*Surgical Considerations: Nasal Stage*

Adapting surgical approaches for unique nasal anatomy and conditions is vital for success. The nasal stage extends from the nostril to the sphenoidal ostium. At the start of surgery, bilateral inferior and middle turbinates, nasal septum, and posterior choana are identified and examined. The posterior nasal septum, superior turbinates, and sphenoidal ostium can be identified with advancement of the endoscope. The nasal cavity should be carefully examined for scarring, polyps, septal spurs, deviations, or perforation. Purulent acute rhinosinusitis, as well as fungal debris, should be ruled out or medically treated before pituitary surgery to reduce the risk of intracranial infections.[23] In contrast, mild-to-moderate chronic rhinosinusitis has not been shown to cause increased adverse complications and should have no impact on proceeding with pituitary surgery.[23] For severe chronic rhinosinusitis, preoperative medical therapy, including topical steroid administration and the use of saline irrigations may reduce inflammation, decrease bleeding, and improve visualization for endoscopic nasal surgery.[24,25] If additional intranasal operative space is required and/or enlarged middle turbinate is encountered, the middle turbinate may be out-fractured and lateralized or partially resected.[8] In the case of septal deviation, typically this can be addressed at the time of pituitary surgery, although it is important to note that nasoseptal flaps may be needed for reconstruction, and active intraoperative preservation of the mucosa will be necessary.

  If reconstruction with a nasoseptal flap is planned, avoiding injury to the septal mucosa as well as the posterior septal branch of the sphenopalatine artery is crucial. A posterior septectomy is often performed for binostril communication. During this stage, the location of the posterior septal artery, a branch of the sphenopalatine artery,

---

**Box 1**
**Special considerations for the nasal, sphenoidal, and sellar stages of pituitary surgery**

Nasal stage
1. Supine reverse Trendelenburg is the best operative position for nasal cavity access.
2. The middle turbinate should be lateralized or partially resected to maximize intranasal visualization.
3. A posterior nasal septectomy may offer additional functional space for accessing the sphenoid sinus.
4. Purulent acute rhinosinusitis should be medically treated before pituitary surgery, whereas mild chronic rhinosinusitis has not been shown to be associated with complications.
5. Actively preserve nasal septal tissue in preparation for potential nasoseptal flap reconstruction.

Sphenoidal stage
1. Great variations exist in sphenoid sinus size, shape, septation, and pneumatization pattern, and preoperative planning is essential to success.
2. Degree of sphenoidal pneumatization is the most important indicator of ease of access to the sella.
3. Maintain midline orientation during the surgery to avoid iatrogenic injuries.
4. Pneumatization patterns, Onodi cells, and the presence of macroadenoma may alter the distance between the sphenoid sinus and neighboring structures.
5. Prevent fracturing of the sphenoidal septum to avoid injury to the ICA.

Sellar stage
1. Angled endoscopes can prove optimal for sellar visualization.
2. Preoperative imaging is essential to rule out "kissing carotids."
3. Micro-Doppler can be used to prevent injury to the ICA.
4. Up to 90% of normal pituitary tissue may be sacrificed with maintenance of normal pituitary function.
5. An extended endonasal approach may be necessary to offer wider access to remove large, fibrous, expanding, or "dumbbell"-shaped tumors.

*Abbreviation:* ICA, internal carotid artery.

---

which is located inferior to the sphenoid ostium, should be identified and protected to avoid inadvertent injury. Sufficient bony septum should be left superiorly and inferiorly as midline markers. The anterior extent of posterior nasal septectomy varies depending on required space, and a large portion of the posterior nasal septum may be removed without adverse effect.[26] Once adequate presphenoid space is achieved, the sphenoidal opening can be expanded for further entry.

### Surgical Considerations: Sphenoidal Stage

Sphenoid sinus anatomy may differ substantially between patients. Preoperative imaging is critical for studying the dimensions of the sphenoid sinus, sellar floor curvature, septation configurations, and pneumatization patterns. The degree of sphenoidal pneumatization is the most important indicator for successful sellar access.[27] Sphenoid sinus pneumatization is generally completed by the age of 10 years and can be divided into conchal, presellar, sellar, and postsellar subtypes in increasing pneumatization order. Conchal and presellar sphenoid sinuses require more extensive drilling to achieve pituitary access and carry higher iatrogenic risks.[27] For macropituitary (≥1 cm) adenomas with conchal or presellar sphenoid subtypes, an open approach should be considered.[27] Conversely, overpneumatization, as seen in the postsellar subtype, may distort normal anatomy, shortening the distances between the operative field and the optic nerves, carotid arteries, and intracranial space.[28]

The intrasphenoidal septum varies greatly in shape, location, and attachment site, with up to 40% of patients having lateral deviation with termination of the septum over the internal carotid artery (ICA).[29] During removal of the septum, fracturing of the septum should be avoided to prevent transferring force to its attaching structures. Onodi cells are posterior ethmoidal air cells located superolateral to the sphenoid sinus, which may distort and narrow the sphenoid face and often require opening surgically before dissecting within the sphenoid sinus to improve access to the pituitary.[30] Up to 10% of patients have a flat or nonprominent sellar floor, and neuronavigation confirmation of operative position is required.[31] In addition, macroadenomas may lead to expansion of the sellar space and thinning of the sellar floor, which should be accounted for before opening the sella.

On entry to the sphenoid sinus, the cavity should be endoscopically inspected. Creating a large opening into the sphenoid with removal of the face of the sphenoid helps substantially with visualization. The intrasphenoidal septum is then identified and resected. The attachment of the intrasphenoidal septum should be identified on preoperative imaging. If it is near or attaches to the ICA, drilling the intersinus septum is preferred to avoid traction injury. Once the sella is visible, the sphenoidal mucosa is removed to visualize the posterior sphenoid sinus wall and the sellar floor. It is important to identify surgical landmarks, including the sellar prominence, tuberculum sphenoidale and planum sphenoidale, clivus, bony prominences of the optic nerve and carotid artery, and the opticocarotid recess.

### Surgical Considerations: Sellar Stage

The sellar floor is often weakened by pituitary adenomas. After access is obtained, it is important to locate the cavernous sinuses and associated contents bilaterally and the anterior intercavernous sinus anteriorly. The average inter-ICA distance is 12 to 30 mm, but some patients may have a shorter distance, and this can be determined preoperatively using imaging studies to decrease potential injury during dissection.[21] The specific course of the ICA may be confirmed and traced with a micro-Doppler intraoperatively.

Patients with bulky, firm, invasive, or "dumbbell"-shaped tumors into supra- and parasellar compartments may need an extended endonasal approach for wide access. In this approach, the tuberculum sellae, planum sphenoidale, opticocarotid recess, and anterior sphenoid sinus wall down to the medial pterygoid plates may be surgically removed. Thirty- and seventy-degree endoscopes are used to provide improved visualization for tumor removal by the neurosurgeon. Although extended exposure techniques carry higher risks for postoperative CSF leak, it allows for direct visualization and exposure, with the potential for rapid hemorrhage control.

### Future Directions

The introduction of endoscopy has significantly enhanced the efficiency and efficacy of pituitary surgery, but limitations exist. Endoscopic vision is monocular, and 3-dimensional (3D) appreciation of the operative field is limited. Recent improvements in technology aim to address these common shortcomings and expand the capabilities of the endoscope. In a recent trial, usage of camera lenses overlying visual fields to provide better 3D depth perception was shown to decrease training time, operative length, and errors for endoscopic surgeries.[32] The incorporation of augmented reality into neuronavigation was additionally used to provide more accurate intraoperative guidance.[33] Huang and colleagues found 3D printed anatomic models to be a valuable resource for visual and tactile learners, and preoperative usage decreased blood loss and operative time in a trial of 20 patients.[34] A multimodality image-guided operating suite combined neuronavigation, micro-Doppler, and intraoperative MRI in one setting, which resulted in 20% higher gross total resection for pituitary macroadenomas.[35]

## SUMMARY

Since its introduction, the endoscope has minimized morbidity in pituitary surgery compared with traditional open techniques and has improved accuracy and curative rates compared with traditional microscopic procedures. Otolaryngologists, with rich experience in endoscopic sinonasal surgery, are naturally suited to assist with endoscopic endonasal pituitary approaches. Although recent advancements have made pituitary surgeries quicker and more effective, mindful presurgical planning and intraoperative attention to detail remain vital components to patient safety.

## CLINICS CARE POINTS

- Careful review of preoperative CT and MRI images is essential to evaluate relevant anatomy, assess tumor size and location, and preemptively identify foreseeable complications.

- In addition to considering extent of surgery, care should be taken to avoid secondary injury to nasal tissue in order to preserve normal sinonasal function. Plans for skull base reconstruction, including the need for a nasoseptal flap, should also be determined before surgical dissection.

- Sphenoid sinus anatomy may differ substantially between patients. Preoperative imaging is critical for studying the dimensions of the sphenoid sinus, sellar floor curvature, septation configurations, and pneumatization patterns.

- Patients with bulky, firm, invasive, or "dumbbell"-shaped tumors into supra- and parasellar compartments may need an extended endonasal approach for wide access.

## REFERENCES

1. Molitch ME. Dopamine resistance of prolactinomas. Pituitary 2003;6(1):19–27.
2. Schloffer H. Erfolgreiche operation eines hypophysentumors auf nasalem Wege. Wien Klin Wochenschr 1907;20:621–4.
3. Kanavel AB. The removal of tumors of the pituitary body by an infranasal route: a proposed operation with a description of the technique. J Am Med Assoc 1909; 53:1704–7.
4. Cushing H. The weir mitchell lecture: surgical experiences with pituitary disorders. J Am Med Assoc 1914;LXIII(18):1515–25. https://doi.org/10.1001/jama.1914.02570180001001.
5. Guiot G, Thibaut B. L'exérèse des adénomes de l'hypophyse par voie trans-sphénoïdale. Adénomes Hypophysaires. Paris: Masson; 1958. p. 165–80.
6. Jankowski R, Auque J, Simon C, et al. Endoscopic pituitary tumor surgery. Laryngoscope 1992;102(2):198–202.
7. Sharma BS, Sawarkar DP, Suri A. Endoscopic pituitary surgery: techniques, tips and tricks, nuances, and complication avoidance. Neurol India 2016;64(4): 724–36.
8. Castaño-Leon AM, Paredes I, Munarriz PM, et al. Endoscopic transnasal transsphenoidal approach for pituitary adenomas: a comparison to the microscopic approach cohort by propensity score analysis. Neurosurgery 2020;86(3):348–56.
9. Dolati P, Eichberg D, Golby A, et al. Multimodal navigation in endoscopic transsphenoidal resection of pituitary tumors using image-based vascular and cranial

nerve segmentation: a prospective validation study. World Neurosurg 2016;95: 406–13.

10. Kahilogullari G, Beton S, Al-Beyati ESM, et al. Olfactory functions after transsphenoidal pituitary surgery: endoscopic versus microscopic approach. Laryngoscope 2013;123(9):2112–9.

11. Zaidi HA, Awad A-W, Bohl MA, et al. Comparison of outcomes between a less experienced surgeon using a fully endoscopic technique and a very experienced surgeon using a microscopic transsphenoidal technique for pituitary adenoma. J Neurosurg 2016;124(3):596–604.

12. Oosmanally N, Paul JE, Zanation AM, et al. Comparative analysis of cost of endoscopic endonasal minimally invasive and sublabial-transseptal approaches to the pituitary. Int Forum Allergy Rhinol 2011;1(4):242–9.

13. O'Malley BW, Grady MS, Gabel BC, et al. Comparison of endoscopic and microscopic removal of pituitary adenomas: single-surgeon experience and the learning curve. Neurosurg Focus 2008;25(6):E10.

14. Stokken JK, Halderman A, Recinos PF, et al. Strategies for improving visualization during endoscopic skull base surgery. Otolaryngol Clin North Am 2016;49(1): 131–40.

15. Douketis JD, Spyropoulos AC, Spencer FA, et al. Perioperative management of antithrombotic therapy: antithrombotic therapy and prevention of thrombosis, 9th ed: american college of chest physicians evidence-based clinical practice guidelines. Chest 2012;141(2 Suppl):e326S–50S.

16. Hodges PJ, Kam PCA. The peri-operative implications of herbal medicines. Anaesthesia 2002;57(9):889–99.

17. Wormald PJ, van Renen G, Perks J, et al. The effect of the total intravenous anesthesia compared with inhalational anesthesia on the surgical field during endoscopic sinus surgery. Am J Rhinol 2005;19(5):514–20.

18. Levine CG, Casiano RR. Revision functional endoscopic sinus surgery. Otolaryngol Clin North Am 2017;50(1):143–64.

19. Cappabianca P, Alfieri A, Colao A, et al. Endoscopic endonasal transsphenoidal surgery in recurrent and residual pituitary adenomas: technical note. Minim Invasive Neurosurg 2000;43(1):38–43.

20. Lobo B, Zhang X, Barkhoudarian G, et al. Endonasal endoscopic management of parasellar and cavernous sinus meningiomas. Neurosurg Clin N Am 2015;26(3): 389–401.

21. Renn WH, Rhoton AL. Microsurgical anatomy of the sellar region. J Neurosurg 1975;43(3):288–98.

22. Dhandapani S, Singh H, Negm HM, et al. Cavernous sinus invasion in pituitary adenomas: systematic review and pooled data meta-analysis of radiologic criteria and comparison of endoscopic and microscopic surgery. World Neurosurg 2016;96:36–46.

23. Nyquist GG, Friedel ME, Singhal S, et al. Surgical management of rhinosinusitis in endoscopic-endonasal skull-base surgery. Int Forum Allergy Rhinol 2015;5(4): 339–43.

24. Ecevit MC, Erdag TK, Dogan E, et al. Effect of steroids for nasal polyposis surgery: a placebo-controlled, randomized, double-blind study. Laryngoscope 2015;125(9):2041–5.

25. Gan EC, Alsaleh S, Manji J, et al. Hemostatic effect of hot saline irrigation during functional endoscopic sinus surgery: a randomized controlled trial. Int Forum Allergy Rhinol 2014;4(11):877–84.

26. Lucas JW, Zada G. Endoscopic surgery for pituitary tumors. Neurosurg Clin N Am 2012;23(4):555–69.
27. Hamid O, El Fiky L, Hassan O, et al. Anatomic variations of the sphenoid sinus and their impact on trans-sphenoid pituitary surgery. Skull Base 2008;18(1):9–15.
28. Sirikci A, Bayazit YA, Bayram M, et al. Variations of sphenoid and related structures. Eur Radiol 2000;10(5):844–8.
29. Sethi DS, Stanley RE, Pillay PK. Endoscopic anatomy of the sphenoid sinus and sella turcica. J Laryngol Otol 1995;109(10):951–5.
30. Otto BA, Bowe SN, Carrau RL, et al. Transsphenoidal approach with nasoseptal flap pedicle transposition: modified rescue flap technique. Laryngoscope 2013; 123(12):2976–9.
31. Zada G, Agarwalla PK, Mukundan S, et al. The neurosurgical anatomy of the sphenoid sinus and sellar floor in endoscopic transsphenoidal surgery. J Neurosurg 2011;114(5):1319–30.
32. Bickerton R, Nassimizadeh A-K, Ahmed S. Three-dimensional endoscopy: the future of nasoendoscopic training. Laryngoscope 2019;129(6):1280–5.
33. Besharati Tabrizi L, Mahvash M. Augmented reality-guided neurosurgery: accuracy and intraoperative application of an image projection technique. J Neurosurg 2015;123(1):206–11.
34. Huang X, Liu Z, Wang X, et al. A small 3D-printing model of macroadenomas for endoscopic endonasal surgery. Pituitary 2019;22(1):46–53.
35. Zaidi HA, De Los Reyes K, Barkhoudarian G, et al. The utility of high-resolution intraoperative MRI in endoscopic transsphenoidal surgery for pituitary macroadenomas: early experience in the Advanced Multimodality Image Guided Operating suite. Neurosurg Focus 2016;40(3):E18.

# Surgical Considerations in Endoscopic Pituitary Dissection for the Neurosurgeon

Chikezie I. Eseonu, MD

## KEYWORDS

• Pituitary • Tumor • Endoscopic • Adenoma • Sella • Endonasal

## KEY POINTS

- Many surgical considerations exist for an endoscopic approach for pituitary surgery for a neurosurgeon.
- Careful surgical planning and evaluation of the patient's anatomy, meticulous surgical technique and sellar reconstruction, and anticipating complications aid in achieving a successful surgical experience.
- Tumor characteristic considerations, such as size, invasiveness, and consistency should all be considered when planning a surgical approach.

## INTRODUCTION

The neurosurgical approach to endoscopic pituitary dissection requires proper surgical planning and identification of relevant anatomic structures. With the introduction of the endoscope for transsphenoidal pituitary tumor surgery, better visualization and more intricate surgical resections are achieved. Whether performing this surgery solo or with the assistance of an otolaryngologist for sinonasal access, the neurosurgeon must consider multiple aspects for this surgical approach. This article focuses on the surgical considerations involving the anatomic regions of the sphenoid sinus and sellar region for endoscopic pituitary dissections.

## POSITIONING

Proper positioning for endoscopic pituitary surgery is essential for optimizing visualization and maintaining a comfortable posture while operating. The patient should be resting in a supine position, with the head maintained in a parallel position to the floor. The head can also be anteriorly translated toward the surgeon to allow for the surgery to be done in a comfortable position.[1] Slight neck flexion can allow for gravity to help

Neurosurgery & Neuroscience Institute, University of Pittsburgh Medical Center Central Pennsylvania, 205 South Front Street, 6th Floor, Suite 6A, Harrisburg, PA 17104, USA
*E-mail address:* eseonuci@upmc.edu

Otolaryngol Clin N Am 55 (2022) 389–395
https://doi.org/10.1016/j.otc.2021.12.009
0030-6665/22/© 2022 Elsevier Inc. All rights reserved.

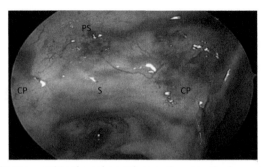

**Fig. 1.** Wide visualization within the sphenoid sinus showing the bony anatomic structures. C, clivus; CP, carotid prominence; OR, opticocarotid recess; PS, planum sphenoidale; S, sella.

bring down any suprasellar components of the tumor.[2] The ipsilateral arm should be tucked by the patient's side, whereas the contralateral arm is tucked or left on an armboard in cases where both surgeons are standing on the ipsilateral side.[3] In cases where the neurosurgeon and otolaryngologist are standing on opposite sides, both arms should be tucked. Additionally, 10° to 15° of flexion is made at the waist and knees to reduce positional pressure at those locations.[2]

**SPHENOID SINUS/SELLA**

Following the nasal exposure done by the otolaryngologist, opening and exposure of the sphenoid sinus and sella are important for determining the extent of visualization that will be available during the tumor resection.

*Sphenoid Sinus Considerations*

The amount of pneumatization of the sphenoid sinus is important to understand, because greater pneumatization allows for easier identification of bony protuberances in the sphenoid sinus, aiding in identifying anatomic structures (**Fig. 1**).[4] Multiple variations of the sphenoid sinus are found; a normal sinus is found in 80% to 86% of the population; a presellar sinus, with minimal pneumatization, is found in 10% to 20%; and a conchal, or no pneumatization is found in 0% to 3% (**Fig. 2**).[5,6] For presellar or conchal sphenoid sinuses, most bony landmarks are not well visualized, which can make it difficult to identify and remove the tuberculum or planum, if additional exposure is needed for a suprasellar lesion. Poor understanding of these structures can put the optic nerves and intracavernous sinus at risk.[4]

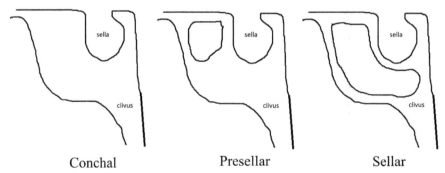

Conchal                    Presellar                    Sellar

**Fig. 2.** Sagittal view showing the types of sphenoid sinus pneumatization in relation to the sella turcica. Conchal has no pneumatization, presellar has pneumatization anterior to the sella, and sellar pneumatization has pneumatization beyond the anterior wall of the sella.

After the opening of the sphenoid sinus, the sella is then exposed. The thickness of the sella bone is assessed to determine whether the drill or a 1- or 2-mm Kerrison rongeur is needed for sellar bone removal. Using the drill and/or Kerrison, the anterior wall of the sella is exposed. The bony opening should expand from one cavernous sinus to the other cavernous sinus laterally, and from the tuberculum sella to the dorsum sella in the anterior-posterior direction. Expansive sellar bony opening allows for full visualization of the intrasellar space during tumor removal.

### Chiasm Considerations

The position of the optic chiasm can influence the surgical approach during sella bone removal. A prefixed chiasm, seen in 5% to 15% of patients, can position the optic chiasm close to the diaphragma sella. This inferior position of the chiasm is at higher risk of injury during the removal of the anterosuperior portion of the sellar floor.[4] For normal and postfixed positioned optic chiasms, the chiasm is located along the posterior aspect of the diaphragma sella, close to or behind the dorsum sellae. This allows for easier access to the suprasellar components of a pituitary tumor given the longer intracranial course of the optic nerves away from the central trajectory used to resect the tumor. The normal and postfixed chiasm positions pose little threat for being damaged during sella bony opening.[4]

Once the sella bone has been removed, the dura mater can then be coagulated using bipolar forceps. The dura can then be incised in a cross shape or circumferentially. If a crossed-shaped incision is used, the incision should start laterally and work medially toward the intersection point to reduce the risk of damaging the laterally placed cavernous sinus.

### TUMOR RESECTION

Once the dura mater of the sella has been removed, tumor removal can begin. Accurate identification of tumor versus normal pituitary tissue is aided by use of gentle suctioning and a ring curette. Oftentimes, tumor tissue is soft with a yellowish white color, whereas the normal anterior pituitary is firm with a pink-orange color and the posterior pituitary is firm with a white color. Pituitary forceps are used for sampling specimens for pathology.[7]

Initial tumor resection should focus on the inferior and posterior component of the tumor to allow for the superior and anterior components of the tumor to descend into the sellar space with the aid of gravity. Angled endoscopes, curved suctions, and angled ring curettes are used as needed for access to these spaces. Next, the lateral borders of the tumor are resected. Care should be taken once the lateral tumor component is removed and the medial wall of the cavernous sinus is exposed. Normal pituitary tissue can begin to be visualized and should be preserved. Next, the rostral portion of the tumor is removed with curved suction and angled ring curettes. As the rostral tumor component is removed, additional pituitary tissue or arachnoid membrane may be visualized descending into the sellar space. Damage to the arachnoid membrane can result in cerebrospinal fluid (CSF) leak.

### Tumor Characteristic Considerations

Pituitary tumor features, such as tumor size, invasiveness, and consistency, greatly influence the operative approach and technique during pituitary surgery.

### Size

For microadenomas, less than 1 cm in diameter, where the normal pituitary tissue covers the tumor during the endonasal approach, the pituitary tissue is sliced to allow dissection of the tumor tissue. A ring curette can subsequently be used to resect the small tumor. For macroadenomas, a suction cannula and curette is used to debulk and resect most soft tumors. If a tumor is fibrotic, a ring curette with a suction or an automated suction-controlled tissue debrider (NICO myriad, NICO Corporation, Indianapolis, IN) is used to debulk the tougher core of the tumor.

### Invasiveness

A tumor found to be invading into the clivus and petrous apex can present additional challenges with the resection and may require combined surgical approaches to achieve a complete resection. Invasion of the pituitary tumor into the cavernous sinus requires an endoscopic approach entering the cavernous sinus through the medial and anterior walls of the cavernous sinus if this invasive component were to be pursued. Tumor resection within the cavernous sinus poses the risk of abducens nerve palsy or postoperative hematoma formation secondary to venous oozing.[8]

### Consistency

The consistency of the pituitary tumor can determine the technique used for resection. Oftentimes, the consistency of the sellar mass is soft; however, in 5% to 36% of cases, the tumor is found to have firmer character.[9–11] The fibrous consistency of the tumor is difficult to mobilize and internally debulk.[10,12–14]

Depending on the consistency of the pituitary mass, either an intracapsular or extracapsular resection of the mass is performed. Oftentimes, a piecemeal intracapsular resection of soft tumors is performed, where the core of the tumor is removed with a ring curette and suctioned from within the pseudocapsule of the tumor. This technique relies on the surgeon's ability to distinguish tumor from normal pituitary gland based on texture, color, and firmness. Resecting the inferior aspects, then lateral parts, and finally superior parts of the tumor is achieved using this technique.[15]

The extracapsular approach for tumor removal is often reserved for fibrous tumors, although soft tumors can also be resected in this manner. A wide opening of the sella is required that extends to the medial wall of the cavernous sinus bilaterally and to the intercavernous sinus anteriorly. The dura is opened, preserving the pseudocapsule of the underlying tumor. The pseudocapsule is then dissected away from the dura. Some internal debulking of the tumor may be required for larger lesions to facilitate dissection of the pseudocapsule from the inferior plane and laterally off the cavernous sinus walls. Following debulking, identifying the pseudocapsule is important to allow for gentle traction to avoid damaging the proximal pituitary, chiasm, and vascular supply.[14] Of note, in cases with significant sinus invasion, a clear plane cannot be established along the lateral aspects of the pseudocapsule. The pseudocapsule is then removed superiorly using a suction and ring curette to separate the remaining tumor from the normal pituitary gland and diaphragma sella.[15]

## SELLA RECONSTRUCTION

The main goal of reconstruction of the sella is to create a watertight reconstruction of the skull base to prevent CSF leakage.[16] Factors that lead to a higher risk for CSF leak following a sellar resection include violation of the arachnoid cistern; large size of the defect; and an irregular shape of the defect formed, whose perimeter is in close proximity to the carotids or optic nerves.[16] For large resection cavities in the sella, fat graft or Gelfoam are used to fill the sellar space to prevent delayed rupture of the arachnoid membrane as a result of excessive Valsalva maneuvers, such as coughing, sneezing, or gaging during extubation, to result in a CSF leak.[7] The sellar graft may also serve as a buttress to prevent downward herniation of the optic chiasm.

Multiple sellar reconstruction methods exist, including intradural reconstruction (inlay), intradural extradural reconstruction (inlay-overlay), and extradural reconstruction (onlay). Various materials are used for the inlay and onlay grafts including synthetic copolymer material, or collagen-based dural substitutes.[16] Fibrin glue can also be applied to help make the barrier watertight.

## COMPLICATION CONSIDERATIONS

Anticipating complications for endoscopic pituitary surgery can best prepare a surgeon during surgical planning. Complications in the sphenoid sinus, sella, para/suprasellar space, internal carotid artery, and pituitary gland are all possibilities that can arise.

Complications in the sphenoid sinus include sinusitis, mucocele formation, or fractures of the sphenoid bone (3%–4% occurrence rate).[17–20] These complications may be reduced by ensuring a wide opening of the sphenoid ostium; avoiding the use of transsphenoidal retractors; and avoiding overpacking the sphenoid sinus, which may interfere with mucociliary clearance.[21]

Complications with the sella are often seen during macroadenoma resections and can present as CSF leak, subarachnoid hemorrhage, tension pneumocephalus, or vasospam (4%–5% occurrence rate).[22] Para/suprasellar complications occur in 2% to 4% of cases, and often present as subarachnoid hemorrhage during an endoscopic approach.[17,22] These risks are reduced with better visualization of the intrasellar, suprasellar, and parasellar space, often with the assistance of an angled endoscope.

Internal carotid artery injury is the most devastating complication during endoscopic endonasal pituitary surgery. Common intraoperative management considerations include packing with a hemostatic agent or muscle patch, bipolar electrocautery, or applying an aneurysm clip.[23] Packing is the first strategy to achieve hemostasis while maintaining a patent internal carotid artery.[24] Harvest sites of a muscle patch include the rectus abdominis, temporalis muscle, retropharyngeal muscles, sternocleidomastoid muscle, or quadriceps.[25–27] Endovascular intervention is then subsequently undertaken after initial control of the bleed and stabilization of the patient.

Manipulation of the pituitary gland during tumor resection can cause endocrine dysfunction postoperatively, with anterior pituitary insufficiency occurring in 10% to 27% of cases and posterior pituitary insufficiency in 15% to 60%.[17] Careful dissection and proper visualization can reduce the extent of pituitary gland manipulation. It is also important to trend relevant laboratory values postoperatively to monitor pituitary function.

## SUMMARY

Many surgical considerations exist during the endoscopic approach for pituitary surgery for a neurosurgeon. Careful surgical planning and evaluation of the patient's anatomy, meticulous surgical technique and sellar reconstruction, and anticipating complications all aid in having a successful surgical experience.

## CLINICS CARE POINTS

- The degree of pneumatization of the sphenoid sinus is important to understand because greater pneumatization allows for easier identification of bony protuberances in the sphenoid sinus, aiding in identifying anatomic structures.

- The position of the optic chiasm can influence the surgical approach to the sella, with a prefixed chiasm being closer to the diaphragma sella, presenting a higher risk of injury during removal of the sella bone.
- Pituitary tumor features, such as size, invasiveness, and consistency, greatly influence the operative approach and technique during pituitary surgery.
- Factors that lead to a higher risk for cerebrospinal fluid leak include violation of the arachnoid cistern, size of the defect, and an irregular shape of the defect whose perimeter is in close proximity to the carotid arteries or optic nerves.
- Potential complications during endoscopic pituitary surgery can occur in the sphenoid sinus, sella, para/suprasellar space, internal carotid artery, or pituitary gland.

## DISCLOSURE

The author has nothing to disclose.

## REFERENCES

1. Jankowski R, Auque J, Simon C, et al. Endoscopic pituitary tumor surgery. Laryngoscope 1992;102(2). https://doi.org/10.1288/00005537-199202000-00016.
2. Jho HD, Ha HG. Endoscopic endonasal skull base surgery: Part 3 - the clivus and posterior fossa. Minimally Invasive Neurosurg 2004;47(1). https://doi.org/10.1055/s-2004-818347.
3. Jho HD, Carrau RL, McLaughlin MR, et al. Endoscopic transsphenoidal resection of a large chordoma in the posterior fossa. Acta Neurochirur (Wein) 1997;139(4). https://doi.org/10.1007/BF01808831.
4. Cavallo LM, de Divitiis O, Aydin S, et al. Extended endoscopic endonasal transsphenoidal approach to the suprasellar area: anatomic considerations - Part 1. Neurosurgery 2008;62(6 SUPPL). https://doi.org/10.1227/01.NEU.0000280005.26449.2D.
5. Hamberger CA, Hammer G, Marcusson G. Experiences in transantrosphenoidal hypophysectomy. Trans Pac Coast Otoophthalmological Soc Annu Meet 1961;42:273–86.
6. Ouaknine GE, Hardy J. Microsurgical anatomy of the pituitary gland and the sellar region: 2. The bony structures. Am Surgeon 1987;53(5):291–7.
7. David J, Diana J, Hae-dong J. Endoscopic Endonasal Pituitary and Skull Base Surgery. Schmidek and Sweet Operative. Chapter 22. Neurosurgical Techniques; 2012. P. 257–79.
8. Fernandez-Miranda JC, Zwagerman NT, Abhinav K, et al. Cavernous sinus compartments from the endoscopic endonasal approach: anatomical considerations and surgical relevance to adenoma surgery. J Neurosurg 2018;129(2). https://doi.org/10.3171/2017.2.JNS162214.
9. Wang S, Lin S, Wei L, et al. Analysis of operative efficacy for giant pituitary adenoma. BMC Surg 2014;14(1). https://doi.org/10.1186/1471-2482-14-59.
10. Pratheesh R, Rajaratnam S, Prabhu K, et al. The current role of transcranial surgery in the management of pituitary adenomas. Pituitary 2013;16(4). https://doi.org/10.1007/s11102-012-0439-z.
11. Cappelletti M, Ruggeri AG, Spizzichino L, et al. Fibrous pituitary macroadenomas: predictive role of preoperative radiologic investigations for proper surgical planning in a cohort of 66 patients. World Neurosurg 2019;121. https://doi.org/10.1016/j.wneu.2018.09.137.

12. Leung GKK, Yuen MMA, Chow WS, et al. An endoscopic modification of the simultaneous "above and below" approach to large pituitary adenomas. Pituitary 2012;15(2). https://doi.org/10.1007/s11102-011-0319-y.

13. Cappabianca P, Cavallo LM, Solari D, et al. Size does not matter. The intrigue of giant adenomas: a true surgical challenge. Acta Neurochirurgica 2014;156(12). https://doi.org/10.1007/s00701-014-2213-7.

14. Maio SDI, Cavallo LM, Esposito F, et al. Extended endoscopic endonasal approach for selected pituitary adenomas: early experience. J Neurosurg 2011;114(2). https://doi.org/10.3171/2010.9.JNS10262.

15. Chamoun R, Takashima M, Yoshor D. Endoscopic extracapsular dissection for resection of pituitary macroadenomas: technical note. J Neurol Surg A Cent Eur Neurosurg 2014;75(1):48–52.

16. Solari D, Villa A, de Angelis M, et al. Anatomy and surgery of the endoscopic endonasal approach to the skull base. Translational Med UniSa 2012;2:36–46. Available at: http://www.ncbi.nlm.nih.gov/pubmed/23905043%0Ahttp://www.pubmedcentral.nih.gov/articlerender.fcgi?artid=PMC3728777.

17. Black McL P, Zervas NT, Candia GL. Incidence and management of complications of transsphenoidal operation for pituitary adenomas. Neurosurgery 1987; 20(6). https://doi.org/10.1227/00006123-198706000-00017.

18. Barrow DL, Tindall GT. Loss of vision after transsphenoidal surgery. Neurosurgery 1990;27(1). https://doi.org/10.1227/00006123-199007000-00008.

19. Herman P, Lot G, Guichard JP, et al. Mucocele of the sphenoid sinus: a late complication of transsphenoidal pituitary surgery. Ann Otology, Rhinology Laryngol 1998;107(9 II). https://doi.org/10.1177/000348949810700905.

20. Kessler L, Legaludec V, Dietemann JL, et al. Sphenoidal sinus mucocele after transsphenoidal surgery for acromegaly. Neurosurg Rev 1999;22(4). https://doi.org/10.1007/s101430050021.

21. Charalampaki P, Ayyad A, Kockro RA, et al. Surgical complications after endoscopic transsphenoidal pituitary surgery. J Clin Neurosci 2009;16(6):786–9.

22. Ciric I, Ragin A, Baumgartner C, et al. Complications of transsphenoidal surgery: results of a national survey, review of the literature, and personal experience. Neurosurgery 1997;40(2). https://doi.org/10.1097/00006123-199702000-00001.

23. Gardner PA, Tormenti MJ, Pant H, et al. Carotid artery injury during endoscopic endonasal skull base surgery: incidence and outcomes. Neurosurgery 2013; 73(SUPPL. 2). https://doi.org/10.1227/01.neu.0000430821.71267.f2.

24. Gardner PA, Snyderman CH, Fernandez-Miranda JC, et al. Management of major vascular injury during endoscopic endonasal skull base surgery. Otolaryngologic Clin North America 2016;49(3). https://doi.org/10.1016/j.otc.2016.03.003.

25. Wang WH, Lieber S, Lan MY, et al. Nasopharyngeal muscle patch for the management of internal carotid artery injury in endoscopic endonasal surgery. J Neurosurg 2020;133(5). https://doi.org/10.3171/2019.7.JNS191370.

26. Morera VA, Fernandez-Miranda JC, Prevedello DM, et al. "Far-medial" expanded endonasal approach to the inferior third of the clivus: the transcondylar and transjugular tubercle approaches. Neurosurgery 2010;66(6 Suppl Operative). https://doi.org/10.1227/01.NEU.0000369926.01891.5D.

27. Wang WH, Abhinav K, Wang E, et al. Endoscopic endonasal transclival transcondylar approach for foramen magnum meningiomas: surgical anatomy and technical note. Oper Neurosurg 2016;12(2):153–61.

# Pituitary Gland Surgical Emergencies
## The Role of Endoscopic Intervention

Mark A. Arnold, MD[a], Juan Manuel Revuelta Barbero, MD[b],
Gustavo Pradilla, MD[b], Sarah K. Wise, MD[a],*

### KEYWORDS

- Pituitary surgery • Pituitary emergencies • Pituitary apoplexy • Vision loss
- Severe Cushing • Cerebrospinal fluid rhinorrhea

### KEY POINTS

- Surgical emergencies in endoscopic transsphenoidal surgery of the pituitary are rare.
- Endoscopic endonasal techniques can manage most surgical emergencies of the pituitary gland with reduced morbidity.
- With appropriate preparation and management, outcomes of surgical emergencies of the pituitary gland are favorable.

### INTRODUCTION

In the era of modern pituitary gland surgery, true surgical emergencies are rare.[1–3] These challenging events can occur throughout the perioperative period and are broadly categorized by the timing of occurrence. Acute indications for pituitary surgery include pituitary apoplexy, vision loss, and severe Cushing presentation. Emergencies can also occur intraoperatively, primarily secondary to bleeding. Postoperative emergencies include epistaxis, pneumocephalus, and intracranial bleeding (**Box 1**). Cerebrospinal fluid (CSF) leak occurs in up to 37.4% of transsphenoidal sellar surgery, yet postoperative CSF leaks are less frequent at approximately 2.6%.[4] As they occur often during pituitary surgery, CSF leaks alone are generally not considered a true surgical emergency unless associated with symptomatic tension pneumocephalus.

Complications leading to a surgical emergency can occur with both endoscopic and microscopic approaches; however, there is evidence to suggest the complication rate may be lower with endoscopic techniques.[5,6] Furthermore, use of the endoscope is poised to manage many of the complications of pituitary gland surgery, as it offers

[a] Department of Otolaryngology–Head and Neck Surgery, Emory Sinus, Nasal and Allergy Center, Emory University School of Medicine, 550 Peachtree Street Northeast, MOT 11th Floor, Atlanta, GA 30308, USA; [b] Department of Neurosurgery, Emory University School of Medicine, Emory Clinic, 1365 Clifton Road Northeast, Building B, Fl 2, Ste 2200, Atlanta, GA 30322, USA
* Corresponding author.
*E-mail address:* skmille@emory.edu

Otolaryngol Clin N Am 55 (2022) 397–410
https://doi.org/10.1016/j.otc.2021.12.016
0030-6665/22/© 2022 Elsevier Inc. All rights reserved.
oto.theclinics.com

---

**Box 1**
**Pituitary gland emergencies**

Preoperative
- Apoplexy
- Acute vision loss
- Severe Cushing presentation

Intraoperative
  Bleeding
  - Nonlocalizable bleeding
  - Intradural arterial injury
  - Cavernous sinus bleeding
  - Carotid artery injury (CAI)

Postoperative
- Epistaxis
- Pneumocephalus
- Intracranial bleeding, hematoma

---

excellent visualization with less morbidity. This article highlights the major pituitary surgical emergencies and the role of endoscopic intervention. With appropriate preparation and experience, the skull base team can maintain favorable outcomes despite a surgical emergency.

### Preoperative Pituitary Gland Emergencies

As a pituitary adenoma is a slow-growing, benign tumor, most patients with a pituitary adenoma develop symptoms slowly. Visual changes are often insidious owing to mass effect and may go unnoticed by the patient.[7] Functioning adenomas, on the other hand, produce a subtle constellation of findings owing to hormone hypersecretion. However, a minority of patients present acutely, warranting urgent medical and surgical management. Although 40% of patients present with visual field loss, acute blindness is exceedingly rare (**Fig. 1**).[8–10] Similarly, Cushing disease, which is discussed elsewhere in this issue, may occasionally present with altered mental status and significant metabolic derangements owing to cortisol excess.[11] Although uncommon, symptoms owing to compressive or obstructive hydrocephalus from a large sellar lesion may warrant urgent surgical treatment (**Fig. 2**). Presentation with acute vision loss, severe Cushing disease, and compressive or obstructive hydrocephalus may warrant urgent surgical intervention, which is often performed via a transnasal endoscopic approach to the sella.

Most acute presentations of pituitary adenomas are due to apoplexy, defined by an abrupt hemorrhage or infarction of the pituitary gland (**Fig. 3**). It is reported that 2% to 12% of patients with a pituitary adenoma experience apoplexy, and most cases arise from nonfunctioning adenomas.[12,13] The underlying cause of apoplexy is unknown in many patients. However, use of anticoagulant medications and significant blood pressure fluctuations during cardiac surgery may be precipitating factors.[12]

Almost all patients with pituitary apoplexy develop sudden headache, secondary to acute expansion and compression of adjacent structures and blood extravasation into the subarachnoid space causing meningeal irritation.[14] The acute expansion may compress nearby cranial nerves, resulting in visual disturbances and ocular palsy. Patients may also present with endocrine dysfunction, manifesting as hyponatremia from SIADH (syndrome of inappropriate antidiuretic hormone secretion) or glucocorticoid insufficiency.[15]

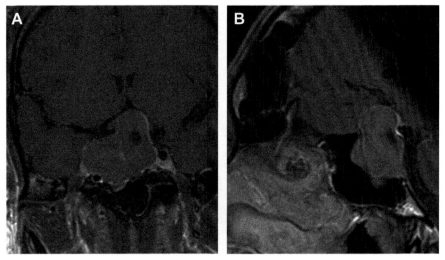

**Fig. 1.** A 30-year-old man with acromegaly presented after acute onset of headache and double vision with partial oculomotor palsies. (*A*) Coronal and (*B*) sagittal T1-weighted postcontrast MRI revealed a large pituitary lesion with suprasellar extension and mass effect on the optic chiasm.

In the acute setting, most patients will undergo an initial computed tomography (CT) to evaluate sudden-onset headaches. CT is diagnostic for apoplexy in only 21% to 28% of cases; however, a sellar mass can be identified in up to 80% of patients.[16] Therefore, an urgent MRI scan should be obtained in patients with suspected apoplexy.

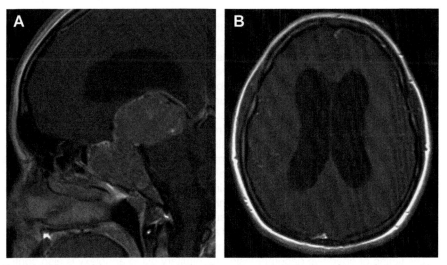

**Fig. 2.** A 22-year-old woman presented with acute on chronic altered mental status, vision changes, and headaches. (*A*) Sagittal and (*B*) axial T1-weighted postcontrast MRI revealed a giant pituitary macroadenoma with complete effacement of the third ventricle and suprasellar cistern with associated obstructive hydrocephalus. After urgent external ventricular drain placement, the patient was taken for endoscopic resection.

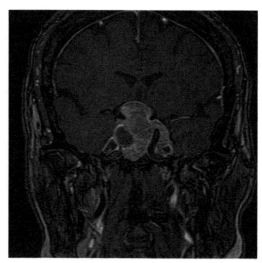

**Fig. 3.** A 79-year-old woman presented with a week of worsening bitemporal hemianopsia. Coronal T1-weighted postcontrast MRI revealed a large solid and cystic hemorrhagic sellar and suprasellar mass, consistent with pituitary apoplexy.

The management of pituitary gland apoplexy is controversial.[1,2,17] Historically, it was regarded as a surgical emergency.[1] Expedient decompression was thought to be necessary to restore or prevent the worsening of cranial neuropathies. Emergent decompression of pituitary gland apoplexy relieves compression of local structures, improving visual and ocular disturbances and mental status. However, urgent decompression not only carries the usual risks associated with pituitary gland surgery but also may incur additional risk if urgently performed by an on-call team, which may lack experience or familiarity with the patient. It is thought that infarction alone portends to better outcomes, compared with hemorrhagic infarction or frank hemorrhage.[17] Significant acute symptoms, including blindness, neurologic decline, and hemodynamic instability, warrant corticosteroid treatment and urgent decompression. However, presentations with this level of acuity are uncommon.[17]

The course of pituitary apoplexy is variable, however, and there are many instances of spontaneous clinical recovery and/or tumor disappearance with nonsurgical management.[2] The evidence for surgery versus conservative management for pituitary apoplexy is limited; most studies are retrospective in nature and nonrandomized.[16,18–20] However, the outcomes are similar and generally result in symptom resolution. When evaluated retrospectively, more severe cases tended toward surgical management. In 2011, guidelines for the management of pituitary apoplexy were developed in the United Kingdom.[16] The investigators established a scoring system to aid in decision making along with monitoring outcomes.[16] The score consists of the Glasgow coma scale, visual acuity, visual field defects, and ocular paresis as parameters, with a maximum score of 10 (**Table 1**).[16] A separate study of 45 patients found that patients with a score of 4 or greater tended toward operative intervention.[21]

The timing of operative decompression for pituitary gland apoplexy is also controversial. Some investigators advocate decompression within 24 hours, whereas others recommend within 3 days.[22] United Kingdom (UK) guidelines recommend intervention within 8 days.[16] These guidelines were based on a review of 35 patients, noting poorer visual outcomes in the group with surgery delayed beyond 8 days.[16,23]

| Table 1<br>Pituitary apoplexy score | |
| --- | --- |
| **Variable** | **Points** |
| Level of consciousness | |
|   Glasgow coma scale, 15 | 0 |
|   Glasgow coma scale, <8–14 | 2 |
|   Glasgow coma scale, <8 | 4 |
| Visual acuity | |
|   Normal[a] | 0 |
|   Reduced, unilateral | 1 |
|   Bilateral | 2 |
| Visual field defects | |
|   Normal | 0 |
|   Unilateral defect | 1 |
|   Bilateral defect | 2 |
| Ocular paresis | |
|   Absent | 0 |
|   Present, unilateral | 1 |
|   Bilateral | 2 |

[a] No change from premorbid visual acuity.

Adapted from Rajasekaran S, Vanderpump M, Baldeweg S, et al. UK guidelines for the management of pituitary apoplexy. Clin Endocrinol (Oxf). 2011;74(1):9-20. https://doi.org/10.1111/j.1365-2265.2010.03913.x.

The principal goal of surgical treatment of pituitary apoplexy is to preserve visual and oculomotor function, and this is accomplished by decompression. If possible, gross total resection of the tumor is preferable. As with other sellar pathologic conditions, endoscopic management of pituitary apoplexy is reported to be successful. Multiple retrospective reviews have demonstrated excellent visual outcomes in endoscopic approaches, with more than 90% of patients having improvements in visual acuity and visual fields.[13,19,20] Endocrine recovery, however, tends to be poor, regardless of the timing of intervention.[24]

### Intraoperative Pituitary Gland Emergencies

Control of bleeding during endoscopic pituitary gland surgery is critical to complete tumor removal while minimizing complications. Bleeding interferes with anatomic visualization, increasing the risk of iatrogenic injury.[25] Furthermore, major bleeding or blood vessel injury itself may be significant enough to warrant additional management and/or early procedure termination. During pituitary surgery, bleeding can occur during any stage and from a variety of sources. Working as a team is essential for managing bleeding. A team-based approach improves visualization, encourages problem solving, and is necessary for addressing any major bleeding event.[26]

As with any approach, meticulous technique with bleeding source control is imperative. Managing nonlocalizable bleeding is the first step to preventing larger bleeding complications. There are multiple studies demonstrating reduced blood loss through use of local injection, topical placement of vasoconstrictors, patient positioning with head elevation, and induced hypotension.[27] In 2 randomized, double-blind, controlled trials of patients undergoing endoscopic sinus surgery, the use of total intravenous anesthesia over inhaled anesthetic resulted in statistically significant improvement in surgical field visualization.[28,29] However, a retrospective review of patients undergoing transsphenoidal surgery found no difference between choice of anesthetic with regards to blood loss or any other clinical parameters.[30] Furthermore, a 2019 randomized trial found that the modality of mechanical ventilation, volume-controlled ventilation versus pressure-controlled, had no impact on bleeding during pituitary surgery.[31]

### Cavernous sinus bleeding

The cavernous sinuses are paired venous cavities on either side of the pituitary fossa, connected by the intercavernous sinuses. Venous bleeding from these areas is considered high flow yet under low pressure. Interestingly, bleeding severity from the cavernous sinuses does not depend on central venous pressure.[32] Although it may be difficult to predict which patient might have significant bleeding, simple therapeutic measures are usually effective in achieving hemostasis. Head of bed elevation greater than 20°, decreasing systemic blood pressure, and decreasing intrathoracic pressure with manual over mechanical ventilation all reduce bleeding. Direct application of hemostatic matrix through dural tears results in partial thrombosis and hemostasis.[26] As these bleeds are low pressure, tamponade tends to be successful with either neurosurgical patties or other dissolvable materials.

### Carotid artery injury

Arterial injuries during pituitary surgery present unique challenges to the skull base team. Intradural arterial injuries are rare but may occur in the setting of large suprasellar adenomas or meningiomas over the sphenoid planum.[33,34] Certainly, internal carotid artery (ICA) injury (CAI) is one of the most feared complications of pituitary gland surgery, but the incidence is low. Single-institution or single-surgeon reviews demonstrated the incidence to be less than 1%.[35–37] Two systematic reviews and meta-analyses determined that CAI incidences are between 0.4% and 3.8%.[3,38] However, because of publication bias, the true incidence may be higher. Interestingly, CAI is more common on the left side, possibly owing to predominantly right-handed surgeons exerting greater force over the lateral wall of the sphenoid, injuring the cavernous ICA.[37] Most of the time, CAI occurs during the tumor removal phase and most commonly at the parasellar segment.[39] Although the overall incidence of CAI is rare, in a survey of skull base surgeons, 20% have experienced CAI during their career.[39] Therefore, knowledge and preparation are essential to minimize morbidity and possible mortality from these injuries.

Patient selection is the first step to minimizing the potential for injury. It is known that tumor involvement or encasement of the ICA increases risk for injury.[37] In a review of 2015 endonasal skull base surgeries at a high-volume center, Gardner and colleagues[36] in 2013 noted 7 cases of CAI. The investigators determined that chondroid tumors were at higher risk, but 2 of the injuries occurred during the 550 adenoma resections, with an incidence of 0.3%. Of these 7 injuries, 4 ICAs were sacrificed intraoperatively or postoperatively without neurologic deficits. One patient died postoperatively owing to cardiac ischemia. Of the 3 ICAs preserved, 1 patient developed pseudoaneurysm and was treated endovascularly.

There are several key aspects of avoiding ICA injury. Not surprisingly, team experience is essential. After building a foundation of success in straightforward cases, higher-risk tumors can be addressed. Image navigation and Doppler localization facilitate understanding of the anatomy. However, given variable sphenoid sinus anatomy and pneumatization, image guidance cannot replace thorough study of preoperative imaging. MRI and CT imaging are complementary in evaluating the course of the

ICA. MRI better delineates the cavernous ICA from the adjacent pituitary gland and/or tumor. CT, on the other hand, details the thin bony anatomy of the sphenoid. Paraclival bony dehiscence of the ICA has been noted in 3.6% of cases, and the sphenoid inter-sinus septum deviates over the ICA in 14% of cases.[40] The protuberances of the ICA into the sphenoid on either side of the sella aids in intraoperative localization, a so-called teddy bear sign.[41] However, in some patients, the topography of the posterior sphenoid is nearly flat without any surface landmarks. Therefore, it is safest to first identify the gland by drilling over the sellar bulge in the midline.[42] Following this, the parasellar anatomy of the ICA is deduced. Similarly, opening of the caudal dura first avoids inadvertent CAI.[35]

CAI during endoscopic pituitary surgery is rare. Consequently, there is limited evidence regarding management.[43] Fortunately, multiple training modules exist to help prepare teams to perform under the pressure of these rapidly evolving and stressful situations.[44–46] The Valentine and Wormald model of CAI features anesthetized sheep that have undergone neck exploration and carotid artery isolation. A synthetic model of the nasal cavity placed over the artery simulates the confined endoscopic environment of a CAI.[47]

Whether training during simulation or managing a live injury, following a protocol optimizes success.[44,47] First, as with any endoscopic surgery, appropriate visualization is critical, and this is first accomplished with ample suctioning. Two surgeons are necessary, with one holding the endoscope, while the other suctions blood away. One suction is placed in the ipsilateral nasal cavity to the bleeding, while the endoscope is placed down the contralateral side, using the septum to shield some blood flow. The primary surgeon next uses a second suction to help clear away blood and to ideally "hover" directly over the site of injury to gain complete visualization. Once the site of injury is localized, there are a few options to attempt hemostasis. Ideally, a muscle patch is harvested quickly and held over the site with enough pressure to stop bleeding but without halting blood flow through the vessel.[44] Gelatin-thrombin matrix, clips, and bipolar cautery are also options, although they may not be sufficient to stop high-pressure bleeding and may risk transforming a small perforation into a larger vessel tear.

Ultimately, vessel sacrifice through endovascular means or direct ligation is the most reliable solution to CAI.[33,34,36] However, perforator or avulsion injuries can be managed by packing or bipolar cautery alone, followed by an angiogram.[48] In some cases, a Willis stent graft may preserve flow across the ICA and circle of Willis, and sacrifice is not necessary.[48]

Given the rarity but potential for catastrophic outcomes, investigators have explored additional management strategies for CAI during endoscopic surgery. Theoretically, if exposed, proximal and distal control of the artery is feasible in cadavers.[49] Neuromonitoring, through somatosensory-evoked potentials and electroencephalography, can accurately detect cerebral hypoperfusion, providing real-time feedback during surgery and predicting outcomes after injury.[50] Although unstudied, the use of intravenous adenosine has long been used by vascular surgeons to temporarily induce asystole.[51] The temporary halting of blood flow can aid in localizing and packing the CAI.

After endoscopic CAI, the outcomes vary from minor to fatal (**Fig. 4**). The sequalae of these injuries include pseudoaneurysm formation, carotid-cavernous fistula, vasospasm, occlusion, and blowout. However, long-term neurologic deficit or mortality is infrequent.[34,36,52] In a case series and literature review of 105 cases, Sylvester and colleagues[52] noted 21.7% of patients had a long-term neurologic deficit. Although immediate postoperative vascular imaging is uniformly recommended, beyond this, the

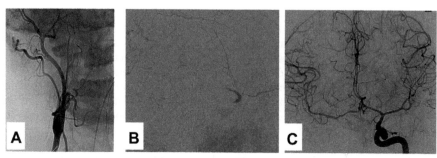

**Fig. 4.** Diagnostic cerebral angiogram of the patient in **Fig. 3** after intraoperative right ICA injury at the cavernous segment, managed with temporary packing and subsequent loss of Doppler signal. Somatosensory-evoked potentials remained stable. (A) Right common carotid angiogram demonstrates little flow of contrast past the proximal cervical segment of the ICA, with normal opacification of the external carotid artery branches. (B) Right common carotid artery angiogram demonstrates distal cavernous right ICA filling from the right ophthalmic artery via external carotid artery collaterals. (C) Left ICA cerebral angiogram demonstrates excellent filling of the right middle cerebral and right anterior communicating artery from the left ICA via the anterior communicating artery. The patient did not suffer any neurologic deficits.

timing of imaging is inconsistent. However, the development of delayed ICA pathologic condition is possible and requires close follow-up.[43] Buerke and colleagues[53] recommend repeat magnetic resonance angiography at 1 week, 6 weeks, 3 months, and 1 year.

## Postoperative Pituitary Gland Surgical Emergencies

### Epistaxis
Epistaxis after endoscopic skull base surgery is uncommon.[54,55] However, multiple algorithms for management exist.[54,56,57] These events can be further divided by their occurrence postoperatively: acute (within 48 hours) or delayed (after day 3).[56] It is important to note that epistaxis after transsphenoidal surgery differs significantly from spontaneous epistaxis. With spontaneous epistaxis, bleeds are usually located at the anterior septum and therefore usually respond to cautery and/or anterior packing. In transsphenoidal surgery, however, the bleeding is more likely posterior in cause owing to trauma and/or manipulation of the distal branches of the internal maxillary artery and ophthalmic artery. Interestingly, men with hypertension, who are at risk for spontaneous epistaxis, are also at higher risk for bleeding after transsphenoidal surgery.[54]

Management of epistaxis begins with initial stabilization with volume resuscitation, laboratory work, transfusion, and airway management as appropriate. Most bleeding episodes, acute or delayed, can be managed initially with bedside packing. Endoscopic evaluation aids both in bleeding localization and in treatment. For acute bleeds that fail to resolve with bedside packing, operative exploration is the next step. The operative field is still fresh, and exposed bleeders are cauterized and covered with hemostatic agents. For delayed bleeds that do not resolve with bedside packing, either operative exploration or angiography with embolization should be considered. As these bleeds most commonly arise from a posterior source, endoscopic sphenopalatine artery ligation should be considered if no obvious bleeder is found. For some patients, however, although rare, bleeding only resolved after bilateral internal maxillary artery or external carotid artery embolization.[56,58] Massive bleeding episodes should raise the suspicion for sentinel bleeding events from major arteries, and angiography should be performed urgently.

A retrospective review by Zimmer and colleagues[57] of 434 consecutive patients undergoing endoscopic transsphenoidal surgery, 42 patients (9.7%) reported epistaxis, with 16 patients presenting to the emergency department. Of these, 8 patients returned to the operating room. Six of these patients had posterior bleeds, requiring cauterization, whereas 2 additionally presented with vision loss and had acute sellar bleeds.[57] Another review by De and colleagues[56] evaluated 551 consecutive patients undergoing transsphenoidal surgery over a 4-year period. Of these, 18 had epistaxis, with 6 occurring in the acute period. Twelve occurred in a delayed fashion at an average of 11 days after surgery. The acute group was managed with bedside packing in 2 patients; the other 4 patients were managed operatively and found to have either mucosal oozing or bleeding from a branch of the sphenopalatine artery. In the delayed group, half were successfully managed bedside, whereas 5 of the 12 patients underwent bilateral internal maxillary artery embolization. One patient developed an anterior ethmoid artery pseudoaneurysm and underwent internal maxillary embolization and balloon tamponade packing.

### Tension pneumocephalus
If air progressively enters the intracranial compartment and is unable to escape, tension pneumocephalus develops. Although a small amount of pneumocephalus is expected after transsphenoidal surgery, large-volume pneumocephalus or increasing pneumocephalus is suggestive of a tension pattern and requires emergent management (**Fig. 5**). The incidence of true tension pneumocephalus after transsphenoidal surgery is rare.[59,60]

The mechanism of tension pneumocephalus is thought to follow 2 patterns. Positive pressure events, such as breathing, coughing, or Valsalva maneuvers, may push air intracranially. However, a CSF leak alone may also produce pneumocephalus. As fluid

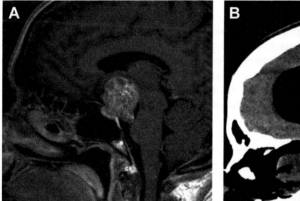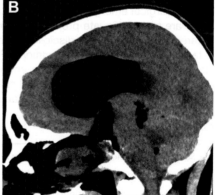

**Fig. 5.** A 45-year-old woman presented with a large cystic pituitary macroadenoma. (*A*) Sagittal T1-weighted postcontrast MRI shows a large pituitary mass with extension into the suprasellar and prepontine cisterns. One month after endoscopic transsphenoidal resection and pedicled nasoseptal flap reconstruction, she presented with altered mental status. Sagittal CT (*B*) demonstrated large-volume intraventricular pneumocephalus and skull base defect at the sella. Reconstruction of the skull base defect with abdominal fat and collagen-based dural grafts was ultimately successful.

leaks out, air enters intracranially, like liquid flowing out of an inverted bottle. Similarly, lumbar drainage may result in pneumocephalus, as it pulls in extradural air.

Pneumocephalus is initially managed conservatively with bed rest and placing the patient in a 30° Fowler position, avoidance of positive pressure events, and use of analgesics and antipyretics.[61,62] In addition, the use of high-flow nasal cannula oxygen has been shown to increase the rate at which air is resorbed.[63] In addressing the above mechanisms, pneumocephalus can also be managed by positive pressure diversion through intubation. Nasal trumpets, if carefully placed, can also divert positive pressure events away from the skull base. Furthermore, clamping the lumbar drain relieves pneumocephalus by halting the "inverted bottle" mechanism as drained CSF is replaced by air. Unless clinically insignificant, all pneumocephalus should be serially evaluated with CT imaging to ensure stability or resolution.

In cases of acute clinical deterioration or progressive pneumocephalus, surgical repair is necessary. Although some cases of pneumocephalus may not be associated with a CSF leak, progressive intracranial air usually stems from a failed skull base repair. Fortunately, urgent endoscopic repair is often successful in resolving progressive pneumocephalus, as evidenced in multiple case series.[64–66]

### Intracranial bleeding

Intracranial bleeding after transsphenoidal surgery is rare, with an incidence of less than 2%.[67,68] Larger tumor diameters greater than 30 mm and suprasellar extension were found to be risk factors for hematoma formation.[68] Additional transcribriform and/or transclival approaches also increase the risk of bleeding. These bleeding events may present in a delayed fashion, with a mean time to evacuation of 4.5 days.[68] Intracranial bleeding, if minimal, may be managed with glucocorticoid therapy alone, and occasionally with endoscopic evacuation.[68,69] Larger hematomas, especially if complicated by brain herniation, require ventriculostomy placement and emergent craniotomy for evacuation.[70]

## SUMMARY

Overall, surgical emergencies in endoscopic transsphenoidal surgery of the pituitary gland are rare. Adequate preparation is essential, as some events may be once-in-a-career occurrence. Multidisciplinary, team-oriented care expands the experience in tackling these difficult complications. Fortunately, most pituitary surgical emergencies can be successfully managed endoscopically, with reduced morbidity. Finally, despite complications that may at first appear to be catastrophic, such as CAI, patient outcomes may remain favorable with appropriate preparedness and management.

## CLINICS CARE POINTS

- Surgical emergencies in endoscopic transsphenoidal pituitary surgery are rare.
- Adequate preparation is essential, as some events may be a once-in-a-career occurrence.
- Multidisciplinary, team-oriented care expands the experience in tackling these difficult complications.
- Most pituitary surgical emergencies can be successfully managed endoscopically with reduced morbidity.
- After pituitary emergencies, patient outcomes remain favorable with appropriate preparedness and management.

## REFERENCES

1. Bonicki W, Kasperlik-Załuska A, Koszewski W, et al. Pituitary apoplexy: endocrine, surgical and oncological emergency. Incidence, clinical course and treatment with reference to 799 cases of pituitary adenomas. Acta Neurochir (Wien) 1993;120(3–4):118–22.
2. Singh TD, Valizadeh N, Meyer FB, et al. Management and outcomes of pituitary apoplexy. J Neurosurg 2015;122(6):1450–7.
3. Ammirati M, Wei L, Ciric I. Short-term outcome of endoscopic versus microscopic pituitary adenoma surgery: a systematic review and meta-analysis. J Neurol Neurosurg Psychiatry 2013;84(8):843–9.
4. Strickland BA, Lucas J, Harris B, et al. Identification and repair of intraoperative cerebrospinal fluid leaks in endonasal transsphenoidal pituitary surgery: surgical experience in a series of 1002 patients. J Neurosurg 2018;129(2):425–9.
5. Cappabianca P, Cavallo LM, Colao AM, et al. Surgical complications associated with the endoscopic endonasal transsphenoidal approach for pituitary adenomas. J Neurosurg 2002;97(2):293–8.
6. Schaberg MR, Anand VK, Schwartz TH, et al. Microscopic versus endoscopic transnasal pituitary surgery. Curr Opin Otolaryngol Head Neck Surg 2010;18(1):8–14.
7. Monteiro MLR, Zambon BK, Cunha LP. Predictive factors for the development of visual loss in patients with pituitary macroadenomas and for visual recovery after optic pathway decompression. Can J Ophthalmol J Can Ophtalmol 2010;45(4):404–8.
8. Ogra S, Nichols AD, Stylli S, et al. Visual acuity and pattern of visual field loss at presentation in pituitary adenoma. J Clin Neurosci 2014;21(5):735–40.
9. Dupont G, Lachkar S, Iwanaga J, et al. Sudden headache and blindness due to pituitary (adenoma) infarction: a case report. Cureus 2019;11(2). https://doi.org/10.7759/cureus.4059.
10. Robinson JL. Sudden blindness with pituitary tumors: report of three cases. J Neurosurg 1972;36(1):83–5.
11. Bello CT, Santos FS, Ferrinhos C, et al. Acute presentation of cushing disease: severe hyperglycemia and refractory hypokalemia. Endocr Abstr 2017;49. https://doi.org/10.1530/endoabs.49.EP951. Bioscientifica.
12. Briet C, Salenave S, Bonneville JF, et al. Pituitary apoplexy. Endocr Rev 2015;36(6):622–45.
13. Gondim JA, de Albuquerque LAF, Almeida JP, et al. Endoscopic endonasal surgery for treatment of pituitary apoplexy: 16 years of experience in a specialized pituitary center. World Neurosurg 2017;108:137–42.
14. Suri H, Dougherty C. Presentation and management of headache in pituitary apoplexy. Curr Pain Headache Rep 2019;23(9):61.
15. Abbara A, Clarke S, Eng PC, et al. Clinical and biochemical characteristics of patients presenting with pituitary apoplexy. Endocr Connect 2018;7(10):1058–66.
16. Rajasekaran S, Vanderpump M, Baldeweg S, et al. UK guidelines for the management of pituitary apoplexy. Clin Endocrinol (Oxf) 2011;74(1):9–20.
17. Semple PL, De Villiers JC, Bowen RM, et al. Pituitary apoplexy: do histological features influence the clinical presentation and outcome? J Neurosurg 2006;104(6):931–7.
18. Zoli M, Milanese L, Faustini-Fustini M, et al. Endoscopic endonasal surgery for pituitary apoplexy: evidence on a 75-case series from a tertiary care center. World Neurosurg 2017;106:331–8.

19. Zhang X, Fei Z, Zhang W, et al. Emergency transsphenoidal surgery for hemorrhagic pituitary adenomas. Surg Oncol 2007;16(2):115–20.
20. Zhan R, Li X, Li X. Endoscopic endonasal transsphenoidal approach for apoplectic pituitary tumor: surgical outcomes and complications in 45 patients. J Neurol Surg B Skull Base 2015;77(1):54–60.
21. Bujawansa S, Thondam SK, Steele C, et al. Presentation, management and outcomes in acute pituitary apoplexy: a large single-centre experience from the United Kingdom. Clin Endocrinol (Oxf) 2014;80(3):419–24.
22. Abdulbaki A, Kanaan I. The impact of surgical timing on visual outcome in pituitary apoplexy: literature review and case illustration. Surg Neurol Int 2017;8(1). https://doi.org/10.4103/2152-7806.199557.
23. Randeva HS, Schoebel J, Byrne J, et al. Classical pituitary apoplexy: clinical features, management and outcome. Clin Endocrinol (Oxf) 1999;51(2):181–8.
24. Rutkowski MJ, Kunwar S, Blevins L, et al. Surgical intervention for pituitary apoplexy: an analysis of functional outcomes. J Neurosurg 2018;129(2):417–24.
25. Maniglia AJ. Fatal and other major complications of endoscopic sinus surgery. Laryngoscope 1991;101(4 Pt 1):349–54.
26. Vaz-Guimaraes F, Su SY, Fernandez-Miranda JC, et al. Hemostasis in endoscopic endonasal skull base surgery. J Neurol Surg Part B Skull Base 2015;76(4):296–302.
27. Alsaleh S, Manji J, Javer A. Optimization of the surgical field in endoscopic sinus surgery: an evidence-based approach. Curr Allergy Asthma Rep 2019;19(1). https://doi.org/10.1007/s11882-019-0847-5.
28. Little M, Tran V, Chiarella A, et al. Total intravenous anesthesia vs inhaled anesthetic for intraoperative visualization during endoscopic sinus surgery: a double blind randomized controlled trial. Int Forum Allergy Rhinol 2018;8(10):1123–6.
29. Brunner JP, Levy JM, Ada ML, et al. Total intravenous anesthesia improves intraoperative visualization during surgery for high-grade chronic rhinosinusitis: a double-blind randomized controlled trial. Int Forum Allergy Rhinol 2018;8(10):1114–22.
30. Gollapudy S, Poetker DM, Sidhu J, et al. Total intravenous versus inhaled anesthesia in transsphenoidal tumor surgery. Am J Otol - Head Neck Med Surg 2018;39(5):567–9.
31. Le Guen M, Paternot A, Declerck A, et al. Impact of the modality of mechanical ventilation on bleeding during pituitary surgery: a single blinded randomized trial. Medicine (Baltimore) 2019;98(38):e17254.
32. Lee HW, Caldwell JE, Wilson CB, et al. Venous bleeding during transsphenoidal surgery: its association with pre- and intraoperative factors and with cavernous sinus and central venous pressures. Anesth Analg 1997;84(3):545–50.
33. Babgi M, Alsaleh S, Babgi Y, et al. Intracranial intradural vascular injury during endoscopic endonasal transsphenoidal surgery: a case report and literature review. J Neurol Surg Rep 2020;81(03):e52–8.
34. Del Carmen A, Romero B, Gangadharan JL, et al. Managing arterial injury in endoscopic skull base surgery: case series and review of the literature. Oper Neurosurg 2017;13(1):138–49.
35. Meyer J, Perry A, Graffeo CS, et al. Carotid artery injury during transsphenoidal pituitary surgery: lessons from a 15-year modern microsurgery cohort. J Neurol Surg Part B Skull Base 2020;81(5):594–602.
36. Gardner PA, Tormenti MJ, Pant H, et al. Carotid artery injury during endoscopic endonasal skull base surgery: incidence and outcomes. Neurosurgery 2013;73(SUPPL. 2). https://doi.org/10.1227/01.neu.0000430821.71267.f2.

37. Chin OY, Ghosh R, Fang CH, et al. Internal carotid artery injury in endoscopic endonasal surgery: a systematic review. Laryngoscope 2016;126(3):582–90.
38. Tabaee A, Anand VK, Barrón Y, et al. Endoscopic pituitary surgery: a systematic review and meta-analysis: clinical article. J Neurosurg 2009;111(3):545–54.
39. Rowan NR, Turner MT, Valappil B, et al. Injury of the carotid artery during endoscopic endonasal surgery: surveys of skull base surgeons. J Neurol Surg Part B Skull Base 2018;79(3):302–8.
40. Dal Secchi MM, Dolci RLL, Teixeira R, et al. An analysis of anatomic variations of the sphenoid sinus and its relationship to the internal carotid artery. Int Arch Otorhinolaryngol 2018;22(2):161–6.
41. Yeung W, Twigg V, Carr S, et al. Radiological teddy bear sign on CT imaging to aid internal carotid artery localization in transsphenoidal pituitary and anterior skull base surgery. J Neurol Surg Part B Skull Base 2018;79(4):401–6.
42. Hamid O, El Fiky L, Hassan O, et al. Anatomic variations of the sphenoid sinus and their impact on trans-sphenoid pituitary surgery. Skull Base 2008;18(1):9–15.
43. Wang EW, Zanation AM, Gardner PA, et al. ICAR: endoscopic skull-base surgery. Int Forum Allergy Rhinol 2019;9(S3):S145–365.
44. Padhye V, Valentine R, Sacks R, et al. Coping with catastrophe: the value of endoscopic vascular injury training. Int Forum Allergy Rhinol 2015;5(3):247–52.
45. Pham M, Kale A, Marquez Y, et al. A perfusion-based human cadaveric model for management of carotid artery injury during endoscopic endonasal skull base surgery. J Neurol Surg Part B Skull Base 2014;75(5):309–13.
46. Ciporen JN, Lucke-Wold B, Mendez G, et al. Endoscopic management of cavernous carotid surgical complications: evaluation of a simulated perfusion model. World Neurosurg 2017;98:388–96.
47. Valentine R, Wormald P-J. A vascular catastrophe during endonasal surgery: an endoscopic sheep model. Skull Base 2011;21(2):109–14.
48. Zhang Y, Tian Z, Li C, et al. A modified endovascular treatment protocol for iatrogenic internal carotid artery injuries following endoscopic endonasal surgery. J Neurosurg 2020;132(2):343–50.
49. Xiao L, Xie S, Tang B, et al. A novel technique to manage internal carotid artery injury in endoscopic endonasal skull base surgery in the premise of proximal and distal controls. Neurosurg Rev 2021. https://doi.org/10.1007/s10143-021-01517-1.
50. Senthamarai Siddharthan YP, Bata A, Anetakis K, et al. Role of intraoperative neurophysiologic monitoring in internal carotid artery injury during endoscopic endonasal skull base surgery. World Neurosurg 2021;148:e43–57.
51. Ley-Urzáiz L, Salge-Arrieta FJ. Letter: safety first: use of adenosine in the management of the injury of the internal carotid artery during endoscopic skull base surgery: a proposal. Neurosurgery 2020;86(6):E591.
52. Sylvester PT, Moran CJ, Derdeyn CP, et al. Endovascular management of internal carotid artery injuries secondary to endonasal surgery: case series and review of the literature. J Neurosurg 2016;125(5):1256–76.
53. Buerke B, Tombach B, Stoll W, et al. Magnetic resonance angiography follow-up examinations to detect iatrogenic pseudoaneurysms following otorhinolaryngological surgery. J Laryngol Otol 2007;121(7):698–701.
54. Thompson CF, Wang MB, Kim BJ, et al. Incidence and management of epistaxis after endoscopic skull base surgery. ORL J Otorhinolaryngol Relat Spec 2012. https://doi.org/10.1159/000345500.

55. Smith TR, Hulou MM, Huang KT, et al. Complications after transsphenoidal surgery for patients with Cushing's disease and silent corticotroph adenomas. Neurosurg Focus 2015;38(2):E12.

56. De KM, Reyes L, Gross BA, et al. Clinical study incidence, risk factors and management of severe post-transsphenoidal epistaxis q. J Clin Neurosci 2015;22: 116–22.

57. Zimmer L, Shikary T, Edwards C. Incidence of epistaxis following endoscopic sellar surgery: proposed treatment algorithm. J Neurol Surg Part B Skull Base 2015;76(S 01):A031.

58. Nishioka H, Ohno S, Ikeda Y, et al. Delayed massive epistaxis following endonasal transsphenoidal surgery. Acta Neurochir (Wien) 2007;149(5):523–6.

59. Iqbal SM, Khan AJ, Zhi C. Tension pneumocephalus: a rare complication of transsphenoidal resection of a pituitary macroadenoma. Cureus 2019;11(5). https://doi.org/10.7759/cureus.4623.

60. Yüceer N, Çakíroğlu K, Erdoğan A, et al. Tension pneumocephalus after transsphenoidal surgery: two case reports. Acta Neurochir (Wien) 1995;137(1–2): 58–61.

61. Li W, Liu Q, Lu H, et al. Tension pneumocephalus from endoscopic endonasal surgery: a case series and literature review. Ther Clin Risk Manag 2020;16:531–8.

62. Das M, Bajaj J. Pneumocephalus. In: StatPearls. StatPearls Publishing; 2021. Available at: http://www.ncbi.nlm.nih.gov/books/NBK535412/. Accessed June 20, 2021.

63. Siegel JL, Hampton K, Rabinstein AA, et al. Oxygen therapy with high-flow nasal cannula as an effective treatment for perioperative pneumocephalus: case illustrations and pathophysiological review. Neurocrit Care 2018;29(3):366–73.

64. Wise SK, Harvey RJ, Patel SJ, et al. Endoscopic repair of skull base defects presenting with pneumocephalus. J Otolaryngol - Head Neck 2009;38(4):509–16.

65. Gâta A, Toader C, Trombitaş VE, Ilyes A, Albu S. Endoscopic skull base repair strategy for CSF leaks associated with pneumocephalus. J Clin Med 2020; 10(1):46.

66. DelGaudio JM, Ingley AP. Treatment of pneumocephalus after endoscopic sinus and microscopic skull base surgery. Am J Otol 2010;31(4):226–30.

67. Agam M, Wedemeyer MA, Carmichael JD, et al. Complications associated with transsphenoidal pituitary surgery: experience of 1171 consecutive cases treated at a single tertiary care pituitary center. Neurosurgery 2017;64(CN_suppl_1):237.

68. Younus I, Gerges MM, Godil SS, et al. Incidence and risk factors associated with reoperation for sellar hematoma following endoscopic transsphenoidal pituitary surgery. J Neurosurg 2020;133(3):702–8.

69. El-Asmar N, El-Sibai K, Al-Aridi R, et al. Postoperative sellar hematoma after pituitary surgery: clinical and biochemical characteristics. Eur J Endocrinol 2016; 174(5):573–82.

70. Zhan R, Zhao Y, Wiebe TM, et al. Acute hemorrhagic apoplectic pituitary adenoma: endoscopic management, surgical outcomes, and complications. J Craniofac Surg 2015;26(6):e510–5.

# Microscopic Transsphenoidal Surgery in the Era of Endoscopy

## Are There Any Advantages?

Robert C. Rennert, MD, Vance L. Fredrickson, MD,
William T. Couldwell, MD, PhD*

## KEYWORDS

• Microscope • Endoscope • Pituitary surgery • Transsphenoidal

## KEY POINTS

• Although the enhanced visualization available with endoscopy has led to its widespread adoption, current outcomes data do not definitively support an endoscopic versus microscopic approach to transsphenoidal surgery.
• Potential advantages of the microscopic approach to transsphenoidal surgery include shorter operative time; an unobstructed, single-surgeon, two-handed technique; and less disruption of the nasal mucosa.
• Limitations in visualization with the microscope can be addressed with endoscope-assisted techniques.

## INTRODUCTION

Surgical attempts to address pituitary disease date back to 1893; they quickly evolved from the earliest lateral transcranial approaches with unacceptably high morbidity to the first successful transsphenoidal approach in 1907.[1–3] Subsequently, despite reduced morbidity with this anterior approach, concerns over infections from cerebrospinal fluid (CSF) leaks combined with limitations in the ability to preoperatively determine the accessibility of larger tumors from below led to an abandonment of this technique by the highly influential Harvey Cushing and a near dormancy of the transsphenoidal approach until the mid-1900s.[3] Interest rekindled in the 1950s when Norman Dott, a previous fellow of Cushing from Scotland who had incorporated a lighted speculum retractor and been successfully using the approach, introduced it to the French neurosurgeon Gerard Guiot, who adapted the technique and added

Department of Neurosurgery, Clinical Neurosciences Center, University of Utah, 175 N Medical Drive East, Salt Lake City, UT 84132, USA
* Corresponding author.
*E-mail address:* neuropub@hsc.utah.edu

Otolaryngol Clin N Am 55 (2022) 411–420
https://doi.org/10.1016/j.otc.2021.12.010
0030-6665/22/© 2021 Elsevier Inc. All rights reserved.

intraoperative fluoroscopy to better define the nasal anatomy.[3,4] The introduction of the operating microscope by Guiot's fellow Jules Hardy in 1967 and the subsequent dramatic increase in visualization was nonetheless the critical innovation that enabled the widespread adaptation of transsphenoidal surgery entering the modern era.[3,4]

The safety of the microsurgical approach to treat pituitary disease was demonstrated immediately, with no deaths or serious morbidities recorded in the first 50 of Hardy's patients treated with this technique.[5] It was therefore used and adapted by neurosurgeons worldwide as the new standard of care for pituitary surgery, with mortality rates between 0% and 1% in subsequent large series confirming the relative safety of the approach.[6–9] Microsurgical exploration beyond the confines of the sella paralleled an increased understanding of regional anatomy and improvements in instrumentation, enabling access to the medial wall of the cavernous sinus via a transmaxillosphenoidal approach[10,11] and to the paraclival and suprasellar regions via expanded transsphenoidal approaches.[12–14]

With the first video demonstrating endoscopic removal of a pituitary tumor by Gerard Guiot in Paris in 1962 and description of its use in pituitary surgery in 1978, the endoscope was the next critical innovation in the field, although it did not gain popularity for this application until the mid-1990s.[4] Given its enhanced panoramic visualization, illumination, and magnification of the sellar and parasellar regions,[15] as well as an increased volume of exposure as compared with the operating microscope,[16] use of the endoscope for transsphenoidal and extended transsphenoidal approaches has dramatically increased since then.[17–20] In a recent survey of United States and European neurosurgeons, a preference for a fully endoscopic versus a microscopic approach, largely in a team-based setting, dramatically increased from 43% in 2010 to 87% in 2020.[21] Database studies reflect this preference, with a fully endoscopic approach now used in most transsphenoidal surgeries performed in the United States.[22,23] This transition occurred despite a lack of high-quality evidence for the superiority of the endoscopic approach, with some data even suggesting higher complication rates and costs associated with this technique.[23]

Although we have clearly entered the endoscopic era, often-discussed potential limitations of a purely endoscopic approach include a lack of stereoscopy, a steep learning curve, and instrument crowding that can limit a 2-handed technique.[24] Conversely, potential advantages of the microscopic- and endoscope-assisted microscopic approaches to pituitary surgery include decreased operative time/increased efficiency, preservation of a single-surgeon, 2-handed technique, and decreased disruption of the nasal mucosa.[24] In this setting, the ongoing role of the microscope in pituitary surgery is discussed herein.

## GOALS OF TRANSSPHENOIDAL SURGERY

The surgical goals for addressing pituitary tumors as defined by Edward Laws include removing the tumor mass, normalizing any hormonal hypersecretion, preserving normal pituitary function, and minimizing tumor recurrence.[25] These goals can be adapted to other pathologies treated through transsphenoidal and extended transsphenoidal approaches to include preservation of cranial nerve and hypothalamic function, as well as avoidance of CSF leaks, infections, disruption of the nasal mucosa, and vascular injuries. Because many of the pathologies addressed through standard and expanded transsphenoidal approaches are benign (adenomas, craniopharyngiomas, meningiomas), incomplete resection with the possibility of secondary radiotherapy for lesions with extension into the cavernous sinus or other high-risk areas is often preferable to a complete resection with an associated permanent neurologic morbidity. Finally, as with any operation, surgical efficiency and limiting operative and anesthetic time are also critical goals.

## TECHNICAL CONSIDERATIONS

Microscopic transsphenoidal surgery involves use of either a sublabial transseptal or a uninaral approach. Although the sublabial approach affords the surgeon a wider operative field, it has largely been abandoned in favor of the simpler, more direct uninaral technique.[3] As practiced by the senior author, this approach involves an incision in the posterior nasal septal mucosa at the junction of the perpendicular plate with the rostrum of the sphenoid sinus, fracture of the perpendicular plate, and mobilization contralaterally. After mobilization of the perpendicular plate of the ethmoid, the dissection is continued in a submucosal manner on the contralateral side, and the keel of the vomer and sphenoid rostrum are identified. With assistance of a bivalve self-retaining speculum, the sphenoid sinus is exposed, the ostia are identified, and the bony floor of the sella is removed. After a wide dural opening, the sellar pathology is removed with ringed curettes and microinstruments. In the absence of an arachnoid breach, closure involves simple reapproximation of the nasal anatomy. In cases with suspected or confirmed arachnoid violation, autologous fascia and fat grafting is used for closure to prevent a CSF fistula.[3,26]

Building on this foundation, the nuances of this technique are then tailored to the specific lesion being treated. For adenomas, extracapsular dissection is generally avoided to minimize risk to the normal pituitary gland and stalk, the location of which can often be determined on preoperative imaging. A Valsalva maneuver or bilateral jugular venous compression can aid in tumor descent during this process. For giant adenomas ($\geq$4 cm) with an intact diaphragma sellae, the senior author removes the lateral and posterior aspects of the tumor first (avoiding early central debulking) to facilitate a posterior to anterior descent of the diaphragma and to minimize tumor residual in the posterior gutter (**Fig. 1**). For giant adenomas with growth beyond the diaphragma sellae, this approach can be less effective, and a transcranial surgery may be considered if it better aligns along the long axis of the tumor. Similarly, adenomas with extension into the oculomotor cistern, which is a transnasal operative blind spot even with endoscopy, can limit tumor descent and require adjuvant radiotherapy and/or a second transcranial approach after transsphenoidal surgery.[27] For Rathke cleft cysts, where recurrence is linked to histology rather than surgical technique,[28] a minimally invasive initial cyst drainage is well suited to the microscopic approach. Recurrences are then treated with more aggressive attempts to remove the capsule with or without marsupialization.

An important adjunct to this approach that the senior author has incorporated over time is the use of an angled endoscope to inspect any areas of concern (ie, behind redundant folds of suprasellar arachnoid or with tumors extending into the cavernous sinus) that may be hidden with a strictly microscopic view (see **Fig. 1**).[3] Identified areas of residual tumor are then typically addressed using the microscope, with subsequent endoscopic visualization to confirm tumor removal. Additional techniques developed by the senior author for tumors with cavernous sinus extension include the toothpaste extraction technique, wherein a Valsalva maneuver forces tumor medially through a breach in the cavernous sinus wall,[29] and pituitary transposition (hypophysopexy), in cases where significant residual postoperative tumor is expected. In the latter technique, the gland is separated from the residual tumor using a fat graft to reduce its effective biological dose of subsequent adjuvant radiation and decrease the likelihood of secondary hypopituitarism.[30–32]

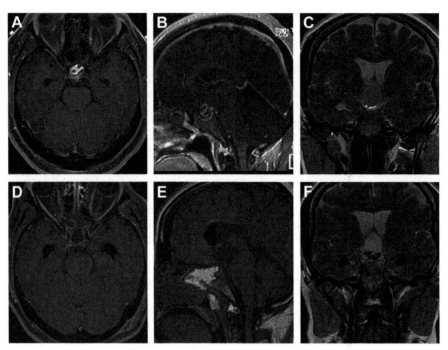

**Fig. 1.** Microscopic transsphenoidal case example. A 36-year-old man with a history of factor XI deficiency underwent workup for progressive bitemporal hemianopsia. He was found to have a 5.6 × 4.2 × 4.1-cm sellar and suprasellar enhancing tumor with compression of the optic chiasm visible on axial (*A*), sagittal (*B*), and coronal (*C*) MRI. A full endocrine workup was unremarkable. He underwent an urgent endonasal transsphenoidal microscopic resection, using a peripheral initial debulking technique to facilitate tumor descent and endoscopic assistance to look within the suprasellar arachnoid folds. The limited disruption of the nasal mucosa required with the microscopic approach helped to minimize blood loss given his factor XI deficiency. The pathologic findings were consistent with a nonfunctioning pituitary adenoma. Postoperative MRI demonstrated a near-total resection with a small amount of residual tumor extending into the right cavernous sinus on axial (*D*), sagittal (*E*), and coronal (*F*) images. At 6-month follow-up, he had moderate improvement in his peripheral vision and did not have any new endocrinopathies.

Extended transsphenoidal approaches can also be successfully performed with the microscope, treating a wide variety of lesions (adenomas with lateral extension, craniopharyngiomas, tuberculum/diaphragma sellae meningiomas, sphenoid sinus mucoceles, clival chordomas, carcinomas, and fibrous dysplasia) extending from the cribriform plate to the inferior clivus in the anteroposterior plane and laterally to the cavernous cranial nerves and optic canal (**Fig. 2**).[33,34] Primary use of the microscope in such cases preserves an unobstructed corridor for fine bimanual microsurgical dissection, with intermittent endoscopic assistance useful for visualizing spaces obscured in the microscopic view to aid in tumor dissection and preservation of critical structures.[35–37]

The relative simplicity of the microsurgical approach and preservation of many of the same skill sets used in other areas of neurosurgery were undoubtedly key aspects to its widespread adaptation, including its demonstrated safety and efficacy in higher-risk populations such as children and the elderly.[38,39] The uninaral microscopic technique may also minimize disruption of the nasal mucosa as compared with the

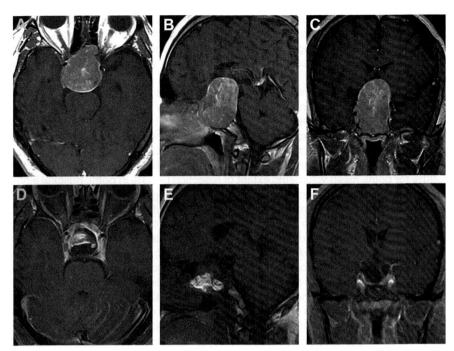

**Fig. 2.** Microscopic extended transsphenoidal case example. Preoperative axial (*A*), sagittal (*B*), and coronal (*C*) MRI scans of a 44-year-old woman who underwent workup for an acute episode of headache, nausea, and vomiting showing a 4.0 × 2.2 × 2.0-cm mixed solid and cystic sellar, suprasellar, and third ventricular adamantinomatous craniopharyngioma. She subsequently underwent an extended endonasal, transsphenoidal complete resection. A bimanual microsurgical technique facilitated by the microscope was critical in dissection of the superior aspect of the tumor from the underside of the optic nerves and chiasm, as well as preservation of the pituitary gland and stalk. The endoscope was used to enhance visualization during removal of the superior aspect of the tumor from the third ventricle. Postoperative imaging [(*D*), axial; (*E*), sagittal; (*F*), coronal] demonstrated the extent of resection. She remained neurologically intact, with short-term hormone replacement therapy ongoing at 1-month follow-up.

commonly used binaral endoscopic approach, wherein portions of the bilateral septal mucosa are removed in some cases to facilitate dispersion of the endoscope and surgical instruments between nostrils and decrease "sword fighting."[40] The hemostatic properties of the open speculum further aid in efficiency and minimization of blood loss by tamponading mucosal hemorrhagic sources. For most pituitary pathologies, this procedure can be performed quickly in experienced hands, avoiding the need to coordinate a cosurgeon's schedule and facilitating the incorporation of a high volume of pituitary cases into a busy neurosurgical practice.[24,41,42] Accordingly, for relatively simple transsphenoidal cases, the senior author can perform multiple transnasal surgeries in 1 day. This practice minimizes surgical wait times, a critical component of running a high-volume neurosurgical department.

## CURRENT EVIDENCE

Although head-to-head analyses of the described endoscope-assisted microscopic technique and fully endoscopic techniques for pituitary surgery do not exist, there have been many studies comparing the outcomes of purely microscopic and purely endoscopic approaches to pituitary tumors. Although important insights can be gained from this literature regarding the relative advantages of each approach, a definitive answer regarding the superiority of one technique versus the other has thus far been elusive.

In the only prospective analysis on the topic, the Transsphenoidal Extent of Resection (TRANSSPHER) study in 2020, Little and colleagues[24] compared the surgical outcomes of purely microscopic versus purely endoscopic transsphenoidal surgery for nonfunctioning pituitary macroadenomas. Encompassing 7 US pituitary centers and 15 surgeons, this work included 82 patients who underwent microscopic surgery and 177 patients who underwent endoscopic surgery. Rates of gross total resection (>80% for both), mean volumetric extent of resection ($\sim$98% in both), hospital length of stay, unplanned readmission rates, and rates of surgical complications including CSF leaks requiring intervention were not significantly different between the 2 groups ($P > .2$). Although operative time was significantly shorter in the microscopic group ($P < .001$), a new hormone deficiency at 6 months was also more likely in this cohort (28.4% vs 9.7%, $P < .001$). Although the surgeons using the microscope in the study were significantly more experienced than their endoscope-using colleagues (in line with national trends), the investigators concluded that both techniques can produce acceptable surgical outcomes in properly trained hands.

For functioning tumors, a smaller retrospective study of 137 patients with Cushing disease found largely comparable surgical complication, hormonal outcome, and early remission (86% vs 83%) rates for microscopic versus endoscopic surgery.[43] Interestingly, despite similar early outcomes data, lower recurrence rates over 10 years were seen in patients in the microscopic surgery cohort (hazard ratio 0.47, 95% confidence interval [CI]: 0.19–1.14), particularly in those with macroadenomas.

Similarly, a single-center retrospective analysis by Agam and colleagues[41] comparing the outcomes of 1153 patients undergoing either microscopic or endoscopic resection of functioning or nonfunctioning pituitary adenomas demonstrated no significant difference in either surgical (6.4% vs 8.8%, $P = .24$) or endocrinologic (11.4% vs 11.8%, $P = .88$) complications between the groups. Although the extent of resection was not reported, a significantly higher rate of delayed epistaxis was seen with endoscopic surgery (2.9% vs 0.8%, $P = .03$), consistent with a higher degree of nasal disruption with this approach.

A meta-analysis by Chen and colleagues[44] of all available worldwide data from 1999 to 2020 comparing endoscopic and microscopic transsphenoidal surgery for the treatment of pituitary adenomas largely supports these findings. In this analysis of 29 retrospective, case-control studies encompassing 7774 patients with both functioning and nonfunctioning adenomas, there were no significant differences in resection rates ($P = .12$), remission rates of excess hormone secretion ($P = .16$), or overall complication rates ($P = .34$) between groups. Endoscopic surgery was nonetheless associated with a lower rate of postoperative diabetes insipidus ($P = .03$).

Studies mining real-world databases provide additional insight into the relative utility of the microscopic versus endoscopic approaches by aggregating data for the entire practicing specialty rather than selected cohort data from likely higher-volume academic centers. A 2017 study of 5886 pituitary surgery cases (54% microscopic, 46% endoscopic spanning from 2010 to 2014) from the US-based Truven MarketScan database demonstrated higher rates of postoperative pituitary dysfunction (22.7% vs 16.0%, $P < .001$), CSF leak/dura tear (13.6% vs 7.6%, $P < .001$), altered mental status (1.1% vs 0.6%, $P = .04$), and fever (0.4% vs 0.1%, $P = .02$) with endoscopic versus microscopic surgery.[23] Similarly, a separate 2017 study of the same database spanning 2007 to 2014 found higher overall complication rates (47% vs 39%, OR 1.37, 95% CI 1.22–1.53), as well as an increased risk of neurologic complications (OR 1.32, 95% CI 1.11–1.55), diabetes insipidus (OR 1.65, 95% CI 1.37–2.00), and CSF leak (OR 1.83, 95% CI 1.07–3.13) with endoscopic versus microscopic approaches.[22]

Although these aggregate data do not clearly support the use of one technique over the other for transsphenoidal pituitary surgery, important insights include the speed of the microscopic technique, largely comparable outcomes in experienced hands despite a smaller visual field with the microscope, and the enhanced optics of the endoscopic approach likely facilitating high resection rates early in a skull base surgeon's career. A critical analysis of the higher complication rates seen in database studies versus retrospective academic data for endoscopic approaches nonetheless highlights the potentially steep initial learning curve with this technique, especially when applied in lower-volume community settings. Regarding endocrinologic outcomes with the microscopic technique, in the senior author's experience of more than 3000 microscopic transsphenoidal surgeries, the incidence of postoperative endocrinologic dysfunction more closely resembles the 11.4% rate reported by Agam and colleagues[41] than the 28% seen in the TRANSSPHER study.[24] This underscores the importance of surgical technique when separating the tumor from the gland, as well as the equipoise in outcomes achievable with either approach.

## SUMMARY

The microscopic transsphenoidal approach is a proven, efficient technique that facilitates an unobstructed corridor for single-surgeon, 2-handed microsurgery with minimal disruption of the nasal mucosa and the potential for expanded access. Endoscopic assistance can be used to overcome associated limitations in visualization as needed. Current data do not definitively support a primarily endoscopic versus microscopic approach to transsphenoidal surgery despite clear trends toward increased use of endoscopy within the field.

## CLINICS CARE POINTS

- Microscopic transsphenoidal surgery can provide rapid access to sellar and parasellar disease with minimal nasal mucosal disruption and comparable outcomes with endoscopic approaches.
- Endoscopic assistance can aid in visualizing areas hidden with a strictly microscopic view.
- The simplicity and speed of the microscopic approach justify its maintenance as a critical skillset for neurosurgeons training within the endoscopic era.

## ACKNOWLEDGMENTS

The authors thank Kristin Kraus, MSc, for editorial assistance with this article.

## DISCLOSURE

The authors have nothing to disclose.

## REFERENCES

1. Cope V. The pituitary fossa, and the methods of surgical approach thereto. Br J Surg 1916;4:107–44.

2. Collins WF. Hypophysectomy: historical and personal perspective. Clin Neurosurg 1974;21:68–78.
3. Couldwell WT. Transsphenoidal and transcranial surgery for pituitary adenomas. J Neurooncol 2004;69(1–3):237–56.
4. Liu JK, Das K, Weiss MH, et al. The history and evolution of transsphenoidal surgery. J Neurosurg 2001;95(6):1083–96.
5. Welbourn RB. The evolution of transsphenoidal pituitary microsurgery. Surgery 1986;100(6):1185–90.
6. Black PM, Zervas NT, Candia GL. Incidence and management of complications of transsphenoidal operation for pituitary adenomas. Neurosurgery 1987;20(6):920–4.
7. Ciric I, Ragin A, Baumgartner C, et al. Complications of transsphenoidal surgery: results of a national survey, review of the literature, and personal experience. Neurosurgery 1997;40(2):225–36 [discussion: 236-237].
8. Laws ER, Kern EB. Complications of trans-sphenoidal surgery. Clin Neurosurg 1976;23:401–16.
9. Wilson CB. A decade of pituitary microsurgery. The Herbert Olivecrona lecture. J Neurosurg 1984;61(5):814–33.
10. Fraioli B, Esposito V, Santoro A, et al. Transmaxillosphenoidal approach to tumors invading the medial compartment of the cavernous sinus. J Neurosurg 1995;82(1):63–9.
11. Sabit I, Schaefer SD, Couldwell WT. Extradural extranasal combined transmaxillary transsphenoidal approach to the cavernous sinus: a minimally invasive microsurgical model. Laryngoscope 2000;110(2 Pt 1):286–91.
12. Kouri JG, Chen MY, Watson JC, et al. Resection of suprasellar tumors by using a modified transsphenoidal approach. Report of four cases. J Neurosurg 2000;92(6):1028–35.
13. Mason RB, Nieman LK, Doppman JL, et al. Selective excision of adenomas originating in or extending into the pituitary stalk with preservation of pituitary function. J Neurosurg 1997;87(3):343–51.
14. Couldwell W, Weiss M. The transnasal transsphenoidal approach. In: Apuzzo M, editor. Surgery of the third ventricle. 2 edition. Baltimore (MD): Williams & Wilkins; 1998. p. 553–74.
15. Jho HD, Carrau RL, Ko Y, et al. Endoscopic pituitary surgery: an early experience. Surg Neurol 1997;47(3):213–22 [discussion: 222-223].
16. Spencer WR, Das K, Nwagu C, et al. Approaches to the sellar and parasellar region: anatomic comparison of the microscope versus endoscope. Laryngoscope 1999;109(5):791–4.
17. Paluzzi A, Fernandez-Miranda JC, Tonya Stefko S, et al. Endoscopic endonasal approach for pituitary adenomas: a series of 555 patients. Pituitary 2014;17(4):307–19.
18. Di Maio S, Cavallo LM, Esposito F, et al. Extended endoscopic endonasal approach for selected pituitary adenomas: early experience. J Neurosurg 2011;114(2):345–53.
19. Juraschka K, Khan OH, Godoy BL, et al. Endoscopic endonasal transsphenoidal approach to large and giant pituitary adenomas: institutional experience and predictors of extent of resection. J Neurosurg 2014;121(1):75–83.
20. Cavallo LM, Frank G, Cappabianca P, et al. The endoscopic endonasal approach for the management of craniopharyngiomas: a series of 103 patients. J Neurosurg 2014;121(1):100–13.

21. Khalafallah AM, Liang AL, Jimenez AE, et al. Trends in endoscopic and microscopic transsphenoidal surgery: a survey of the international society of pituitary surgeons between 2010 and 2020. Pituitary 2020;23(5):526–33.
22. Azad TD, Lee YJ, Vail D, et al. Endoscopic vs. microscopic resection of sellar lesions-A matched analysis of clinical and socioeconomic outcomes. Front Surg 2017;4:33.
23. Asemota AO, Ishii M, Brem H, et al. Comparison of complications, trends, and costs in endoscopic vs microscopic pituitary surgery: analysis from a US Health Claims Database. Neurosurgery 2017;81(3):458–72.
24. Little AS, Kelly DF, White WL, et al. Results of a prospective multicenter controlled study comparing surgical outcomes of microscopic versus fully endoscopic transsphenoidal surgery for nonfunctioning pituitary adenomas: the Transsphenoidal Extent of Resection (TRANSSPHER) Study. J Neurosurg 2019;132(4): 1043–53.
25. Laws ER. Pituitary surgery. Endocrinol Metab Clin North Am 1987;16(3):647–65.
26. Couldwell WT, Kan P, Weiss MH. Simple closure following transsphenoidal surgery. Technical note. Neurosurg Focus 2006;20(3):E11.
27. Hoang N, Tran DK, Herde R, et al. Pituitary macroadenomas with oculomotor cistern extension and tracking: implications for surgical management. J Neurosurg 2016;125(2):315–22.
28. Kinoshita Y, Tominaga A, Usui S, et al. The long-term recurrence of Rathke's cleft cysts as predicted by histology but not by surgical procedure. J Neurosurg 2016; 125(4):1002–7.
29. Baker C, Karsy M, Couldwell WT. Resection of pituitary tumor with lateral extension to the temporal fossa: the toothpaste extrusion technique. Cureus 2019; 11(10):e5953.
30. Couldwell WT, Rosenow JM, Rovit RL, et al. Hypophysopexy technique for radiosurgical treatment of cavernous sinus pituitary adenoma. Pituitary 2002;5(3): 169–73.
31. Taussky P, Kalra R, Coppens J, et al. Endocrinological outcome after pituitary transposition (hypophysopexy) and adjuvant radiotherapy for tumors involving the cavernous sinus. J Neurosurg 2011;115(1):55–62.
32. Liu JK, Schmidt MH, MacDonald JD, et al. Hypophysial transposition (hypophysopexy) for radiosurgical treatment of pituitary tumors involving the cavernous sinus. Technical note. Neurosurg Focus 2003;14(5):e11.
33. Couldwell WT, Weiss MH, Rabb C, et al. Variations on the standard transsphenoidal approach to the sellar region, with emphasis on the extended approaches and parasellar approaches: surgical experience in 105 cases. Neurosurgery 2004;55(3):539–47 ; [discussion: 547-550].
34. Chakrabarti I, Amar AP, Couldwell W, et al. Long-term neurological, visual, and endocrine outcomes following transnasal resection of craniopharyngioma. J Neurosurg 2005;102(4):650–7.
35. Ikeda H, Gotoh H, Watanabe K. Outcome of endoscopy-assisted microscopic extended transsphenoidal surgery for suprasellar adult craniopharyngiomas. Front Endocrinol (Lausanne) 2012;3:25.
36. Kim EH, Ahn JY, Kim SH. Technique and outcome of endoscopy-assisted microscopic extended transsphenoidal surgery for suprasellar craniopharyngiomas. J Neurosurg 2011;114(5):1338–49.
37. Catapano D, Sloffer CA, Frank G, et al. Comparison between the microscope and endoscope in the direct endonasal extended transsphenoidal approach: anatomical study. J Neurosurg 2006;104(3):419–25.

38. Abunimer AM, Abou-Al-Shaar H, Azab MA, et al. Transsphenoidal approaches for microsurgical resection of pituitary adenomas in pediatric patients. World Neurosurg 2019;123:e186–93.
39. Azab MA, O'Hagan M, Abou-Al-Shaar H, et al. Safety and outcome of transsphenoidal pituitary adenoma resection in elderly patients. World Neurosurg 2019; 122:e1252–8.
40. Elhadi AM, Hardesty DA, Zaidi HA, et al. Evaluation of surgical freedom for microscopic and endoscopic transsphenoidal approaches to the sella. Neurosurgery 2015;11(Suppl 2):69–78 [discussion: 78-79].
41. Agam MS, Wedemeyer MA, Wrobel B, et al. Complications associated with microscopic and endoscopic transsphenoidal pituitary surgery: experience of 1153 consecutive cases treated at a single tertiary care pituitary center. J Neurosurg 2018;1–8.
42. Jane JA, Laws ER. The surgical management of pituitary adenomas in a series of 3,093 patients. J Am Coll Surg 2001;193(6):651–9.
43. Broersen LHA, van Haalen FM, Biermasz NR, et al. Microscopic versus endoscopic transsphenoidal surgery in the Leiden cohort treated for Cushing's disease: surgical outcome, mortality, and complications. Orphanet J Rare Dis 2019;14(1):64.
44. Chen X, Huang W, Li H, et al. Comparison of outcomes between endoscopic and microscopic transsphenoidal surgery for the treatment of pituitary adenoma: a meta-analysis. Gland Surg 2020;9(6):2162–74.

# Anesthesia for Pituitary Surgery

Jinu Kim, MD[a],*, Ross Scott-Miller, MD[b]

## KEYWORDS

- Anesthesia • Pituitary • Diabetes insipidus • Pituitary surgery • Cushing disease
- Acromegaly • SIADH

## KEY POINTS

- Anesthesia planning should begin in the preoperative period and incorporate aspects specific to the type of pituitary tumor the patient is presenting with.
- Various pituitary syndromes pose specific anesthetic challenges that should be addressed during preoperative planning.
- A smooth extubation is important at the end of the procedure and can be accomplished through a variety of methods.

## INTRODUCTION

Transsphenoidal pituitary surgery is the most common treatment for pituitary masses. In this article, the authors review the anesthetic concerns for pituitary surgery in the preoperative, intraoperative, and postoperative periods.

Anesthesia for pituitary tumor resection requires careful preoperative planning, considering the physiologic and anatomic consequences of pituitary lesions. Tumors may present as an excess or deficiency of hormones depending on the type of tumor and the degree of compression caused by the tumor. With the exception of pituitary apoplexy, hemorrhage, or vision loss owing to compression, most pituitary tumor resection surgery is performed electively, and an appropriate workup is available before surgery.

Intraoperative anesthetic management of pituitary surgery revolves around maintaining stable hemodynamics, immobility, and preparedness for major hemorrhage. During emergence from anesthesia, great care is taken to ensure a smooth rapid emergence with minimal bucking to facilitate a postoperative neurologic examination in the operating room.

[a] Department of Anesthesia, Albert Einstein College of Medicine, 111 East 210 Street, Bronx, NY 10467, USA; [b] Department of Anesthesia, Montefiore Medical Center, 111 East 210 Street, Bronx, NY 10467, USA
* Corresponding author.
E-mail address: jinkim@montefiore.org

Otolaryngol Clin N Am 55 (2022) 421–430
https://doi.org/10.1016/j.otc.2022.01.003
0030-6665/22/© 2022 Elsevier Inc. All rights reserved.
oto.theclinics.com

Recognition and treatment of metabolic and hormonal abnormalities are the focus of postoperative care. In addition, prevention of nausea and vomiting is especially important for pituitary surgery patients, as the associated Valsalva movements could cause epistaxis or cerebrospinal fluid (CSF) leak at the surgical site.

## PREOPERATIVE ASSESSMENT

Patients undergoing elective pituitary surgery should have standard preoperative laboratory evaluation, which, if recently performed during the initial workup, need not be repeated. This typically includes complete blood counts, basic metabolic and coagulation profile, as well as a type and screen owing to the rare but potentially catastrophic possibility of intracranial vascular injury. Electrocardiograms and more extensive cardiac testing should be obtained if appropriate to the patient's age and medical condition. Electrolyte abnormalities especially in patients with secretory pituitary tumors should be addressed.[1]

Approximately 40% of pituitary tumors are nonsecretory, and the anesthetic concerns focus mainly on the effect of the tumor on intracranial pressure (ICP). The standard anesthetic precautions for increased ICP include maintaining cerebral perfusion and oxygenation by avoiding periods of hypotension and keeping the arterial line transducer at the level of the tragus as opposed to the heart. In the case of very large tumors, the surgical approach may be a bicoronal craniotomy, as opposed to endonasal transsphenoidal necessitating the standard precautions for a supratentorial craniotomy, such as seizure prophylaxis and steroids to reduce brain edema. Large, nonfunctional tumors may be highly vascularized, and preparations should be made for significant hemorrhage, such as additional large-bore intravenous access and intra-arterial blood pressure (BP) monitoring.[2]

Anesthetic concerns for secretory pituitary tumors revolve around the type of hormone secreted and are discussed in **Table 1**.

## ACROMEGALY

Acromegaly, the syndrome of overabundant growth hormone (GH) secretion, causes numerous changes, which are relevant to the anesthesiologist. These changes include difficult airway morphology, sleep apnea, cardiac disturbances, and diabetes mellitus. In a small study, cardiac abnormalities and hypertension were present in 50% of patients, and obstructive sleep apnea (OSA) was present in 37.5% of patients.[3]

The airway changes associated with acromegaly include macroglossia, maxillary and mandibular hypertrophy, soft palate and pharyngeal swelling, true and false vocal cord thickening, vocal cord paresis, tracheal compression, and hypertrophy of the epiglottis.[4] These changes bring a dramatically increased risk of difficult direct laryngoscopy in 9% to 40% of patients when compared with the general population (2%–6%), irrespective of Mallampati score, thyromental distance, or mouth opening.[5–9] In a small case series, video intubation was required for 21.9% and fiberoptic intubation was required for 12.5% of patients. Overall failure rate for the first intubation technique was 12.5%.[3] The advent of video laryngoscopy has made management of the difficult airway more routine, but preparations for alternative methods for securing the airway, such as fiberoptic intubation, should still be made.

OSA is very common, with up to 70% prevalence among patients with acromegaly. The postoperative use of bilevel positive airway pressure and constant positive airway pressure devices is typically recommended postoperatively for patients with OSA but generally avoided in patients post transsphenoidal pituitary resection, as the positive pressure could cause pneumocephalus.[10] This presents a clinical dilemma as the

**Table 1**
**Perioperative assessment of disease states**

| Disease | Features | Physical Examination | Preoperative Considerations |
|---|---|---|---|
| Acromegaly | Swelling and hypertrophy of peripharyngeal tissues, HTN, CAD, DM2, cardiomegaly, diastolic cardiac dysfunction, OSA, ulnar artery compromise | Macroglossia, mandibular and maxillary hypertrophy. Facial bone hypertrophy. Elevated blood pressure. ± Hoarse voice (secondary to tracheal compression), S4 or S3 heart sounds, peripheral edema, jugular vein distention, enlarged hands | Video or fiberoptic intubation, consider rapid sequence intubation if decreased gastric emptying. If exercise intolerance, consider cardiac workup. Consider bedside point-of-care ultrasound to assess global cardiac function. If history consistent with OSA, consider sleep study. Basic metabolic panel if metabolically active tumor. Allen test to assess for radial artery collateral flow |
| Cushing disease | Exophthalmos, OSA secondary to obesity and myopathy of oropharyngeal muscles, HTN, CAD, DM2, increased risk of MI and VTE, hypercortisolism, osteoporosis, truncal obesity, myopathies, friable skin | Truncal obesity, moon facies, "buffalo hump", striae, proximal muscle weakness | Consider video intubation with rapid sequence intubation if history findings consistent with delayed gastric emptying. May be difficult to mask ventilate. If exercise intolerance, follow American Heart Association guidelines. Basic metabolic panel. Consider sleep study for suspected OSA. Metabolic panel. Withhold perioperative steroids |
| Thyrotropic adenomas | May present as euthyroid, hyperthyroid, or | Hyperthyroid: exophthalmos, tachycardia, | Depending on the degree of thyroid function, may be |

*(continued on next page)*

| Disease | Features | Physical Examination | Preoperative Considerations |
|---------|----------|---------------------|----------------------------|
| | hypothyroid, with features consistent as such. Depends if the patient has undergone thyroid ablation | hyperactivity, arrhythmias. Hypothyroid: bradycardia, diastolic hypertension, and delayed relaxation of deep tendon reflexes | more or less susceptible to anesthesia agents. Basic metabolic panel. Thyroid function tests |
| Prolactinoma | Infertility, galactorrhea, amenorrhea | Decreased visual fields, orthostatic hypotension | Often treated with dopamine agonists, therefore susceptible to orthostatic hypotension, consider slow vertical movement in preoperative and postoperative settings. Basic metabolic panel |
| Nonfunctioning macroadenoma | Panhypopituitarism | Decreased visual fields | Depending on size and vascularity: type and screen, additional intravenous access, ± large-bore intravenous access. Arterial line |

*Abbreviations:* CAD, coronary artery disease; OSA, obstructive sleep apnea; MI, myocardial infarction; DM2, diabetes mellitus type 2; HTN, hypertension; VTE, venous thromboembolism.

goals of avoiding bucking at the end of a procedure, as well as having the patient awake enough to maintain a non-obstructive breathing pattern are in opposition. As in most dilemmas in clinical medicine, the risks and benefits must be weighed with respect to each individual patient.

Hypertension is common in acromegalic patients (35%), the degree of which correlates to the extent of GH secretion. Hypertension in acromegalic patients is characterized by a higher diastolic BP as compared with the other patients with hypertension. The cause of this hypertension is multifactorial and includes sodium and water retention, insulin resistance, OSA, and increased arterial stiffness.

Cardiac hypertrophy is common and increases with the duration of untreated disease. Approximately 20% of patients with acromegaly under the age of 20 years may have cardiac hypertrophy on echocardiographic examination. In older acromegalic patients, the prevalence increases to 70% in those with normotension and to 90% in those with hypertension. Acromegaly typically causes concentric biventricular hypertrophy, which may be subclinical at first but progresses often to heart failure by the age of 60 years if left untreated. The structural changes are multifactorial; it is suggested that both direct effect of GH on the heart, hypertension, glucose tolerance, and growth hormone/insulin growth factor 1 oversecretion contribute to left ventricular hypertrophy. Cardiomyopathy initially begins with subclinical diastolic dysfunction. Premature coronary artery disease and arrhythmias are also resultant from the effects of excess GH.[4,10]

## CUSHING DISEASE

Cushing disease can present with a spectrum of morphologic changes, typically dependent on the progression of disease and the degree of steroid secretion. In terms of airway assessment, central obesity, moon facies, and buffalo hump may increase the difficulty of laryngoscopy.

Patients can also present with OSA secondary to obesity and myopathy of oropharyngeal muscles. The risk of coronary artery disease, along with hypertension, hyperlipidemia, risk of stroke, myocardial infarction, and venous thromboembolism, is greatly increased. Hyperglycemia and metabolic derangements are also seen with Cushing disease.

## THYROID-STIMULATING HORMONE

A patient presenting with thyroid-stimulating hormone–secreting tumor can be euthyroid, hyperthyroid, or hypothyroid, depending on whether their thyroid has been ablated.[11] There is a prevailing thought that patients with hyperthyroidism may have increased sensitivity to catecholamines, secondary to in vitro evidence of increased beta-adrenergic receptor density in cardiac tissue.[2,12,13] There is also evidence that despite this increased density, there is decreased responsiveness to catecholamines caused by intracellular changes.[14] Overall, these counteracting effects result in normal catechol responsiveness.

## PROLACTIN

Prolactin-secreting tumors are commonly treated with dopamine agonists, such as bromocriptine, which are associated with orthostatic hypotension. Care should be maintained in these patients during position changes.

**Electrolyte Abnormalities:** Pituitary tumors can be associated with central diabetes insipidus (DI), which usually occurs postoperatively but can occur pre and intraoperatively. The syndrome of inappropriate antidiuretic hormone secretion (SIADH) is also common postoperatively.[14–16] Pre-operatively, all electrolyte abnormalities should be corrected, and the medications for DI should be continued on the day of surgery.

## INTRAOPERATIVE MANAGEMENT

Standard monitors, including pulse oximetry, electrocardiogram, BP, temperature, and capnography, should be applied. Invasive arterial monitoring may help with BP management and can be placed based on the surgeon's and patient's needs. The decision for invasive arterial BP measurement is dependent on either need for close monitoring of BP for highly vascularized tumors with risk of hemorrhage, a relevant history of significant cardiac disease, or the need for frequent blood sampling, such as in patients with severe diabetes mellitus or electrolyte abnormalities. In a small study, patients with acromegaly carried a higher likelihood of having a positive Allen test, therefore a higher risk of ischemia with arterial line placement. Brachial, axillary, or dorsalis pedis artery cannulation may be preferred if the Allen test is positive.[17]

Induction of anesthesia may proceed with precautions for a difficult airway if the patient has acromegaly, in which case an awake fiberoptic intubation may be warranted. Large pituitary tumors have the potential for increased ICP; thus, hypotension should be avoided in these patients to maintain cerebral perfusion. Additional large-bore intravenous access and a crossmatch for blood transfusion should be obtained should vascular injury occur intraoperatively.

Premedication may be administered to alleviate the patient's anxiety. A short-acting benzodiazepine, such as midazolam, is often used. In addition, the administration of ERAS (early recovery after surgery) protocols should be considered, which may be included in institutional policies as well. Considerations if not otherwise contraindicated include oral acetaminophen.

Intubation may proceed as routine, with special considerations for a possible difficult airway in acromegalic patients. The endotracheal tube should be taped to the side of the mouth according to the surgeon's preference. If the surgeon is standing on the right side of the patient during the procedure, the tube is usually taped to the contralateral side.

## MAINTENANCE OF ANESTHESIA

Although transsphenoidal pituitary surgery is not generally painful, there are portions which can be very stimulating. Use of local anesthetic with epinephrine and less often cocaine can be associated with arrhythmias and hypertension. In a retrospective review of 100 hypophysectomy patients at a single institution, 58% had a 50% increase of systolic BP after injection, and 33% had a 50% increase of systolic BP during emergence. There was no correlation regarding history of Cushing disease, acromegaly, hypertension, diabetes, prior pituitary surgery, gender, age, surgeon, perioperative usage of beta-adrenergic, or calcium channel blocker. In addition, there was no correlation with magnitude of hypertension and the dose of epinephrine used in the surgical field.[18]

Drilling of the sphenoid bone may require deepening of anesthesia with propofol or possibly administering a short-acting beta-antagonist. Maintaining paralysis during surgery is helpful to prevent patient movement during increased periods of stimulation. BP is usually maintained on the lower end of normal to minimize bleeding, as the surgery is performed with small endoscopes, through which even small amounts of bleeding can obscure the view of the surgical site and increase the risk of complications.

Intraoperative agents used during anesthesia maintenance should be chosen with the goal of a rapid emergence at the termination of surgery so that a neurologic exam can be performed reliably. Short-acting opioids, such as remifentanil, and judicious use of paralytics should be titrated so that the patient is able to cooperate with a neurologic examination shortly after extubation.

Although there are strict guidelines for perioperative blood glucose management, an intraoperative nominal blood glucose of 110 to 180 is acceptable, as the incidence of iatrogenic hypoglycemia with strict glucose control is higher with the tighter protocol.

CSF leak is a complication of endoscopic pituitary surgery, and surgeons often will ask for a Valsalva maneuver to be performed to check the integrity of their closure. This is accomplished by manually performing the Valsalva maneuver and maintaining airway pressure around 20 mm Hg for 10 to 15 seconds.

Prevention of postoperative nausea and vomiting (PONV) is crucial, as vomiting and retching can increase venous pressure, leading to disruption of hemostasis. Standard medications for PONV prophylaxis include ondansetron or dexamethasone; however, the use of dexamethasone should be discussed with the surgical team, as it can suppress cortisol and confound postoperative laboratory investigation.[19] At the termination of transsphenoidal surgery, an orogastric tube should be used to suction blood that may collect in the oropharynx and stomach from the surgical site, even if a throat pack is used. This may be done once the procedure is completed, before the start of emergence. It is imperative that the tube be placed through the mouth, as a nasogastric tube may inadvertently enter the brain after transsphenoidal surgery.

## EMERGENCE

Rapid and smooth emergence from anesthesia is preferred, as it allows for a prompt neurologic examination and vision assessment. The physiologic response to an endotracheal tube is typically characterized as "bucking," which increases intracranial venous pressure and may cause epistaxis. In addition, there is the risk of potential migration of nasopharyngeal flora to the CSF resulting in meningitis.

Techniques to consider for smooth extubation include administration of intravenous or endotracheal lidocaine, avoidance of external stimulation, exchange of an endotracheal tube for a supraglottic airway while the patient is still deeply anesthetized (Bailey maneuver), and maintenance of a low-dose (0.05 µg/kg/min) remifentanil infusion until extubation. These precautions may be forgone if the patient was a difficult airway at the time of intubation and the risks/benefits favor standard extubation criteria. Positioning the patient with the head up minimizes the risk of aspiration of remnant blood and secretions, as well as relieves airway obstruction.

Control of BP during emergence is also desired; typically, surgeons may request systolic BP to not exceed 140 mm/Hg. Labetalol is often used in titrated doses to achieve this, but other agents, such as short-acting calcium blockers like nicardipine and nimodipine, are also adequate.

A rare but dreaded surgical complication is hemorrhage from the internal carotid artery or its branches owing to the proximity of the pituitary to the circle of Willis. Deliberate hypotension may be requested to assist in control of the hemorrhage and may be achieved by deepening the level of anesthesia or using a short-acting antihypertensive, such as nimodipine or nitroglycerin. If control of the hemorrhage cannot be obtained, emergent embolization by neurointerventional radiology or craniotomy may be required.

Emergency pituitary resection is rare and typically occurs in the setting of pituitary apoplexy or infarction from Sheehan syndrome. If the patient has pituitary apoplexy, vasoconstrictor-refractory hypotension should be expected owing to cortisol deficiency. These patients should be treated preemptively with a glucocorticoid, such as hydrocortisone. Postoperative pituitary apoplexy can be difficult to manage and carries a high rate of mortality.[20]

## POSTOPERATIVE MANAGEMENT

Transsphenoidal surgery is not typically painful, and postoperative pain can be managed with acetaminophen. If necessary, a long acting opioid-like hydromorphone can be given with fentanyl for short-term pain management. The use of nonsteroidal anti-inflammatory drugs (NSAIDs) is almost entirely at the surgeon's discretion. Given the difficult areas to achieve hemostasis, NSAIDs are generally avoided because of concern for postoperative bleeding.

Postoperative hormonal changes can vary with both the type and the size of the tumor. Regarding new-onset hormonal deficiencies, GH-secreting adenomas, prolactinomas, and nonfunctional tumors carry a 5% to 10% incidence. If the patient has preexisting Cushing disease, the incidence is 25%, thus requiring long-term steroid replacement therapy.[21]

In addition, the risk of incidence of hormonal changes is linked to the location, size, consistency, degree of resection, and the surgeon's experience. If the pituitary stalk is resected or damaged, there is a 10% to 20% likelihood of transient postoperative SIADH and 2% to 7% risk of permanent disease.[22,23]

Sodium and water derangements can occur from either hypernatremia secondary to central DI or hyponatremia from cortisol deficiency, SIADH, or cerebral salt wasting (CSW). Diagnosis of DI, SIADH, or CSW relies on urine and plasma osmolarity investigations and is imperative as the treatment for the various causes can be diametrically opposed. Intraoperative DI is rare, and recognition and treatment of such may not be able to wait for typical laboratory test results. In this case, a urine output of greater than 2 mL/kg/h is highly suggestive, and intravenous/subcutaneous desmopressin (DDAVP) may be given.

The patient with SIADH who is awake can be permitted free access to water; however, if the patient is obtunded or otherwise unable to self-regulate free access to water, DDAVP may be indicated. In the patient who is euvolemic and hyponatremic, conservative measures of watchful waiting and restricting free access to water are the preferred approach.[24]

## SUMMARY

Anesthesia for endoscopic pituitary surgery can be straightforward, but there are many pitfalls that can be avoided. Preoperatively, there are considerations for secretory pituitary tumors that can affect airway and maintenance of anesthesia and must be addressed. Intraoperatively, the choice of anesthetic agents is carefully tailored to ensure smooth extubation and rapid return to consciousness so an accurate neurologic examination can be obtained quickly. Postoperatively, concerns for metabolic and endocrine responses to tumor resection are the primary focus.

## CLINICS CARE POINTS

---

- Acromegaly requires a careful preoperative examination of the airway and preparations for difficult intubation. In addition, a thorough cardiac and obstructive sleep apnea assessment should be made.

- Cushing disease requires assessment of potential electrolyte abnormalities, difficult airway, and possible obstructive sleep apnea.

- A smooth emergence and extubation is important to limit the possibility of bucking and postoperative bleeding. Bag mask ventilation after extubation should be avoided, as it can cause pneumocephalus.

- Although rare, the potential for catastrophic hemorrhage during pituitary surgery does occur, and preparations should be made preoperatively.

---

## DISCLOSURE

The authors have nothing to disclose.

## REFERENCES

1. Fleisher LA, Fleischmann KE, Auerbach AD, et al. 2014 ACC/AHA guideline on perioperative cardiovascular evaluation and management of patients undergoing

noncardiac surgery: a report of the American College of Cardiology/American Heart Association Task Force on practice guidelines. J Am Coll Cardiol 2014; 64(22):e77–137.

2. Osuna PM, Udovcic M, Sharma MD. Hyperthyroidism and the heart. Methodist Debakey Cardiovasc J 2017;13(2):60–3.

3. Friedel ME, Johnston DR, Singhal S, et al. Airway management and perioperative concerns in acromegaly patients undergoing endoscopic transsphenoidal surgery for pituitary tumors. Otolaryngol Head Neck Surg 2013;149(6):840–4.

4. Colao A, Ferone D, Marzullo P, et al. Systemic complications of acromegaly: epidemiology, pathogenesis, and management. Endocr Rev 2004;25(1):102–52.

5. Schmitt H, Buchfelder M, Radespiel-Tröger M, et al. Difficult intubation in acromegalic patients: incidence and predictability. Anesthesiology 2000;93(1):110–4.

6. Ali Z, Bithal PK, Prabhakar H, et al. An assessment of the predictors of difficult intubation in patients with acromegaly. J Clin Neurosci 2009;16(8):1043–5.

7. Seidman PA, Kofke WA, Policare R, et al. Anaesthetic complications of acromegaly. Br J Anaesth 2000;84(2):179–82.

8. Lee H-C, Kim M-K, Kim YH, et al. Radiographic predictors of difficult laryngoscopy in acromegaly patients. J Neurosurg Anesthesiol 2019;31(1):50–6.

9. Nemergut EC, Zuo Z. Airway management in patients with pituitary disease: a review of 746 patients. J Neurosurg Anesthesiol 2006;18(1):73–7.

10. Vitale G, Pivonello R, Lombardi G, et al. Cardiovascular complications in acromegaly. Minerva Endocrinol 2004;29(3):77–88. https://www.ncbi.nlm.nih.gov/pubmed/15282442.

11. Dyer MW, Gnagey A, Jones BT, et al. Perianesthetic management of patients with thyroid-stimulating hormone-secreting pituitary adenomas. J Neurosurg Anesthesiol 2017;29(3):341–6.

12. Nabbout LA, Robbins RJ. The cardiovascular effects of hyperthyroidism. Methodist Debakey Cardiovasc J 2010;6(2):3–8.

13. Vargas-Uricoechea H, Bonelo-Perdomo A, Sierra-Torres CH. Effects of thyroid hormones on the heart. Clin Investig Arterioscler 2014;26(6):296–309.

14. Ojamaa K, Klein I, Sabet A, et al. Changes in adenylyl cyclase isoforms as a mechanism for thyroid hormone modulation of cardiac beta-adrenergic receptor responsiveness. Metabolism 2000;49(2):275–9.

15. Kanda M, Omori Y, Shinoda S, et al. SIADH closely associated with nonfunctioning pituitary adenoma. Endocrinol J 2004;51(4):435–8.

16. Sato H, Takahashi H, Kanai G, et al. Syndrome of inappropriate secretion of antidiuretic hormone caused by pituitary macroadenoma with hemangiomatous stroma. Tokai J Exp Clin Med 2011;36(4):128–33. https://www.ncbi.nlm.nih.gov/pubmed/22167496.

17. Campkin TV. Radial artery cannulation. Potential hazard in patients with acromegaly. Anaesthesia 1980;35(10):1008–9.

18. Pasternak JJ, Atkinson JLD, Kasperbauer JL, et al. Hemodynamic responses to epinephrine-containing local anesthetic injection and to emergence from general anesthesia in transsphenoidal hypophysectomy patients. J Neurosurg Anesthesiol 2004;16(3):189–95.

19. Burkhardt T, Rotermund R, Schmidt N-O, et al. Dexamethasone PONV prophylaxis alters the hypothalamic-pituitary-adrenal axis after transsphenoidal pituitary surgery. J Neurosurg Anesthesiol 2014;26(3):216–9.

20. Kurwale NS, Ahmad F, Suri A, et al. Post operative pituitary apoplexy: preoperative considerations toward preventing nightmare. Br J Neurosurg 2012;26(1):59–63.

21. Roelfsema F, Biermasz NR, Pereira AM. Clinical factors involved in the recurrence of pituitary adenomas after surgical remission: a structured review and meta-analysis. Pituitary 2012;15(1):71–83.
22. Ciric I, Ragin A, Baumgartner C, et al. Complications of transsphenoidal surgery: results of a national survey, review of the literature, and personal experience. Neurosurgery 1997;40(2):225–36.
23. Nemergut EC, Zuo Z, Jane JA Jr, et al. Predictors of diabetes insipidus after transsphenoidal surgery: a review of 881 patients. J Neurosurg 2005;103(3):448–54.
24. de Vries F, Lobatto DJ, Verstegen MJT, et al. Postoperative diabetes insipidus: how to define and grade this complication? Pituitary 2021;24(2):284–91.

# Complications in Endoscopic Pituitary Surgery

Joshua Vignolles-Jeong, BA[a], Daniel Kreatsoulas, MD[b],*, Saniya Godil, MD[b],
Bradley Otto, MD[c], Ricardo Carrau, MD[b,c], Daniel Prevedello, MD[b,c]

## KEYWORDS

- Pituitary surgery • Pituitary adenoma • Complications
- Endonasal endoscopic approach • EEA

## KEY POINTS

- Complication avoidance begins in the planning and preoperative setup of the surgery. Optimizing operating room setup, utilizing navigation, and considering various pharmacologic adjuncts will aid in preventing mishaps.
- Careful review of patient factors including preoperative imaging, extent of tumor invasion, and prior operations/recurrences will aid in complication avoidance.
- Intraoperative complications can be minimized by ensuring proper visualization, using micro-Doppler or other multimodal monitoring, and determining protocols in advance for when major complications arise.
- Cerebrospinal fluid leak can be minimized by taking advantage of advanced closure or reinforcement techniques intraoperatively.
- Postoperatively, a rigorous medical and postsurgical protocol can be used to streamline patient discharge without significant endocrinologic, rhinologic, or neurologic complications.

## INTRODUCTION

Pituitary tumors constitute approximately 10% to 15% of all intracranial lesions.[1,2] Common sellar pathologies include pituitary adenomas, craniopharyngiomas, and Rathke cleft cysts.[2] Pituitary adenomas are the most common sellar lesion and the third most common intracranial tumor with a prevalence rate of 25 cases per 100,000 population.[3,4] Over the past several decades, the endoscopic endonasal approach (EEA) has emerged as the primary surgical intervention to address sellar/suprasellar pathologies.[5,6] The EEA offers superior visualization compared with the traditional

[a] The Ohio State University College of Medicine, 370 W 9th Avenue, Columbus, OH 43210, USA;
[b] Department of Neurological Surgery, The Ohio State University Wexner Medical Center, 410 W 10th Avenue, Columbus, OH 43210, USA; [c] Department of Otolaryngology–Head and Neck Surgery, The Ohio State University Wexner Medical Center, 410 W 10th Avenue, Columbus, OH 43210, USA
* Corresponding author.
E-mail address: Daniel.Kreatsoulas@osumc.edu

Otolaryngol Clin N Am 55 (2022) 431–448
https://doi.org/10.1016/j.otc.2021.12.011
0030-6665/22/© 2022 Elsevier Inc. All rights reserved.

| Abbreviations | |
|---|---|
| CSF | cerebrospinal fluid |
| CT | computed tomography |
| DI | diabetes insipidus |
| EEA | endoscopic endonasal approach |
| GTR | gross total resection |
| ICA | internal carotid artery |
| ICU | intensive care unit |
| MRI | magnetic resonance imaging |
| OR | operating room |
| PRES | posterior reversible encephalopathy syndrome |
| SIADH | syndrome of inappropriate antidiuretic hormone |

microscopic transsphenoidal approach, allowing for a panoramic view of the target tissue and surrounding neurovascular structures.[6–10] The enhanced visualization, technological advances in image guidance, angled endoscopes, and use of Doppler probes have improved the safety and efficacy of this approach, resulting in lower complication rates when compared with the microscopic approach.[1,6,10,11,12]

Despite these advances, the EEA has its limitations in cases where the pathology crosses neurovascular structures and requires mobilization of cranial nerves or dissection around a major vessel.[13] Invasion of the cavernous sinus presents an additional obstacle to achieving maximal resection. Aggressive resection attempts in these lateral compartments have been shown to be associated with higher rates of morbidity.[14,15] In these instances, adjuvant treatment modalities such as radiosurgery and medical management or a combination of transcranial and endoscopic approaches may be indicated.[12,16,17] In short, the EEA is not a replacement for, but

**Table 1**
**Review of intraoperative complications in endonasal pituitary surgery according to published series**

| Study | Number of Cases | Vascular Injury (%) | STR (%) |
|---|---|---|---|
| Cappablanca et al.[87] (2002) | 146 | 0.68 | 37.7 |
| Kabil et al. (2005) | 300 | 0 | 7.0 |
| Frank et al.[36] (2006) | 418 | 0 | 23.1 |
| Rudnik et al. (2007) | 70 | - | 30 |
| Dehdashti et al. (2008) | 200 | 0 | 12 |
| Charalampaki et al. (2009) | 150 | 0.7 | 6 |
| Gondim et al. (2010) | 301 | 1 | 22.6 |
| Zada et al.[40] (2010) | 169 | 0.6 | - |
| Berker et al. (2012) | 624 | 0.16 | - |
| Karppinen et al. (2015) | 41 | 0 | 44 |
| Lopez et al. (2021) | 80 | 0 | 29.5 |
| Ouyang et al. (2021) | 102 | 2 | 29.4 |
| Younus et al. (2020)—JNS | 1000 | 0.6 | 33.5 |
| Younus et al. (2020)—Acta Neurochirurgica | 600 | 0.16 | 32 |

Abbreviations: CSF, cerebrospinal fluid; JNS, journal of neurosurgery; STR, subtotal resection.

**Table 2**
**Review of postoperative endocrine complications in endonasal pituitary surgery according to published series**

| Study | Number of Cases | Anterior Pituitary Deficiency (%) | Pan-hypopituitarism (%) | Transient Diabetes Insipidus (%) | Permanent Diabetes Insipidus (%) | SIADH (%) |
|---|---|---|---|---|---|---|
| Cappablanca et al. (2002) | 146 | 13.7 | - | 5.48 | 3.42 | - |
| Kabil et al. (2005) | 300 | 2.7 | - | 4 | 1.33 | - |
| Frank et al.[36] (2006) | 418 | 2.8 | 7.4 | - | 1.4 | 7.6 |
| Rudnik et al. (2007) | 70 | 11.4 | - | 5.7 | 0 | - |
| Dehdashti et al. (2008) | 200 | 3 | 11 | 2.5 | 1 | - |
| Charalampaki et al. (2009) | 150 | 7.5 | - | 6.7 | 1.3 | - |
| Gondim et al. (2010) | 301 | 11.6 | - | 4.98 | 1.32 | - |
| Zada et al.[40] (2010) | 169 | - | - | 3 | 0 | 2 |
| Berker et al. (2012) | 624 | 1.9 | 0.16 | 4.6 | 0.48 | 1.1 |
| Karppinen et al. (2015) | 41 | - | - | 4.9 | 0 | - |
| Lopez et al. (2021) | 80 | - | 1.25 | 2.5 | 3.75 | - |
| Ouyang et al. (2021) | 102 | 2.9 | - | - | 2 | - |
| Younus et al. (2020)—JNS | 1000 | - | - | - | - | - |
| Younus et al. (2020)—Acta Neurochirurgica | 600 | - | 4.6 | - | - | - |

*Abbreviations:* JNS, journal of neurosurgery; SIADH, syndrome of inappropriate antidiuretic hormone.

rather a complement to traditional transcranial techniques.[18–20] Patient safety and the avoidance of complications is of paramount importance in surgery. In this article, we will describe the common complications of endonasal pituitary surgery with an additional focus on complication avoidance and management strategies. A summary of our review of the literature regarding endonasal approach pituitary surgery complications is shown in **Tables 1–3**. For comparison, our group's recent experience in complications is shown in **Table 4**.[21]

## PREOPERATIVE EVALUATION AND CASE SETUP

Complication avoidance begins when the surgeon meets the patient. Preoperative neurologic examination, as well as ophthalmologic and endocrinologic evaluation,

**Table 3**
Review of postoperative nonendocrine complications in endonasal pituitary surgery according to published series

| Study | Number of Cases | Meningitis (%) | Sphenoid Sinusitis (%) | CSF Leak (%) | Epistaxis (%) | Vascular (%) | Tumor Recurrence (%) | Mortality (%) |
|---|---|---|---|---|---|---|---|---|
| Cappablanca et al. (2002) | 146 | 0.68 | 2.05 | 2.05 | 1.4 | - | - | 0.68 |
| Kabil et al. (2005) | 300 | 0 | - | 1.7 | 1.3 | 0.7 | - | 0 |
| Frank et al.[36] (2006) | 418 | 0.4 | 0 | 0.97 | 0.7 | 0.72 | - | 0 |
| Rudnik et al. (2007) | 70 | 1.4 | - | 2.8 | 1.4 | - | - | 0 |
| Dehdashti et al. (2008) | 200 | 1 | 0 | 3.5 | 1 | 0.5 | - | 0 |
| Charalampaki et al. (2009) | 150 | 0 | 2 | 3.3 | 0.7 | 1.3 | - | 0.7 |
| Gondim et al. (2010) | 301 | 0.66 | 1.66 | 2.65 | 2 | 0.66 | - | 0 |
| Zada et al.[40] (2010) | 169 | - | - | 1 | 3 | - | - | 0 |
| Berker et al. (2012) | 624 | 0.8 | 0.48 | 1.3 | 0.6 | - | - | 0 |
| Karppinen et al. (2015) | 41 | 0 | - | 2.4 | 0 | 0 | 12.2 | 0 |
| Lopez et al. (2021) | 80 | 1.25 | - | 12.5 | 6.25 | 3.75 | 2.5 | 0 |
| Ouyang et al. (2021) | 102 | - | - | 5.9 | - | - | 5.9 | 0 |
| Younus et al. (2020)—JNS | 1000 | 0.6 | 0 | 2 | - | - | - | 0.2 |
| Younus et al. (2020)—Acta Neurochirurgica | 600 | - | - | 1.5 | - | - | - | 0.16 |

*Abbreviations:* CSF, cerebrospinal fluid; JNS, journal of neurosurgery.

| Table 4 Review of endonasal pituitary adenoma resection complications at the author's institution | |
|---|---|
| Total operations | 392 |
| Intraoperative complications | 0 (0%) |
| Postoperative CSF leak | 14 (3.6%) |
| Postoperative hematoma | 3 (7.7%) |
| Endocrine complications | Transient DI: 34 (11.5%) Permanent DI: 0 (0%) SIADH: 16 (4.1%) Hypopituitarism: 7 (1.8%) |
| Neurologic complications | CN palsy: 1 (0.26%) Hydrocephalus: 0 (0%) Seizure: 2 (0.52%) PRES: 1 (0.26%) Vasospasm: 1 (0.26%) |
| Infection, all types | Meningitis: 1 (0.26%) Sinusitis: 1 (0.26%) |
| Medical complication | 18 (4.6%) |

Structural complications are defined as: significant epistaxis requiring intervention; postoperative pneumocephalus requiring oxygen or evacuation; postoperative intracranial hematoma. Neurologic complications are defined as: new-onset seizures; cranial nerve deficits; hydrocephalus postoperatively; cerebral vasospasm; and posterior reversible encephalopathy syndrome.

*Abbreviations:* CN, cranial nerve; CSF, cerebrospinal fluid; DI, diabetes insipidus; PRES, posterior reversible encephalopathy syndrome; SIADH, syndrome of inappropriate antidiuretic hormone.

*Data from* Hardesty DA, Montaser A, Kreatsoulas D, Shah VS, VanKoevering KK, Otto BA, Carrau RL, Prevedello DM. Complications after 1002 endoscopic endonasal approach procedures at a single center: lessons learned, 2010-2018. J Neurosurg. 2021 Aug 6:1-12. https://doi.org/10.3171/2020. 11.JNS202494. Epub ahead of print. PMID: *34359021.*

to determine the baseline status of the patient in these characteristics, is vital to ensuring that appropriate mitigating steps are performed before surgery and to safeguard patient safety in the operating room (OR). Next, with regard to the individual tumor, deciding whether the lesion seen on magnetic resonance imaging (MRI) or computed tomography (CT) scan can safely be approached with an EEA is a key factor in the overall success of the surgery. A keen knowledge and understanding of sinonasal and anterior skull base anatomy is important. Key orienting landmarks in pituitary surgery include the sphenoid sinus, the sphenoid ostium, and the inferior and middle turbinates. Landmark recognition helps surgeons orient themselves during surgery and to know how far outside the sellar region they can dissect and where key areas to avoid are located. This is most useful in small lesions that are contained entirely within the pituitary gland or within the sella turcica proper. However, with larger lesions, there can be significant blurring or entire destruction/distortion of known anatomic landmarks, making it difficult for surgeons to orient themselves. Obtaining preoperative imaging is paramount to successful endoscopic endonasal surgery, as there are anatomic factors that can affect the approach and resection. For example, a study of 100 adults' preoperative imaging found that 62% had a deviated septum, 18% had bony carotid dehiscence, 24% had sphenoid septation overlying the carotid, and there was over a 1.5 cm range in distance from the sphenoid ostium to the skull base.[22] In a morphometric study from 2020, the authors detailed that patients with acromegaly secondary to growth hormone-secreting tumors had sphenoid ostia located further from the midline and more superior, in addition to larger intracavernous carotid diameters and smaller intercarotid distances.[23] Pneumatization of the sphenoid sinus helps determine the success of an EEA, with extensive sellar pneumatization being the most favorable variant. In this type, the sphenoid sinus extends posteriorly below the sella as far as the clival margin with the anterior sellar wall frequently measuring less than 1 mm in thickness.[24] Lack of pneumatization is more common in younger patients, but this has not been shown to negatively affect outcomes when the EEA is performed by experienced surgeons.[25,26] These studies highlight the need for keen preoperative planning in all endonasal pituitary cases, as failure to do so can cause a loss of anatomic orientation and serious consequent complications.

Endoscopic endonasal surgery has a steep learning curve, given the significant variability in anatomic parameters and the need for learning new instruments and surgical skills. It has been highlighted in the literature that the surgeon's experience can improve overall outcomes. Qureshi and colleagues demonstrated that 9 cases performed together by a multidisciplinary team helped decrease OR times and reduce postoperative cerebrospinal fluid (CSF) leak rates.[27] Another group determined that surgeons' skills and outcomes continue to improve even when they cross into the realm of hundreds of cases performed. Younus and colleagues examined 1000 EEA cases performed after an initial 200 cases, splitting the 1000 cases into a first and second half, and found that over time, fewer lumbar drains were used postoperatively, gross total resection (GTR) rates increased from 60% to 73%, and hormonal cure rates improved in functional pituitary tumors from 83% to 89%.[28] Younus and colleagues also divided their 600 consecutive cases into quartiles and demonstrated similar results: intraoperative CSF leak rates decreased from 60% to 33% between first and last quartile, GTR rates improved from 55% to 79%, and hormonal remission rates improved from 68% to 90%.[29] All these studies demonstrate that although the slope of the initial learning curve is very steep, it does not plateau with the number of cases a group performs together. This is an important consideration when developing a practice, and determining which cases are amenable to an EEA based on where one group is in their learning curve.

Preoperative antibiotics at the time of incision have been demonstrated to be one of the most important factors in avoiding infectious complications in most surgical fields. Given the lack of ability to fully sterilize the sinonasal mucosal membranes for an EEA, a preoperative wash with betadine can help improve antibiosis. In addition, preoperative antibiotics are used in a high number of centers, with 81% of respondents to one survey stating they used either penicillin or cephalosporin antibiotics perioperatively to prevent meningitis and sinusitis.[30] Another survey by Smith and Stringer found that over 90% of respondents used preoperative intravenous antibiotics for infection control.[31] A recent systematic review of antibiotic use in pituitary surgery reported no clear practice guidelines, with overall limited evidence and varying protocols used by surgeons around the world.[32] Best practices would indicate that preoperative antibiotics are suitable to cover skin flora, with postoperative antibiotics used on a case-by-case basis. At our institution, we use cefepime as a standard preoperative antibiotic except in the cases of anaphylactic allergic reactions. We also swab each patient's nose at a preoperative anesthesia clearance visit, usually 1 to 2 weeks before surgery, for methicillin-resistant *Staphylococcus aureus* and if positive, use vancomycin as an additional antibiotic. During setup, a betadine wash of the nasal cavities and nasopharynx is also used. Using this protocol, we have observed a 0.5% rate of infections in our patients.

The last preoperative step in which the surgeon can help prevent complications is the patient setup. The patients are positioned supine, in a horseshoe headrest, with a facial landmark mask placed sterilely, to allow for stereotactic navigation. The patient undergoes arterial line placement for blood pressure monitoring, and if needed,

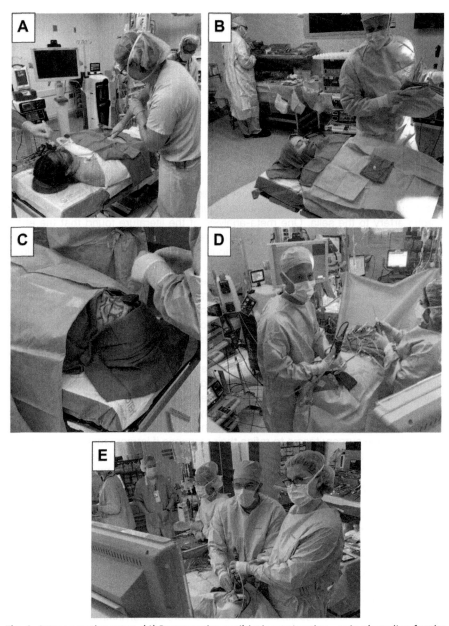

**Fig. 1.** Intraoperative setup. (*A*) Preoperative antibiotic preparation—using betadine for the face and chlorhexidine-based antiseptic for the abdomen, both sites are prepped sterilely. (*B*) Draping—the superior portion of the face is left undraped for placement of the stereotactic landmark mask to be used for navigation. (*C*) Close-up view of the stereotactic landmark mask. This communicates with a separate navigation computer and must remain visible. (*D*) Final draping—one surgeon operating. (*E*) Four-hand technique.

neurophysiologic monitoring of cranial nerves, depending on the tumor characteristics. We position the patient with the head slightly rotated (about 15°) to the right, anteriorly translated, and slightly laterally cocked, to facilitate ergonomic surgeon access with the instruments. Several monitors are used to display the feed from the endoscope, allowing various viewing angles. The patient's abdomen and right lateral thigh are prepped to allow for harvesting of a fat graft or fascia lata/muscle graft at the end of the case for repair of the skull base defect if needed. Our typical preoperative setup is shown in **Fig. 1.**

## INTRAOPERATIVE COMPLICATIONS

There are several intraoperative complications during endoscopic pituitary surgery reported in the literature. One of the most feared complications of endoscopic endonasal surgery is intraoperative vascular injury, given the close proximity of the carotid artery to the sella. One meta-analysis of the literature found that the endoscopic approach was associated with a higher rate of vascular complications than transcranial approaches. This may be attributable to the more extensive sphenoid sinus exposure, as well the lack of 3-dimensional perception in this technique.[33] Most of these complications involve internal carotid artery (ICA) injury, posterior cerebral artery injury, midbrain stroke, and hemorrhage of intracerebral and mesencephalic vasculature.[34–37] ICA injury is difficult to manage because of obscured visualization of the operative field, restricted access to the sphenoid sinus, and inability to directly repair the arterial injury via endonasal approach.[38] Steps can be taken to mitigate the risk of ICA injury during EEA skull base surgery. The position of the carotid artery can be confirmed with micro-Doppler intraoperatively before making incisions into the dura.[7,39,40] In addition, well-calibrated image guidance can be used to confirm landmarks and positioning of the ICA. Although, one must keep in mind that once the lesion is debulked, shifting of adjacent structures may alter the anatomy, eliminating the accuracy of the image guidance system.[41] ICA injury simulation models can be used to train skull base surgery teams to refine their response if intraoperative ICA injury occurs.[42–46] Furthermore, the location of the sphenopalatine artery must also be considered when performing mucosal dissection in the region of the middle and superior meatus. Management of bleeding from this vessel includes nasal tamponade, cauterization, or even endovascular occlusion of the vessel.[11,34,47]

We have previously published a comprehensive management protocol regarding ICA injury.[48] In our institution, the initial actions taken in the event of a suspected or confirmed ICA injury are to call the attention of all staff in the room and key them into the dire situation at hand, and ensure silence other than absolutely required communication. Simultaneously, the anesthesia team is notified to activate a massive transfusion protocol for possible blood transfusion and asked to manage the blood pressure to ensure continued cerebral perfusion. Immediate efforts are made to control the field and ensure visualization with 2 large-bore suction instruments, performed using the four-hand technique. It is vital to quickly identify the area of injury, secure the prior harvested repair graft or flap away from the working area, and place nasal packing with only enough pressure to staunch the bleeding and not occlude the lumen of the vessel. The best repair strategy is use of a muscle graft under direct pressure. The team should quickly harvest a large muscle graft from the thigh, temporalis, or other preprepared site. The harvested graft is bluntly smashed to release cytokines and then quickly placed against the site of injury, then a large amount of packing material—both synthetic and biological, potentially a fat graft if it can be harvested quickly enough—is placed until the bleeding is managed. Once the bleeding can be managed more easily, the endovascular neurosurgery team is notified and the patient is taken from the OR to the angiography suite to determine if any actionable pathology is present, and if so, to manage it in a timely fashion.

After angiography, the patient is taken to the neurocritical care unit, where they are kept deeply sedated overnight to allow for vascular healing. Blood pressure is monitored via the arterial line and the patient is kept with systolic pressures that are slightly hypertensive to ensure adequate cerebral perfusion. Intracranial imaging is obtained as per routine and for any changes in vitals or neurologic examination. A special notice is placed in the patient's room and an electronic chart indicating that they have a potential emergent condition, and supplies are kept bedside in the event of reopening of the ICA injury and requirement for emergency packing of the nares and oropharynx. The patient is then slowly brought out of sedation after stabilization, and postoperative neurologic examinations are performed to ensure no ischemia occurred secondary to the carotid injury. An intensive care unit (ICU) level of nursing care is kept for at least 7 days postinjury. After 7 days, the patient is taken back to the angiography suite to have a repeat evaluation of their cerebral vasculature to rule out pseudoaneurysm and other sequelae of vascular injury. This is the final post-ICA injury step in the protocol we have developed.

Although the EEA can provide good visualization of the sellar/parasellar region, several factors can prevent achieving GTR of lesions in this area. If a tumor is located more laterally, initial dissection and exposure around the cavernous sinus and ICA is challenging. For example, a tumor located in the lateral cavernous sinus may not be readily accessible with a midline endoscopic approach and higher rates of complications are associated with aggressive attempts at resecting these lesions located in the lateral compartment.[14–16] These are cases in which a partial endonasal resection followed by transcranial resection or radiotherapy may be required to avoid complications. However, this can lead to residual tumor and higher chances of tumor progression or recurrence. Multiple studies have found that tumor recurrence and progression have a negative impact on the extent of re-resection.[16,49–51] This may be explained by the formation of scar tissue and changes that occur in the patient's normal anatomy following initial resection.[50,52] To address the possibility of leaving residual tumor behind, intraoperative MRI can be used to obtain real-time images of the patient's anatomy and to gain a more complete assessment of the extent of resection, ultimately leading to higher rates of GTR.[53,54]

One of the most common complications in the EEA is intraoperative CSF leaks. The initial rates of CSF leaks reported following EEA procedures were unacceptably high. The description of the vascularized nasoseptal flap by Haddad and colleagues in 2006 was a turning point in the field of endoscopic endonasal skull base surgery as rates of postoperative CSF leaks were dramatically reduced following its introduction.[55] One large review of endoscopic skull base tumor resections revealed a drop from 27.8% to 13.5% with the use of nasoseptal flaps compared with free grafts, a testament to the durability of this repair.[56] Although this repair method is a significant improvement from prior repair methods, there are limitations to its use. Although very rare, necrosis of the nasoseptal flap due to compromise of the vascularized pedicle has been reported to occur in less than 1% of cases.[49,57] This has led to the development of many other repair strategies. The gasket seal repair technique involves the insertion of an autologous fat graft to seal up intracranial dead space, followed by an autologous fascia lata graft to cover up the skull base defect. This is then sealed by a bone graft or synthetic polyethylene implant. The gasket seal technique can be used in conjunction with a vascularized nasoseptal flap. Garcia-Navarro et al reported a CSF leak rate of 4.7% when the 2 repair methods were used concurrently.[58] The bilayer button technique, originally described by Luginbuhl and colleagues, uses a bilayer fascia lata graft with a piece slightly larger than the bony defect serving as an onlay sutured to a much larger piece serving as an inlay in addition to a nasoseptal flap.[59] In some instances, a pedicled nasoseptal flap is not available, such as in cases where prior reconstruction involved a nasoseptal flap or in the setting of malignancy invading the nasal septum.[60] In these cases, alternative vascularized options include a lateral nasal wall flap supplied by the lateral nasal wall artery or an inferior turbinate flap. These flaps cover a smaller surface area compared to nasoseptal flaps and may have a greater propensity to migrate from their intended positions.[61] Avascular repair method can also be used in the setting where a vascularized flap is not accessible. This often involves middle turbinate free mucosal grafts, which can be used with high rates of success and low morbidity.[62]

## POSTOPERATIVE COMPLICATIONS

Numerous complications can occur in the postoperative period after endoscopic endonasal pituitary surgery. The most frequent postoperative complication encountered after an EEA is CSF leak.[1,6,12,19] A key factor in avoiding persistent leaks is identifying their origin in the individual patient. CSF leaks are considered high-flow when they are a result of a cisternal or ventricular opening defect and low-flow when they produce a few drops as a result of increased intracranial pressure.[59] The majority of leaks associated with the EEA in the sellar compartment are low-flow.[63] The higher incidence of CSF leak associated with the EEA compared with the traditional microscopic approach may be related to the increased exposure and larger sellar floor and dural openings that the endoscopic approach can provide.[1,8,64,65] Unfortunately, CSF leaks require return to the OR, as failure to repair the leak can lead to additional subsequent complications including bacterial meningitis, intracranial hypotension, pneumocephalus, and increased length and cost of hospital stay.[66] Increased frequency of CSF leak is associated with patients with prior surgery, patients with macroadenomas compared with microadenomas, and tumors with suprasellar extension.[19,36,64,67] Although smaller, low-flow defects of the skull base can be adequately managed using a wide range of avascular or noncellular methods, larger defects with high-flow CSF egress require more fortified repair methods such as the use of vascularized flaps.[57] As mentioned earlier, the introduction of the pedicled nasoseptal flap for the reconstruction of skull base defects following endoscopic endonasal procedures dramatically reduces the incidence of postoperative CSF leaks.[55,68–70]

Although CSF leak is relatively common, infectious complications after the EEA are surprisingly rare. It may be secondary to the use of prophylactic perioperative antibiotics, frequent intraoperative irrigation of the nasal cavity and surgical site, as well as the use of vascularized flaps for skull base defect reconstruction.[20] Several studies have indicated that postoperative CSF leak is associated with the development of subsequent intracranial infections.[71–74] Postoperative pneumocephalus has also been found to be associated with intracranial infection after the EEA.[75] Overall, appropriately managing CSF leaks during and after surgery is the most important factor in avoiding postoperative infections.

Tumor recurrence is another complication that can arise after endoscopic endonasal pituitary surgery. One factor that has been found to be associated with tumor recurrence after the EEA is size of the initial tumor, with larger sizes having higher rates of recurrence.[76] In non-EEA series, a strong relationship has been found between postoperative residual tumor and recurrence rates.[77–79] A meta-analysis by Roelfsema and colleagues reported that patients with prolactinomas have a higher rate of recurrence compared with patients with Cushing disease or acromegaly and that most recurrences occurred between 1 and 5 years after initial resection.[80] Tumor recurrence requiring revision surgery may present with additional complications. One large study of 1000 revision transsphenoidal surgeries reported higher rates of meningitis, postoperative diabetes insipidus (DI), CSF leak, and length of hospital stay.[81] Intraoperative MRI and experience of the surgeon are also key factors in achieving GTR during surgery and reducing rates of recurrence.

Postoperative epistaxis as a result of injury to the sphenopalatine artery or from one of the septal branches is a well-described complication.[1,34,36] One preventative measure against postoperative epistaxis includes meticulous bilateral cauterization of the posterior nasal branch of the sphenopalatine artery.[82] Subarachnoid hemorrhage (SAH) is a rare complication after transsphenoidal surgery that has been documented to occur at rates of 0.1% to 0.7%.[37,82–84] This can occur as a result of bleeding from suprasellar vessels due to operative trauma or from hemorrhage of residual tumor that is in contact with suprasellar structures. Patients presenting with postoperative SAH should be admitted to the ICU and monitored for signs of vasospasm, hydrocephalus, or ischemic complications.[66]

Finally, hormonal complications can arise after endoscopic endonasal pituitary surgery. Transient DI is thought to be caused by surgical trauma of the pituitary gland or hypothalamic-pituitary axis leading to dysfunction of vasopressin-producing neurons.[82,84,85] However, a well-known triple-phase reaction can occur postoperatively as well, proceeding from DI to syndrome of inappropriate antidiuretic hormone (SIADH), then progressing back to permanent DI. This is thought to be secondary to initial injury of the posterior pituitary/hypothalamic cells (transient DI) progressing to cell death and sudden release of ADH (SIADH), which when cleared by the body results in permanent DI.[86] Intraoperative injury to the anterior pituitary lobe can also result in hormonal disturbances. Maneuvers resulting in excessive manipulation or resection of the gland or heat damage due to bipolar coagulation of the sellar cavity can cause anterior lobe dysfunction.[84] Of note, macroadenomas can expand against and cause thinning of normal pituitary tissue, making it difficult to tell the two apart leading to damage of pituitary tissue during tumor resection.[84] SIADH and DI require close monitoring of sodium and urine outputs and may warrant ICU admission, with a slow transition to outpatient endocrinology follow-up. Prevention and appropriate management of hormonal disturbances require multidisciplinary care and close preoperative and postoperative evaluation and monitoring by endocrinologists.

**CASE ILLUSTRATION**

A patient presented with bitemporal hemianopsia and was noted to have a worse vision on the right. Imaging demonstrated a pituitary lesion and the patient subsequently underwent an EEA for resection of the tumor. Intraoperatively, the tumor was found to be extremely firm. There was extension of the tumor beyond the right optic nerve that was inaccessible and therefore some residual tumor was left. In the immediate postoperative period, the patient had significant improvement in vision. However, 10 hours after surgery, he had an acute decline in vision on the right. Emergent CT was performed and there was a concern for apoplexy (**Fig. 2**). The patient was taken to the OR for evacuation and resection of the residual tumor. Initially, an EEA was used but it was impossible to completely decompress the optic nerves and remove the tumor as the residual tumor itself had bled. Therefore, a right pterional

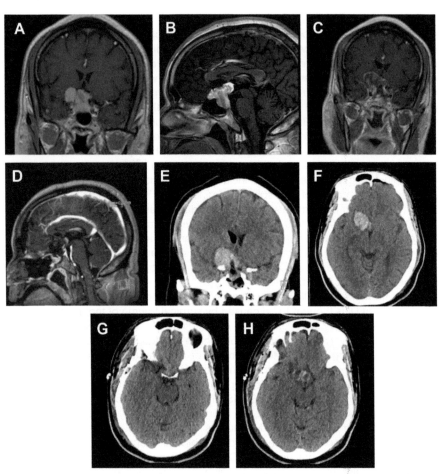

**Fig. 2.** Preoperative and postoperative images. (*A*) & (*B*) preoperative MRI images demonstrating large pituitary lesion with significant extension on the right around the optic nerves. (*C*) & (*D*) Postoperative MRI demonstrating the resection bed with residual tumor. (*E*) & (*F*) HCT postoperatively after decline in vision on the right demonstrating hemorrhage in the resection cavity and pituitary apoplexy. (*G*) & (*H*) Postoperative HCT after pterional craniotomy demonstrating good resection of tumor and evacuation of postoperative hemorrhage.

approach was performed and hemorrhage was evacuated and residual tumor was removed. At the end of the resection, both optic nerves appeared healthy and intact. However, the patient did not have significant recovery of vision on the right side in the postoperative period. He did have 20/20 vision and normal visual fields on the left side.

## SUMMARY

EEAs have revolutionized pituitary surgery, with excellent tolerability and ever-improving rates of GTR and complications for varying pathologies. With the development of new techniques comes the surfacing of new complications, and the EEA is no different. Although CSF leak, subtotal resection, endocrine dysfunction, and vascular injuries are possible in the EEA, there are strategies that can be used to decrease their likelihood and to manage them appropriately if they do occur. Attention to detail during preoperative planning and patient setup, as well as knowledge of intraoperative and postoperative complication avoidance and management techniques, can help improve patient outcomes. Over time, the importance of multidisciplinary team effort in the medical and surgical management of pituitary pathologies has been recognized and implemented, which promises continued and improving safety and efficacy of endoscopic surgery into the future.

## DISCLOSURE

Dr. Prevedello has consulting relationships with Stryker, Integra, and BK Medical. He also receives royalties from technologies with KLS Martin, ACE Medical, and Mizuho. None of the other authors have disclosures.

## REFERENCES

1. Gondim JA, Almeida JC, Alberquerque LA, et al. Endoscopic endonasal approach for pituitary adenoma: surgical complications in 301 patients. Pituitary 2011;14:174–83.
2. Pennacchietti V, Garzaro M, Grottoli S, et al. Three-Dimensional Endoscopic Endonasal Approach and Outcomes in Sellar Lesions: A Single-Center Experience of 104 Cases. World Neurosurg 2016;89:121–5.
3. Ezzat S, Asa SL, Couldwell WT, et al. The prevalence of pituitary adenomas: a systematic review. Cancer 2004;101:613–9.
4. Fernandez A, Karavitaki N, Wass JA. Prevalence of pituitary adenomas: a community-based, cross-sectional study in Banbury (Oxfordshire, UK). Clin Endocrinol (Oxf) 2010;72:377–82.
5. Rolston JD, Han SJ, Aghi MK. Nationwide shift from microscopic to endoscopic transsphenoidal pituitary surgery. Pituitary 2016;19:248–50.
6. Gao Y, Zhong C, Wang Y, et al. Endoscopic versus microscopic transsphenoidal pituitary adenoma surgery: a meta-analysis. World J Surg Oncol 2014;12:94.
7. Karppinen A, Kivipelto L, Satu V, et al. Transition From Microscopic to Endoscopic Transsphenoidal Surgery for Nonfunctional Pituitary Adenomas. World Neurosurg 2015;84:48–57.
8. Goudakos JK, Markou KD, Georgalas C. Endoscopic versus microscopic transsphenoidal pituitary surgery: a systematic review and meta-analysis. Clin Otolaryngol 2011;36:212–20.
9. O'Malley BW Jr, Grady MS, Gabel BC, et al. Comparison of endoscopic and microscopic removal of pituitary adenomas: single-surgeon experience and the learning curve. Neurosurg Focus 2008;25:E10.
10. Jho HD, Carrau RL, Ko Y, et al. Endoscopic pituitary surgery: an early experience. Surg Neurol 1997;47:213–22.
11. Tabaee A, Anand VK, Barron Y, et al. Endoscopic pituitary surgery: a systematic review and meta-analysis. J Neurosurg 2009;111:545–54.
12. Koutourousiou M, Gardner P, Fernandez-Miranda J, et al. Endoscopic endonasal surgery for giant pituitary adenomas: advantages and limitations. J Neurosurg 2013;118:621–31.
13. Kasemsiri P, Carrau RL, Ditzel Filho L, et al. Advantages and limitations of endoscopic endonasal approaches to the skull base. World Neurosurg 2014;82: S12–21.

14. Woodworth GF, Patel KS, Shin B, et al. Surgical outcomes using a medial-to-lateral endonasal endoscopic approach to pituitary adenomas invading the cavernous sinus. J Neurosurg 2014;120:1086–94.

15. Ferreli F, Turri-Zanoni M, Canevari FR, et al. Endoscopic endonasal management of non-functioning pituitary adenomas with cavernous sinus invasion: a 10- year experience. Rhinology 2015;53:308–16.

16. Tajudeen BA, Mundi J, Suh JD, et al. Endoscopic endonasal surgery for recurrent pituitary tumors: technical challenges to the surgical approach. J Neurol Surg B Skull Base 2015;76:50–6.

17. Shin SS, Gardner PA, Ng J, et al. Endoscopic Endonasal Approach for Adreno-corticotropic Hormone-Secreting Pituitary Adenomas: Outcomes and Analysis of Remission Rates and Tumor Biochemical Activity with Respect to Tumor Invasiveness. World Neurosurg 2017;102:651–8.e651.

18. Kassam AB, Prevedello DM, Carrau RL, et al. Endoscopic endonasal skull base surgery: analysis of complications in the authors' initial 800 patients. J Neurosurg 2011;114:1544–68.

19. Paluzzi A, Fernandez-Miranda J, Stefko ST, et al. Endoscopic endonasal approach for pituitary adenomas: a series of 555 patients. Pituitary 2014;17:307–19.

20. Snyderman CH, Pant H, Carrau RL, et al. What are the limits of endoscopic sinus surgery?: the expanded endonasal approach to the skull base. Keio J Med 2009;58:152–60.

21. Hardesty DA, Montaser A, Kreatsoulas D, et al. Complications after 1002 endoscopic endonasal approach procedures at a single center: lessons learned, 2010-2018. J Neurosurg 2021;1–12.

22. Twigg V, Carr SD, Balakumar R, et al. Radiological features for the approach in trans-sphenoidal pituitary surgery. Pituitary 2017;20:395–402.

23. Rajagopal N, Thakar S, Hegde V, et al. Morphometric Alterations of the Sphenoid Ostium and other Landmarks in Acromegaly: Anatomical Considerations and Implications in Endoscopic Pituitary Surgery. Neurol India 2020;68:573–8.

24. García-Garrigós E, Arenas-Jimenez J, Monjas-Canovas I, et al. Transsphenoidal Approach in Endoscopic Endonasal Surgery for Skull Base Lesions: What Radiologists and Surgeons Need to Know. Radiographics 2015;35:1170–85.

25. Gallieni, M., Zaed, I., Fahlbusch, R., et al Transsphenoidal approach in children with partially or minimally developed sphenoid sinus. Childs Nerv Syst 37, 131-136, doi:).

26. Kuan EC, Kaufman AC, Lerner D, et al. Lack of Sphenoid Pneumatization Does Not Affect Endoscopic Endonasal Pediatric Skull Base Surgery Outcomes. Laryngoscope 2019;129:832–6.

27. Qureshi T, Chaus F, Fogg L, et al. Learning curve for the transsphenoidal endoscopic endonasal approach to pituitary tumors. Br J Neurosurg 2016;30:637–42.

28. Younus I, Gerges MM, Uribe-Cardenas R, et al. How long is the tail end of the learning curve? Results from 1000 consecutive endoscopic endonasal skull base cases following the initial 200 cases. J Neurosurg 2020;1–11.

29. Younus I, Gerges M, Uribe-Cardenas R, et al. The slope of the learning curve in 600 consecutive endoscopic transsphenoidal pituitary surgeries. Acta Neurochir (Wien) 2020;162:2361–70.

30. Little AS, White WL. Prophylactic antibiotic trends in transsphenoidal surgery for pituitary lesions. Pituitary 2011;14:99–104.

31. Smith EJ, Stringer S. Current perioperative practice patterns for minimizing surgical site infection during rhinologic procedures. Int Forum Allergy Rhinol 2014;4: 1002–7.
32. Moldovan ID, Agbi C, Kilty S, et al. A Systematic Review of Prophylactic Antibiotic Use in Endoscopic Endonasal Transsphenoidal Surgery for Pituitary Lesions. World Neurosurg 2019;128:408–14.
33. Ammirati M, Wei L, Ciric I. Short-term outcome of endoscopic versus microscopic pituitary adenoma surgery: a systematic review and meta-analysis. J Neurol Neurosurg Psychiatr 2013;84:843–9.
34. Cappabianca P, Cavallo LM, Colao A, et al. Surgical complications associated with the endoscopic endonasal transsphenoidal approach for pituitary adenomas. J Neurosurg 2002;97:293–8.
35. Senior BA, Ebert CS, Bednarski KK, et al. Minimally invasive pituitary surgery. Laryngoscope 2008;118:1842–55.
36. Frank G, Pasquini E, Farneti G, et al. The endoscopic versus the traditional approach in pituitary surgery. Neuroendocrinology 2006;83:240–8.
37. Charalampaki P, Reisch R, Ayad A, et al. Endoscopic endonasal pituitary surgery: surgical and outcome analysis of 50 cases. J Clin Neurosci 2007;14:410–5.
38. Chin OY, Ghosh R, Fang CH, et al. Internal carotid artery injury in endoscopic endonasal surgery: A systematic review. Laryngoscope 2016;126:582–90.
39. Dusick JR, Esposito F, Malkasian D, et al. Avoidance of carotid artery injuries in transsphenoidal surgery with the Doppler probe and micro-hook blades. Neurosurgery 2007;60:322–8.
40. Zada G, Du R, Laws ER. Defining the "edge of the envelope": patient selection in treating complex sellar-based neoplasms via transsphenoidal versus open craniotomy. J Neurosurg 2011;114:286–300.
41. AlQahtani A, London Jr. NR, Castelnuovo P, et al. Assessment of Factors Associated With Internal Carotid Injury in Expanded Endoscopic Endonasal Skull Base Surgery. JAMA Otolaryngol Head Neck Surg 2020;146:364–72.
42.. Donoho DA, Johnson CE, Hur KT, et al. Costs and training results of an objectively validated cadaveric perfusion-based internal carotid artery injury simulation during endoscopic skull base surgery. Int Forum Allergy Rhinol 2019;9: 787–94.
43.. Maza G, VanKoevering KK, Yanez-Siller JC, et al. Surgical simulation of a catastrophic internal carotid artery injury: a laser-sintered model. Int Forum Allergy Rhinol 2019;9:53–9.
44. Muto J, Carrau RL, Oyama K, et al. Training model for control of an internal carotid artery injury during transsphenoidal surgery. Laryngoscope 2017;127:38–43.
45. Pham M, Kale A, Marquez Y, et al. A Perfusion-based Human Cadaveric Model for Management of Carotid Artery Injury during Endoscopic Endonasal Skull Base Surgery. J Neurol Surg B Skull Base 2014;75:309–13.
46. van Doormaal TPC, Diederen SJH, van der Zwan Albert, et al. Simulating Internal Carotid Artery Injury during Transsphenoidal Transclival Endoscopic Surgery in a Perfused Cadaver Model. J Neurol Surg B Skull Base 2018;79:161–6.
47. Pádua FG, Voegels RL. Severe posterior epistaxis-endoscopic surgical anatomy. Laryngoscope 2008;118:156–61.
48. AlQahtani A, Castelnuovo P, Nicolai P, et al. Injury of the Internal Carotid Artery During Endoscopic Skull Base Surgery: Prevention and Management Protocol. Otolaryngol Clin North Am 2016;49:237–52.
49. Chabot JD, Chakraborty S, Imbarrato G, et al. Evaluation of Outcomes After Endoscopic Endonasal Surgery for Large and Giant Pituitary Macroadenoma:

A Retrospective Review of 39 Consecutive Patients. World Neurosurg 2015;84: 978–88.

50. Ouyang T, Zhang N, Xie S, et al. Outcomes and Complications of Aggressive Resection Strategy for Pituitary Adenomas in Knosp Grade 4 With Transsphenoidal Endoscopy. Front Oncol 2021;11:693063.

51. Bao X, Deng K, Liu X, et al. Extended transsphenoidal approach for pituitary adenomas invading the cavernous sinus using multiple complementary techniques. Pituitary 2016;19:1–10.

52. Negm HM, Al-Mafoudh R, Pai M, et al. Reoperative endoscopic endonasal surgery for residual or recurrent pituitary adenomas. J Neurosurg 2017;127: 397–408.

53. Berkmann S, Schlaffer S, Nimsky C, et al. Intraoperative high-field MRI for transsphenoidal reoperations of nonfunctioning pituitary adenoma. J Neurosurg 2014; 121:1166–75.

54. Ogiwara T, Hori T, Fujii Y, et al. Effectiveness of the intraoperative magnetic resonance imaging during endoscopic endonasal approach for acromegaly. Pituitary 2021. https://doi.org/10.1007/s11102-021-01144-5.

55. Hadad G, Bassagasteguy L, Carrau RL, et al. A novel reconstructive technique after endoscopic expanded endonasal approaches: vascular pedicle nasoseptal flap. Laryngoscope 2006;116:1882–6.

56. Fraser S, Gardner PA, Koutsourousiou M, et al. Risk factors associated with postoperative cerebrospinal fluid leak after endoscopic endonasal skull base surgery. J Neurosurg 2018;128:1066–71.

57. Thorp BD, Sreenath SB, Ebert CS, et al. Endoscopic skull base reconstruction: a review and clinical case series of 152 vascularized flaps used for surgical skull base defects in the setting of intraoperative cerebrospinal fluid leak. Neurosurg Focus 2014;37:E4.

58. Garcia-Navarro V, Anand VK, Schwartz TH. Gasket seal closure for extended endonasal endoscopic skull base surgery: efficacy in a large case series. World Neurosurg 2013;80:563–8.

59. Luginbuhl AJ, Campbell PG, Evans J, et al. Endoscopic repair of high-flow cranial base defects using a bilayer button. Laryngoscope 2010;120:876–80.

60. Hannan CJ, Kelleher E, Javadpour M. Methods of Skull Base Repair Following Endoscopic Endonasal Tumor Resection: A Review. Front Oncol 2020;10:1614.

61. Lavigne P, Belen Vega M, Ahmed OH, et al. Lateral nasal wall flap for endoscopic reconstruction of the skull base: anatomical study and clinical series. Int Forum Allergy Rhinol 2020;10:673–8.

62. Fishpool SJ, Amato-Watkins A, Hayhurst C. Free middle turbinate mucosal graft reconstruction after primary endoscopic endonasal pituitary surgery. Eur Arch Otorhinolaryngol 2017;274:837–44.

63. Zhan R, Chen S, Xu S, et al. Postoperative Low-Flow Cerebrospinal Fluid Leak of Endoscopic Endonasal Transsphenoidal Surgery for Pituitary Adenoma–Wait and See, or Lumbar Drain? J Craniofac Surg 2015;26:1261–4.

64. Rotenberg B, Tam S, Ryu WH, et al. Microscopic versus endoscopic pituitary surgery: a systematic review. Laryngoscope 2010;120:1292–7.

65. Cho DY, Liau WR. Comparison of endonasal endoscopic surgery and sublabial microsurgery for prolactinomas. Surg Neurol 2002;58:371–5.

66. Magro E, Graillon T, Lassave J, et al. Complications Related to the Endoscopic Endonasal Transsphenoidal Approach for Nonfunctioning Pituitary Macroadenomas in 300 Consecutive Patients. World Neurosurg 2016;89:442–53.

67. Berker M, Burcu Hazer D, Yucel T, et al. Complications of endoscopic surgery of the pituitary adenomas: analysis of 570 patients and review of the literature. Pituitary 2012;15:288–300.
68. Kessler RA, Garzon-Muvdi T, Kim E, et al. Utilization of the Nasoseptal Flap for Repair of Cerebrospinal Fluid Leak after Endoscopic Endonasal Approach for Resection of Pituitary Tumors. Brain Tumor Res Treat 2019;7:10–5.
69. Horridge M, Jesurasa A, Olubajo F, et al. The use of the nasoseptal flap to reduce the rate of post-operative cerebrospinal fluid leaks following endoscopic trans-sphenoidal surgery for pituitary disease. Br J Neurosurg 2013;27:739–41.
70. Lopez S, Jerves M, Santillan F, et al. Endoscopic endonasal approach for pituitary adenomas: Results from a multidisciplinary management. Interdisciplinary Neurosurgery 2021;25.
71. Dumont AS, Nemergut EC, Jane JA, et al. Postoperative care following pituitary surgery. J Intensive Care Med 2005;20:127–40.
72. van Aken MO, de Marie S, ven der Lely AJ, et al. Risk factors for meningitis after transsphenoidal surgery. Clin Infect Dis 1997;25:852–6.
73. Conger A, Zhao F, Wang X, et al. Evolution of the graded repair of CSF leaks and skull base defects in endonasal endoscopic tumor surgery: trends in repair failure and meningitis rates in 509 patients. J Neurosurg 2018;130:861–75.
74. Ivan ME, Iorgulescu JB, El-Sayed I, et al. Risk factors for postoperative cerebrospinal fluid leak and meningitis after expanded endoscopic endonasal surgery. J Clin Neurosci 2015;22:48–54.
75. Guo K, Heng L, Zhang H, et al. Risk factors for postoperative intracranial infections in patients with pituitary adenoma after endoscopic endonasal transsphenoidal surgery: pneumocephalus deserves further study. Neurosurg Focus 2019;47:E5.
76. Bodhinayake I, Kalinin P, Kutin M, et al. Results and risk factors for recurrence following endoscopic endonasal transsphenoidal surgery for pituitary adenoma. Clin Neurol Neurosurg 2014;119:75–9.
77. Brochier S, Galland F, Kujas M, et al. Factors predicting relapse of nonfunctioning pituitary macroadenomas after neurosurgery: a study of 142 patients. Eur J Endocrinol 2010;163:193–200.
78. Chang EF, Zada G, Kim S, et al. Long-term recurrence and mortality after surgery and adjuvant radiotherapy for nonfunctional pituitary adenomas. J Neurosurg 2008;108:736–45.
79. Losa M, Mortini P, Barzaghi R, et al. Early results of surgery in patients with nonfunctioning pituitary adenoma and analysis of the risk of tumor recurrence. J Neurosurg 2008;108:525–32.
80. Roelfsema F, Biermasz NR, Pereira AM. Clinical factors involved in the recurrence of pituitary adenomas after surgical remission: a structured review and meta-analysis. Pituitary 2012;15:71–83.
81. Jahangiri A, Wagner J, Han SW, et al. Morbidity of repeat transsphenoidal surgery assessed in more than 1000 operations. J Neurosurg 2014;121:67–74.
82. Dehdashti AR, Ganna A, Karabatsou K, et al. Pure endoscopic endonasal approach for pituitary adenomas: early surgical results in 200 patients and comparison with previous microsurgical series. Neurosurgery 2008;62:1006–15.
83. Halvorsen H, Ramm-Pettersen J, Josefsen R, et al. Surgical complications after transsphenoidal microscopic and endoscopic surgery for pituitary adenoma: a consecutive series of 506 procedures. Acta Neurochir (Wien) 2014;156:441–9.
84. Wang F, Zhou T, Wei S, et al. Endoscopic endonasal transsphenoidal surgery of 1,166 pituitary adenomas. Surg Endosc 2015;29:1270–80.

85. Ciric I, Ragin A, Baumgartner C, et al. Complications of transsphenoidal surgery: results of a national survey, review of the literature, and personal experience. Neurosurgery 1997;40:225–36.
86. Kruis RWJ, Schouten-van Meeteren AYN, Finken MJJ, et al. Management and consequences of postoperative fluctuations in plasma sodium concentration after pediatric brain tumor surgery in the sellar region: a national cohort analysis. Pituitary 2018;21:384–92.
87. Cappablanca P, Cavallo LM, Colao A, et al. Surgical complications associated with the endoscopic endonasal transsphenoidal approach for pituitary adenomas. J Neurosurg 2002;97(2):293–8. https://doi.org/10.3171/jns.2002.97.2.0293. In press.

# Reconstruction of Skull Base Defects in Pituitary Surgery

Cassidy Anderson, BS[a], Nadeem Akbar, MD[b], Patrick Colley, MD[b],*

## KEYWORDS

- Skull base reconstruction • Pituitary adenoma defect repair • Nasoseptal flap
- Free nasal mucosal graft

## KEY POINTS

- Following pituitary tumor resections via the endoscopic transsphenoidal approach, defects are graded based on intraoperative cerebrospinal fluid leak flow and/or diaphragm sellae appearance.
- Defects graded from 0 to 3 are each approached with a variety of reconstructive methods, including allograft underlays, intrasellar packing, synthetic dural grafts, free nasal mucosal grafts, rigid buttresses, and nasoseptal flaps.
- This review synthesizes several practiced methods of repairing skull base defects following pituitary surgery.

## INTRODUCTION

Transnasal pituitary surgery was first developed by Schloffer in 1906 and further refined by Cushing shortly afterward. In the 1960s, Hardy began using the operative microscope during the procedure, which became the workhorse approach for removal of sellar tumors. Then, in the 1990s, the endoscopic transsphenoidal approach was developed and grew in popularity along with advances in endoscopic technology. The endoscopic approach to the sella has many reported advantages over the microscopic or transcranial approaches. First, it provides improved visualization of the operative field in comparison to the microscope's view and allows surgeons to look into the lateral portions of the sella. In addition, the endoscopic approach reduces the traction placed on cranial nerves and parenchyma, while allowing for improved rates of gross total resection as opposed to transcranial approaches.[1–4] Because of these advantages, the use of the endoscopic approach has been expanded beyond pituitary tumor resections and is now used commonly to treat tumors that involve

[a] Albert Einstein College of Medicine, 1300 Morris Park Avenue, Bronx, NY 10461, USA; [b] Department of Otolaryngology, Albert Einstein College of Medicine, 3400 Bainbridge Avenue, Bronx, NY 10467, USA
* Corresponding author. Department of Otolaryngology, Montefiore Medical System, 3400 Bainbridge Ave, Bronx, NY 10467.
E-mail address: pcolley@montefiore.org

Otolaryngol Clin N Am 55 (2022) 449–458
https://doi.org/10.1016/j.otc.2022.01.004
0030-6665/22/© 2022 Elsevier Inc. All rights reserved.

adjacent areas of the anterior skull base.[2,3,5] Despite these advances in endoscopic surgery, there continues to be a significant risk of cerebrospinal fluid (CSF) leaks.

The main goal of sellar reconstruction following pituitary surgery is to create a stable, watertight partition between the sinonasal and intracranial cavities. Despite advances within the field of endoscopic endonasal skull base surgery, CSF leaks owing to a failure to secure a watertight closure of the dura remain one of the most common postoperative complications. Patients with CSF leaks are susceptible to serious, often fatal conditions, including symptomatic pneumocephalus and meningitis.[2,5-7] A graded repair approach following transsphenoidal surgery can be used to guide operative decision making based on the degree of intraoperative CSF leak detected and thickness of the diaphragm sellae.[2,8] This review outlines the current grading system of intraoperative CSF leaks and the corresponding repairs described in the literature.

## DISCUSSION
### Grade 0

Grade 0 is defined by the absence of intraoperative CSF leak. This is typically seen in cases of intrasellar microadenomas, macroadenomas without suprasellar extension, or macroadenomas with incompletely resected suprasellar extension.[2,7,9] Sellar floor reconstruction is typically unnecessary when no intraoperative CSF leakage has occurred, but some investigators advocate for repair to prevent structural complications, such as arachnoid prolapse or chiasmal defect, into the empty tumor space.[2,7] A range of repairs is described: no repair,[9] synthetic underlay grafts,[7,8,10,11] a combination of overlay and underlay grafts with abdominal fat,[12] or underlay synthetic material with free mucosal grafts.[13-16]

### Synthetic closure

Esposito and colleagues[7,8] advocated placing only a collagen sponge (Helistat-Collagen Hemostatic Sponge; Integra Lifesciences Corp, Plainsboro, NJ, USA; or Instat Collagen Absorbable Hemostat; Ethicon, Inc, Johnson & Johnson, Somerville, NJ, USA). Similarly, Jandali and colleagues[10] closed the sella with absorbable hemostatic material (Surgicel; Ethicon, Cincinnati, OH, USA) and stabilized this with a layer of dural sealant (DuraSeal; Integra LifeSciences, Plainsboro, NJ). Dehdashti and colleagues[11] reconstructed using a single layer of Surgicel (Ethicon, Johnson and Johnson Co., Somerville, NJ, USA), several layers of fibrin glue (Evicel; Ethicon, Johnson and Johnson Co., Somerville, NJ, USA), and Gelfoam (Pharmacia and Upjohn Co, Kalamazoo, MI, USA). On the contrary, Wang and colleagues[7] only placed resorbable gelatin sponge (Spongostan; Ethicon, UK) into the bony margins of the tumor defect without tissue sealant or placement into the extradural space. Zeden and colleagues[2] similarly closed the defect solely with gelatin foam (tradename not available).

### Combination of synthetic underlay and autologous fat graft

Conger and colleagues[12] discussed placing an intrasellar autologous fat graft into large sellar defects and using an onlay collagen sponge (Helistat absorbable collagen hemostatic sponge; Integra LifeSciences Corp, Princeton, NJ, USA) over the diaphragm, followed by positioning the sphenoidal mucosa over the sella. Another collagen sponge is then placed over the mucosa, and the whole apparatus is sealed with tissue glue (Tisseel fibrin sealant; Baxter International, Inc, Deerfield, IL, USA).

### Free nasal mucosal graft

Several other investigators use free nasal mucosal grafts to facilitate closure of the sella. These grafts can be harvested from the inferior meatus, nasal floor, middle turbinate, or occasionally nasal septum. Care must be taken to lay the graft flat with the mucosal side facing toward the nasal cavity to prevent postoperative mucocele formation.[14–17] Scagnelli and colleagues[14] and Peris-Celda and colleagues[15] use an underlay of collagen allograft (Durarepair; Medtronic, Minneapolis, MN, USA) that is laid against the diaphragm before the mucosal graft. These investigators also stabilize the graft with oxidized cellulose (Surgicel; Ethicon, Somerville, NJ, USA) and/or tissue sealant (polyethylene glue or Tisseel; Baxter International Inc) (**Fig. 1**).[14,15,17] Other investigators add a bolster of either a 14F Foley catheter in the nasal cavity[13] or Gelform (Pfizer Inc, New York, NY, USA) in the sphenoid sinus to further stabilize the graft during postoperative healing.[17]

### Grade 1

Grade 1 intraoperative CSF leaks have small or "weeping" CSF flow without a visible diaphragm defect.[7,8] Wang and colleagues[7] further differentiate grade 1 leaks into grade 1a, in which the leak originates superiorly from the diaphragm, or grade 1b, in which the leak occurs at the anterior bony border of the planum sphenoidale. Patients with a body mass index greater than 30 or thin diaphragm sellae upon inspection are repaired in a grade 1 manner.[2,12,13] The repair for grade 1 leaks may be composed of synthetic allograft underlays and overlays with an intrasellar pack of autologous

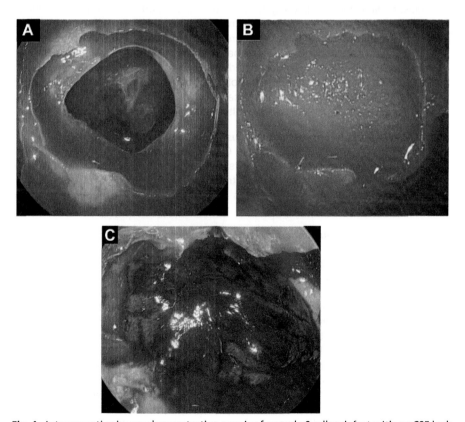

**Fig. 1.** Intraoperative image demonstrating repair of a grade 0 sellar defect with no CSF leak (*A*). Dural substitute graft used as an epidural inlay (*B*). Free mucosal graft used as an only graft over the dural substitute with mucosal surface inked (*C*).

abdominal fat or heterologous material, with or without a rigid buttress.[2,8,11,12,18,19] Other investigators use free nasal mucosal grafts as described in the previous section.[13-17]

### Synthetic allografts, intrasellar synthetic packing, without rigid buttress

Wang and colleagues[7] close the intrasellar defect with a hemostatic gelatin sponge to fill the tumor cavity and cover the sponge with hydrogel sealant (Duraseal; Confluent Surgical Inc, Waltham, MA, USA). For grade 1a leaks, most of the sponge fills the tumor cavity, and the remainder covers the bony portion of the pituitary fossa. In grade 1b leaks, a similar repair is performed; however, the gelatin sponge fills the defect and is placed extradurally on the floor of the anterior cranial fossa to provide counterforce to the arachnoid defect.

Seiler and Mariani[18] repaired defects based on the suprasellar extension of the macroadenoma. In cases without suprasellar extension, the sellar cavity was packed with gelatin foam (Spongostan; Johnson & Johnson Medical Ltd, Skipton, UK) previously soaked in fibrin glue (Tissucol, Baxter AG, Vienna, Austria), and the closure had a covering of fibrin glue–soaked Vicryl patch (polyglactin 910/poly-$p$-dioxanone, Ethisorb dura patch; Ethicon, Inc, Somerville, NJ, USA). In cases with suprasellar extension, the fibrin glue–soaked Vicryl patch is used as an inlay against the diaphragm sellae; the sella turcica is packed with the gelatin foam soaked in fibrin glue and closed with another fibrin glue–soaked Vicryl patch. Although other studies have recommended using a rigid reconstructive material to stabilize the sellar packing,[2,19] Seiler and Mariani[18] found no increase in postoperative complications using solely fibrin glue as a stabilizer, as only 2 patients of the 376 cases reviewed had postoperative CSF leaks (0.5%). Dehdashti and colleagues[11] place several underlay grafts beginning with Surgicel and fibrin glue followed by Alloderm (LifeCell Corp, Woodlands, TX, USA) that is placed flat on the sellar floor. This is then covered with a single layer of fibrin glue and several layers of alternating Gelfoam and fibrin glue.

### Synthetic allografts, intrasellar autologous fat graft, without rigid buttress

In a review of 170 cases of sellar repair, Cappabianca and colleagues[9] packed the sella in cases of intraoperative CSF leaks or invasive macroadenoma. In this technique, an underlay or overlay dural graft (tradename not available) is placed intradurally, followed by packing the autologous fat graft, and then closed with fibrin glue (tradename not available).

### Synthetic and autologous underlay and overlay grafts, intrasellar synthetic packing, or autologous fat graft, with rigid buttress

Kuan and colleagues[13] placed an autologous abdominal fat graft within the empty sella with a rigid Resorb-X plate (KLS Martin, Tuttlingen, Germany) or harvested nasal septal bone if the dura is thin and has increased tension. A posterior septal free mucosal graft is placed, and a 14F Foley catheter holds the graft in place and is removed on postoperative day 3. Zeden and colleagues[2] lay collagen matrix (tradename not specified) that is stabilized with fibrin glue (tradename not specified) and place polydioxanone foils (Ethicon Inc, Somerville, NJ, USA) extradurally within the bony opening with roughly 1 to 2 mm of overlap. Conger and colleagues[12] perform the aforementioned grade 0 repair with the addition of a solid buttress, either harvested nasal septum bone or synthetic (Medpor TSI; Stryker Corporation Kalamazoo, MI, USA), that is placed in the extradural space within the bony margin. An additional layer of abdominal fat, collagen sponge, and tissue glue within the posterior sphenoid is used to further bolster the repair. Reconstruction with abdominal fat or collagen matrix filling the empty tumor space and closure with free nasal mucosa graft is adequate for repairing grade 1 leaks if the patient is not at high risk for developing a postoperative CSF leak.[16]

## Grade 2

Esposito and colleagues[8] define grade 2 intraoperative CSF leaks as moderate leaks with a visible diaphragmatic defect or tear. As this is not considered high flow, a lumbar drain to control intracranial pressure is not usually advised.[8,20,21] To repair a moderate leak, more robust repairs are required. Reconstruction commonly involves multilayered approaches, including use of an allograft underlay; intrasellar packing; with or without a rigid buttress; synthetic onlay graft, free mucosal graft overlay, or nasoseptal flap (NSF); and tissue sealant.[2,8,11–14,16,18] Some approaches include packing the sphenoid sinus to reinforce the watertight closure of the sella and other bolsters.[9,11,12]

### Allograft underlay, intrasellar packing, and rigid buttress

Seiler and Mariani[18] repaired defects based on the suprasellar extension of the adenoma and used the same closure technique as described above with their grade 1 repairs. Peris-Celda and colleagues[15] repaired pituitary adenoma resection defects with free mucosal grafts regardless of the status of intraoperative CSF leakage. Depending on patient preoperative likelihood of developing postoperative CSF leakage, Perez-Lopez and colleagues[16] placed an underlay of collagen (tradename not specified) with an intrasellar fat graft with a free mucosal overlay graft held with tissue sealant (tradename not specified) in cases of low risk but intraoperative grade 2 leak.

Esposito and colleagues[8] recommend an intrasellar autologous abdominal fat graft, layered with a collagen sponge and intrasellar titanium mesh buttress (0.2-mm Micro Mesh; Stryker Leibinger, Kalamazoo, MI, USA). A fat graft is also added into the sphenoid sinus. BioGlue, a tissue sealant (CryoLife, Inc, Atlanta, GA, USA), is added to stabilize the graft. Conger and colleagues[12] use the same approach as Esposito and colleagues. Cappabianca and colleagues[9] add an intradural underlay dural graft (tradename not specified) followed by abdominal fat graft that is closed with fibrin glue (tradename not specified). The sphenoid sinus is further packed in cases of insufficiency of sellar packing to maintain watertight closure but is often avoided to prevent postoperative sphenoid mucocele complications.

### Nasoseptal flap

The NSF, first described by Hadad and colleagues[22] in 2006, is the "workhorse" of skull base reconstructive surgery and has allowed for the increased extent of endoscopic endonasal skull base procedures.[3,6,20,22,23] The NSF is a pedicled, mucoperichondrial/periosteal flap from the nasal septum supplied by the posterior septal branch of the sphenopalatine artery. As a vascularized flap, the NSF can close larger defects, spanning as far as the frontal sinus to the sella and between the medial orbital walls.[3,22] Currently, the postoperative rate of CSF leak complications for endoscopic endonasal skull base reconstructions is 0.0% to 2.9%.[14,16]

The NSF can be used on its own or in combination with an underlay/inlay graft of collagen and autologous fat graft (**Fig. 2**).[3,20–22] Hadad and colleagues[22] use collagen matrix (tradename not specified) as an inlay subdural graft and fill the intrasellar space with abdominal fat or an onlay of autologous fascial graft. The NSF is placed over the fat graft or directly over the dural inlay and is secured with fibrin glue. The flap is stabilized with a bolster of nasal packing or a 12F Foley catheter with silicone splints to protect the nasal septum. Eloy and colleagues[20] will similarly add an intrasellar packing of acellular dermal allograft before positioning the NSF to

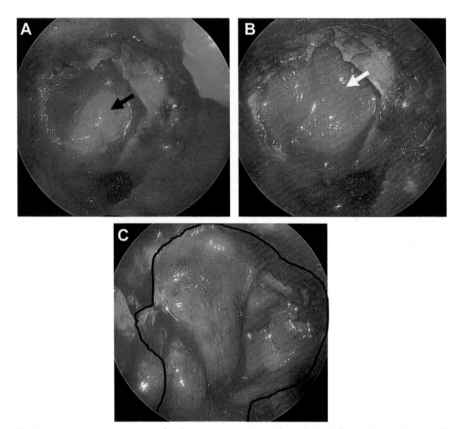

**Fig. 2.** Intraoperative images of sellar reconstruction of grade 2 defect with moderate CSF leak after resection. Abdominal fat graft (*black arrow*) packed into the empty sella (*A*). Synthetic dural onlay membrane (*white arrow*) placed over autologous fat graft (*B*). NSF (*outlined in black line*) harvested from left nasal septum and placed against the defect (*C*).

close the defect. Fibrin glue (Tisseel; Baxter Healthcare Corp) is used to hold the NSF in place. In another study by Eloy and colleagues,[24] they established that the use of dural sealant for NSF repairs does not result in decreased postoperative CSF leaks. Therefore, dural sealant is not required for NSF repairs of high-grade pituitary defects. Dehdashti colleagues[11] pack the intrasellar space with fat graft and Alloderm, place the NSF with the mucosal side facing anteriorly, stabilize with fibrin glue and Gelfoam, and temporarily use a 14F Foley catheter for 1 day postoperatively. Conger and colleagues[12] will cover the fat graft with collagen sponge and stabilize with a bony or synthetic buttress before placing the NSF. Kuan and colleagues[13] place a Resorb-X plate over the abdominal fat graft inside the empty sella and fortify the closure with an NSF for grades 2 and 3 leaks. The flap is held in place by a 14F Foley catheter for 3 postoperative days.

### Grade 3

Grade 3 intraoperative leaks are high-flow CSF leaks with a large, visible diaphragm tear, often owing to an extended transsphenoidal approach through the clival or

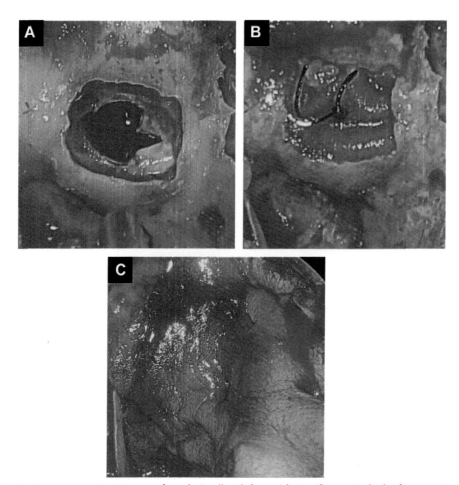

**Fig. 3.** Intraoperative images of grade 3 sellar defect with significant CSF leak after tumor resection and subsequent reconstruction. Grade 3 defect with large diaphragmatic defect and high-flow leak (*A*). Autologous fat with stitch through the dermal fat to fill the dead space and used as an underlay (*B*). NSF harvested from left nasal septum and placed over the defect (*C*).

supradiaphragmatic dura.[8,16] The repair for grade 3 leaks is equivalent to grade 2 repairs, but lumbar drains are often added to decrease intracranial pressure and localize the leak origin intraoperatively.[8,20,21] Use of an NSF is recommended over free nasal mucosal grafts for suprasellar adenomas and grade 3 leaks.[14] Multilayered approaches as previously described are used with additional abdominal fat graft and collagen matrix extending extradurally.[8] Autologous tissue, such as the tensor fascia lata grafts, can be used in place of collagen matrix. Last, solid buttress support (whether nasal septal bone or a synthetic material) placed flush with the intrasellar bony margin can also be used to support repairs when there is significantly elevated intracranial pressure.[2,8,12] The NSF has revolutionized the endoscopic endonasal approach by allowing for closure of large defects, such as those with grade 3 CSF leaks with a much higher success rate (**Fig. 3**).[3,22]

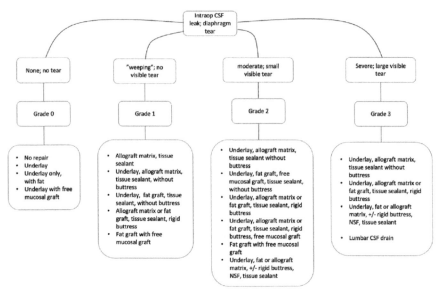

**Fig. 4.** Repair approaches as determined by intraoperative CSF leaking and presence of diaphragm defect. Intraop, intraoperative.

## SUMMARY

Postoperative CSF leak is a common complication following transsphenoidal pituitary surgery.[25] However, developments within the endoscopic skull base surgery field have allowed for more complex procedures with better reassurance of sellar repair. Many surgeons have effective repair approaches following tumor resection, but a standard guideline for repair has not yet been determined. Agreement on a standard algorithm for repair can help decrease the steep learning curve of endoscopic skull base surgery (**Fig. 4**).

## CLINICS CARE POINTS

- Following pituitary tumor resections via the endoscopic endonasal transsphenoidal approach, sellar defects are evaluated based on the flow of the intraoperative cerebrospinal fluid leak and appearance of the diaphragm sellae.

- Grade 0 defects have no intraoperative cerebrospinal fluid leaks. Repairs range from no repair, underlay of allograft material, underlay grafts with intrasellar packing, or overlay-free mucosal grafts.

- Grade 1 defects have minimal, "weeping" cerebrospinal fluid flow intraoperatively and/or thin diaphragm sellae. These defects are repaired using underlay grafts, intrasellar packing, overlay grafts, with or without rigid buttress support.

- Grade 2 defects have moderate intraoperative cerebrospinal fluid flow with a small, visible diaphragm tear. Grade 2 defects are reconstructed with multilayered allograft approaches with or without rigid buttress support; free nasal mucosal overlay grafts with intrasellar packing and rigid buttress support; or nasoseptal flaps.

- Grade 3 defects have high intraoperative cerebrospinal fluid flow with large tears in the diaphragm. These defects are repaired in the same manner as grade 2 defects. A lumbar drain can be performed to further decrease intracranial pressure to stabilize the repair postoperatively.

## DISCLOSURE

The authors have no funding, financial relationships, or conflicts of interest to disclose.

## REFERENCES

1. Jankowski R, Auque J, Simon C, et al. How I do it: head and neck and plastic surgery: endoscopic pituitary tumor surgery. Laryngoscope 1992;102(2):198–202.
2. Zeden J-P, Baldauf J, Schroeder HW. Repair of the sellar floor using bioresorbable polydioxanone foils after endoscopic endonasal pituitary surgery. Neurosurg Focus 2020;48(6):E16.
3. Hannan CJ, Kelleher E, Javadpour M. Methods of skull base repair following endoscopic endonasal tumor resection: a review. Front Oncol 2020;10.
4. Rolston JD, Han SJ, Aghi MK. Nationwide shift from microscopic to endoscopic transsphenoidal pituitary surgery. Pituitary 2016;19(3):248–50.
5. Ivan ME, Iorgulescu JB, El-Sayed I, et al. Risk factors for postoperative cerebrospinal fluid leak and meningitis after expanded endoscopic endonasal surgery. J Clin Neurosci 2015;22(1):48–54.
6. Lai LT, Trooboff S, Morgan MK, et al. The risk of meningitis following expanded endoscopic endonasal skull base surgery: a systematic review. J Neurol Surg B: Skull Base 2014;75(01):018–26.
7. Wang YY, Kearney T, Gnanalingham KK. Low-grade CSF leaks in endoscopic trans-sphenoidal pituitary surgery: efficacy of a simple and fully synthetic repair with a hydrogel sealant. Acta neurochirurgica 2011;153(4):815–22.
8. Esposito F, Dusick JR, Fatemi N, et al. Graded repair of cranial base defects and cerebrospinal fluid leaks in transsphenoidal surgery. Oper Neurosurg 2007; 60(suppl_4). ONS-295-ONS-304.
9. Cappabianca P, Cavallo LM, Esposito F, et al. Sellar repair in endoscopic endonasal transsphenoidal surgery: results of 170 cases. Neurosurgery 2002;51(6): 1365–72.
10. Jandali D, Shearer S, Byrne R, et al. Assessment of post-operative healing following endoscopic, transnasal, transsphenoidal pituitary surgery without formal sellar grafting. Am J Otol 2020;41(2):102306.
11. Dehdashti AR, Stofko D, Okun J, et al. Endoscopic endonasal reconstruction of skull base: repair protocol. J Neurol Surg 2016;77(03):271–8.
12. Conger A, Zhao F, Wang X, et al. Evolution of the graded repair of CSF leaks and skull base defects in endonasal endoscopic tumor surgery: trends in repair failure and meningitis rates in 509 patients. J Neurosurg 2018;130(3):861–75.
13. Kuan EC, Yoo F, Patel PB, et al. An algorithm for sellar reconstruction following the endoscopic endonasal approach: a review of 300 consecutive cases. J Neurol Surg 2018;79(02):177–83.
14. Scagnelli RJ, Patel V, Peris-Celda M, et al. Implementation of free mucosal graft technique for sellar reconstruction after pituitary surgery: outcomes of 158 consecutive patients. World Neurosurg 2019;122:e506–11.
15. Peris-Celda M, Chaskes M, Lee DD, et al. Optimizing sellar reconstruction after pituitary surgery with free mucosal graft: results from the first 50 consecutive patients. World Neurosurg 2017;101:180–5.

16. Perez-Lopez C, Palpan AJ, Zamarrón Á, et al. Free mucosal graft for reconstruction after nonfunctional pituitary adenoma surgery. Asian J Neurosurg 2020; 15(4):946.
17. Fishpool SJ, Amato-Watkins A, Hayhurst C. Free middle turbinate mucosal graft reconstruction after primary endoscopic endonasal pituitary surgery. Eur Arch Oto-Rhino-Laryngology. 2017;274(2):837–44.
18. Seiler RW, Mariani L. Sellar reconstruction with resorbable Vicryl patches, gelatin foam, and fibrin glue in transsphenoidal surgery: a 10-year experience with 376 patients. J Neurosurg 2000;93(5):762–5.
19. Arita K, Kurisu K, Tominaga A, et al. Size-adjustable titanium plate for reconstruction of the sella turcica. J Neurosurg 1999;91(6):1055–7.
20. Eloy JA, Kalyoussef E, Choudhry OJ, et al. Salvage endoscopic nasoseptal flap repair of persistent cerebrospinal fluid leak after open skull base surgery. Am J Otol 2012;33(6):735–40.
21. Kassam AB, Thomas A, Carrau RL, et al. Endoscopic reconstruction of the cranial base using a pedicled nasoseptal flap. Oper Neurosurg 2008;63(suppl_1): ONS44–53.
22. Hadad G, Bassagasteguy L, Carrau RL, et al. A novel reconstructive technique after endoscopic expanded endonasal approaches: vascular pedicle nasoseptal flap. Laryngoscope 2006;116(10):1882–6.
23. Chabot JD, Patel CR, Hughes MA, et al. Nasoseptal flap necrosis: a rare complication of endoscopic endonasal surgery. J Neurosurg 2017;128(5):1463–72.
24. Eloy JA, Kuperan AB, Friedel ME, et al. Endoscopic nasoseptal flap repair of skull base defects: is addition of a dural sealant necessary? J Neurol Surg Part B: Skull Base 2012;73(S 01):A021.
25. Rizvi ZH, Ferrandino R, Luu Q, et al. Nationwide analysis of unplanned 30-day readmissions after transsphenoidal pituitary surgery. Int Forum Allergy Rhinol 2019;322–9.

# Postoperative Care from the Rhinologic and Neurological Perspectives

Stella E. Lee, MD[a],*, Carl H. Snyderman, MD[b],
Paul A. Gardner, MD[c]

## KEYWORDS

- Pituitary • Transsphenoidal surgery • Postoperative management • Hyponatremia
- Diabetes insipidus • CSF leak • Epistaxis

## KEY POINTS

- Postoperative management following pituitary surgery ideally includes a multidisciplinary team well versed in the comprehensive care of these patients, including neurosurgery, endocrinology, ophthalmology, otolaryngology, and critical care medicine.
- Most patients undergoing endoscopic transsphenoidal surgery for pituitary tumors have excellent outcomes with minimal morbidity.
- The most common medical complication following transsphenoidal surgery is hyponatremia, which is one of the most common reasons for hospital readmission.
- The most common surgical complication following transsphenoidal surgery is cerebrospinal fluid leak, which often requires surgical intervention.

## INTRODUCTION

Pituitary tumors are one of the most common intracranial tumors, but patients present with diverse and heterogenous clinical and pathologic presentations requiring a multidisciplinary team approach including neurosurgery, otolaryngology, endocrinology, ophthalmology, and radiology. With advances in endoscopic endonasal approaches, technology, anatomic knowledge, and technique, most patients have excellent outcomes with low morbidity and mortality. However, early identification and management of postoperative complications is crucial. The most common postoperative complications following transsphenoidal surgery (TSS) include hyponatremia,

[a] Division of Otolaryngology—Head & Neck Surgery, Brigham and Women's Hospital, Harvard Medical School, 45 Francis Street, Boston, MA 02115, USA; [b] Department of Otolaryngology—Head & Neck Surgery, University of Pittsburgh School of Medicine, 200 Lothrop Street, Suite 500, Pittsburgh, PA 15213, USA; [c] Department of Neurological Surgery, University of Pittsburgh School of Medicine, 200 Lothrop Street, Suite B400, Pittsburgh, PA 15213, USA
* Corresponding author:
E-mail address: slee192@bwh.harvard.edu

Otolaryngol Clin N Am 55 (2022) 459–467
https://doi.org/10.1016/j.otc.2021.12.012
0030-6665/22/© 2021 Elsevier Inc. All rights reserved.

cerebrospinal fluid (CSF) leak, hypopituitarism, and nasal crusting. Patients often require long-term postoperative follow-up for surveillance and management of neurologic, endocrinologic, and sinonasal concerns.

## HYPONATREMIA AND DIABETES INSIPIDUS

Hyponatremia can result from multiple causes including syndrome of inappropriate secretion of antidiuretic hormone (SIADH), adrenal insufficiency, and cerebral salt wasting. Rates of hyponatremia after TSS for pituitary tumors range from 4% to 12% in the literature.[1] Hyponatremia is a common cause of readmission to the hospital, and in a series of 1240 patients undergoing TSS, the readmission rate was approximately 8.5% at a median of 11 days postdischarge. Hyponatremia was the most common cause, comprising 29.5% of the cohort.[2] A recent study of readmission for hyponatremia from the same group reported a rate of 2.5%, with a significant drop after implementing fluid restriction of 1 liter (L) per day for 1 week following surgery.[3]

In a review of 928 patients and 1023 surgeries, a standardized protocol has been developed for all patients regardless of underlying pathology.[4] As discussed earlier, patients restrict oral fluid intake to 1 L daily until 1 week postoperatively and are encouraged to only drink when thirsty. In the immediate postoperative period, assessments of serum sodium and urine specific gravity are checked every 6 hours and serum cortisol daily in the fasted state in the early morning (7–8 AM).[4] SIADH, which has a described peak incidence on the seventh postoperative day, presents with hyponatremia that can be severe and symptomatic.[5] Symptoms include nausea, vomiting, lethargy, delirium, and seizure. Management with fluid restriction is generally effective with close postoperative monitoring. It is important to properly diagnose SIADH by measuring fluid status, serum electrolytes, BUN/creatinine/glucose/cortisol, and serum and urine osmolality. Correction with hypernatremic fluids may be ineffective and is generally avoided. Interestingly, machine learning algorithms in the future may be helpful to predict postoperative hyponatremia using several preoperative and intraoperative clinical features.[6]

Conversely, diabetes insipidus (DI) is characterized by production of excessive inappropriately dilute urine, which can lead to hypernatremia. DI should be suspected in patients who have urine output greater than 240 mL/h for at least 2 consecutive hours, urine-specific gravity less than 1.005, and serum sodium greater than 145 mEq/L. It is generally treated with intravenous or subcutaneous desmopressin initially and converted to oral administration as needed. The nasal spray form is usually avoided, given inconsistent absorption in the postoperative period. Most patients can maintain adequate fluid intake to achieve euvolemia, but desmopressin therapy is required for select patients and may also be added for patient comfort in the setting of extreme thirst or nocturia. As such, desmopressin treatment is usually reserved for patients with a sodium level greater than 145 mEq/L and inability to achieve adequate fluid intake. In a series of 700 patients undergoing TSS, the overall rate of postoperative DI was 14.7% (n = 103 patients) with permanent DI in 4.6% (n = 16 patients) with a median follow-up of 10.7 months (range 0.2–136.6) and at least 1 year for evaluation of permanent DI.[7] Compared with patients with pituitary adenoma, postoperative DI was more likely to develop in patients with Rathke cleft cyst (odds ratio [OR] = 2.2, $P = .009$) and craniopharyngioma (OR = 7.0, $P \leq .001$).

## HYPOPITUITARISM

New-onset hypopituitarism is rare in experienced hands[8] and occurs more frequently in patients with large or invasive lesions and in patients with functioning adenomas who may experience significant hormonal shifts postoperatively. Depending on the pituitary axis deficiency, lifelong hormonal replacement may be required for some patients, and this potential outcome should be discussed with patients before surgery.[4] Deficiencies of cortisol, thyroid, growth hormone, testosterone, estrogen, and ADH should be considered and appropriately replaced. It is critical that patients understand the symptoms of adrenal insufficiency including fatigue, nausea, syncope, as well as the increased need for hydrocortisone/prednisone during illness/physiologic stress in order for replacement to be given appropriately.[4]

In patients with a diagnosis of Cushing disease, cortisol is checked every 6 hours and replacement is started when cortisol levels reach levels less than 5 $\mu$g/dL with symptoms of adrenal insufficiency or a nadir less than 2 $\mu$g/dL at any time point.[4] For patients with acromegaly, growth hormone (short half-life) can be measured on the first postoperative day and insulin-like growth factor 1 (long half-life) at the 3-month follow-up. For patients with prolactinomas, serum prolactin (short half-life) is measured on the first postoperative day and then at 6-week follow-up.

Strategies to assess anterior and posterior pituitary function and treatment with appropriate replacement therapy is important in patients with axis deficiencies. In general, long-term follow-up with evaluation of pituitary function in conjunction with pituitary imaging is helpful for all patients who have undergone surgery, regardless of hormone status.

## CEREBROSPINAL FLUID LEAK AND MENINGITIS

The incidence of CSF leak following TSS is typically 1% to 4% (range 0.6%–12%) with advances in technique and increased experience. Several repair methods have been described including autologous fat, mucosa, fascia, nasoseptal flaps, dural substitutes, and fibrin glues. In a series of 1166 patients with 806 (69.1%) patients with macroadenoma and 115 (10%) giant adenomas, reconstruction was performed with Duragen (Integra, Plainsboro, NJ, USA), Duraform, and Bio Glue (Cryolife, Inc., Kennesaw, GA, USA) with an overall incidence of postoperative leak of 0.6% (n = 7).[9] Of these 7 patients, 6 did not have an observable CSF leak at the primary surgery.

Although the best way to prevent a postoperative CSF leak is to identify the leak intraoperatively, there are variations in management strategies reported. In a series of 1002 patients, postoperative CSF leak was identified in 26 patients (2.6%), including 13 patients who had no evidence of apparent intraoperative leak (1.3%).[10] Seven of the thirteen patients had a macroadenoma with visible arachnoid suggesting the possibility of a delayed leak. In a review of 334 patients, multivariate analysis indicated an increased risk of CSF leak with history of radiotherapy to the skull base (OR = 8.67, $P < .05$). Elevated body mass index and hydrocephalus were identified as predictors of postoperative CSF leaks in a study of 806 patients undergoing TSS with a rate of 2.6% (n = 21 patients).[11] Another study of 492 patients undergoing TSS for resection of pituitary adenoma found that fibrous tumors and larger tumor size were associated with intraoperative CSF leak.[12] Delayed postoperative CSF leak has been reported as the most common reason for reoperation (3.7%).[2] CSF leak has also been associated with higher rates of postoperative DI ($P = .040$), intracerebral hemorrhage (OR = 17.44, $P < .05$), and postoperative intracranial infection (OR = 28.73, $P < .05$) leading to increased length of hospitalization.[13] A retrospective review of 658 patients undergoing endoscopic TSS for the resection of pituitary adenoma revealed that intraoperative CSF leak and use of continuous positive airway pressure (CPAP) predicted a prolonged hospital stay defined as greater than 4 days (n = 72). Postoperative CSF leak, DI or hypopituitarism, or need for revision surgery were also additional reasons for prolonged hospitalization.[14]

Postoperatively, patients are advised to avoid strenuous activity and nose blowing, which can lead to disruption of reconstruction, pneumocephalus, and bacterial infection. CSF rhinorrhea can manifest as watery drainage into the nasopharynx, causing a salty/metallic taste and cough. Testing of this fluid for beta-2 transferrin or obtaining a computed tomography (CT) scan to evaluate for new pneumocephalus can help confirm a CSF leak. If a leak is suspected, head of bed elevation and CSF diversion can be helpful although prompt reexploration and repair is preferable over lumbar drainage unless the leak is questionable or very minor. The rate of drainage is generally 5 to 15 mL/h for 5 days, and close monitoring to prevent excessive drainage is important to avoid meningeal inflammation, pneumocephalus, and low-pressure headache, among other symptoms. In addition, prolonged CSF diversion can lead to an increased risk of meningitis and intracranial abscess and therefore should be avoided.[4]

The overall incidence of meningitis after TSS ranges from 0% to 9%, with most series reporting in the range of 1%. There should be a low threshold for spinal fluid sampling, however, in patients with suspected meningitis.

In rare cases, nasoseptal flap necrosis due to inadequate vascular supply to the flap can present with delayed onset of meningitis in the absence of a CSF leak. These patients benefit from early debridement of the necrotic tissue and secondary reconstruction, if necessary, in addition to medical treatment of meningitis.[15]

## PNEUMOCEPHALUS

Patients with symptoms of mental status change, nausea/vomiting, new-onset or worsening headache, and seizures should be assessed for pneumocephalus with a head CT. Depending on the degree of pneumocephalus, initial management includes head of bed elevation, bed rest, supplemental oxygen, taking care to avoid introduction of positive pressure, and pain management. If there is evidence of tension pneumocephalus or failure of conservative measures, surgical exploration should be performed expeditiously. New or increased pneumocephalus should be treated in the same fashion and with the same urgency as a CSF leak with the exception that CSF diversion should be avoided before reexploration. Obese patients and patients with obstructive sleep apnea may be at increased risk for developing pneumocephalus.[16] Although clinical studies are lacking, in the authors' opinion, CPAP can generally be resumed safely at 2 weeks following surgery. Placement of a nasal trumpet at the time of surgery may alleviate the symptoms of sleep apnea and decrease the risk of pneumocephalus.

## VISUAL COMPLICATIONS

Patients who report visual changes postoperatively should be evaluated immediately for possible nerve injury, ischemia, or compression. Vision should be assessed in each eye separately because some patients may not notice a unilateral or peripheral field loss and may confuse binocular diplopia for "blurred" vision. Loss of an afferent pupillary reflex may indicate compromise of a unilateral optic nerve. The inability to detect the color red may be an early sign of optic nerve compression.[16] Visual fields can also be assessed at the bedside postoperatively. Bitemporal hemianopsia can occur from chiasmal compression, which can occur due to hematoma in the tumor bed. If there is concern regarding visual loss, expedited and thorough evaluation by ophthalmology is recommended and followed closely by fine-cut CT or MRI. Overinflation of a balloon catheter or overpacking can cause optic nerve compression and should be promptly deflated or removed. Surgical exploration may be indicated to relieve compression secondary to a hematoma or fat graft. A sudden unilateral loss of vision due to hemorrhage and retroorbital hematoma is an ophthalmologic emergency with a low threshold for lateral canthotomy and cantholysis to relieve pressure on the optic nerve. Other measurements that are concerning include intraocular pressure greater than 40 mm Hg, proptosis, and severe pain.

## SINONASAL MORBIDITY AND QUALITY OF LIFE

In a study of 83 patients in which no formal grafting or reconstruction was performed after TSS, mean time to mucosalization was 119 days, with smoking found to be associated with prolonged time to full mucosalization.[17] Nasal crusting was the most common problem after TSS, seen in 61% of patients. A systematic review also found that nasal crusting was the most common sinonasal morbidity (50.8%) followed by nasal discharge (40.4%), nasal blockage (40.1%), and olfactory dysfunction (26.7%).[18] A prospective study evaluating risk factors for development of nasal crusting and discharge found that surgical complexity was a risk for nasal discharge (OR = 5.17), although no risk factors could be identified for crusting in their patient cohort.[19] Disruption and removal of ciliated mucosa also contributes to crusting and nasal discharge, and therefore the decision to remove turbinates or mucociliary lining should be done with care.[18]

Evaluation of patient-reported outcome measures is important, and various tools have been used to evaluate postoperative quality of life. Using the Sinonasal Outcome Test (SNOT)-22, a systematic review showed significant postoperative improvements in quality of life at the 6-month and 1-year time points. Interestingly, patients who had preoperative SNOT-22 scores less than 20 did not worsen postoperatively.[20] In another series of 148 patients undergoing TSS, patients had worsened quality of life based on SNOT-22 in the 1-month follow-up period, which returned to preoperative levels at 2 to 4 months.[21] Patients with Cushing disease, however, may have greater impairments in health-related quality of life compared with patients with other pituitary disorders. In a prospective longitudinal case-control study (n = 10 with Cushing disease, n = 10 with nonfunctioning pituitary adenoma, and n = 20 healthy matched controls), patients with Cushing disease had greater psychological and cognitive impairments compared with patients with nonfunctioning pituitary adenomas as measured by the Short Form Health Survey SF-36, Beck Depression Inventory-II, and the Minnesota Multiphasic Personality Inventory-II.[22] A Cushing disease–specific quality of life questionnaire with items generated by patients, caregivers, and health care providers has also been recently validated, consisting of 56 items that are more specific and relevant to this population including headache, anxiety, and mood changes.[23]

Olfactory dysfunction can cause significant morbidity in the postoperative period in patients undergoing skull base surgery, and a discussion with the patient as well as testing before and after may be helpful to guide postoperative management. A study of 161 patients evaluated smell disturbance after TSS for pituitary surgery, showing that 67.1% of patients following surgery had transient severe olfactory dysfunction (hyposmia or anosmia) and 14.9% had long-term olfactory dysfunction. Preoperative nasal disease and smoking were risk factors for long-term olfactory dysfunction.[24] In another series of 18 patients, preoperative and postoperative University of Pennsylvania Smell Identification Test scores were not significantly different for patients undergoing TSS for pituitary tumors or for patients who had nasoseptal flaps (29.4 vs 28.6,

$P = .87$).[25] Identification and preservation of the olfactory epithelium (olfactory strip-sparing technique) while harvesting a nasoseptal flap has shown to be helpful in preserving olfaction.[26]

## OTHER POSTOPERATIVE COMPLICATIONS

If patients develop respiratory compromise after surgery, a low threshold for intubation with the avoidance of positive pressure mask ventilation is critical. Patients with acromegaly can be at risk for airway compromise due to tongue hypertrophy, and appropriate preoperative discussion with anesthesia and postoperative monitoring is key. Although some small degree bloody nasal discharge after skull base surgery is expected, high-flow brisk bleeding is uncommon and can suggest a pseudoaneurysm of the internal carotid artery, cavernous fistula, or injury to the sphenopalatine artery. Bleeding from the ethmoidal arteries is less common and can be seen associated with traumatic injuries of the skull base. If a significant bleed is encountered, the airway should be first secured followed by prompt evaluation with a CT angiogram, angiography, or endovascular techniques for internal carotid artery injuries. Overall, significant epistaxis is rare and in a systematic review, the reported incidence ranged from 0% to 3%.[18]

A study of more than 15,000 patients undergoing pituitary surgery found a small incidence of pneumonia (n = 98, 0.68%) postoperatively.[27] Older age, male sex, and a transfrontal surgical approach were associated with increased risk. Prolonged intubation may place patients at a higher risk of pneumonia. Patients with pneumonia had a significantly higher mortality and incurred more than 4 times the hospital charges and 5 times lengthier hospital stays compared with patients without pneumonia.

Monitoring and prophylaxis for thromboembolism is important for all patients undergoing surgery but especially in patients with lengthier procedures. Early mobilization is important. Patients with Cushing disease can have a hypercoagulative state that can lead to increased risk of venous thromboembolic events.[28] Early mobilization and early and prolonged chemical prophylaxis for deep venous thrombosis is key to preventing thromboembolic complications.[29,30]

## PRACTICAL CONSIDERATIONS

At the University of Pittsburgh Medical Center, postoperative head CT is performed on the day of surgery if intradural dissection was performed (ie, intraoperative CSF leak). Uncomplicated cases do not require intensive care unit (ICU) care, and step-down units may be used if monitoring of intake and output can be done frequently. Specific guidelines from another tertiary care institution indicate admission to neurosurgical ICU for the following conditions: evidence of hemorrhagic lesions with risk for hematoma, need for frequent monitoring of vision, severe medical comorbidities, and presence of tumors that exhibit suprasellar extension.[4]

Monitoring and regulation of blood pressure is important to avoid hypertension but ensure adequate perfusion especially in patients with visual loss and inadequate blood flow to the optic chiasm and optic nerves. Care is taken to ensure systolic blood pressure is maintained at less than 150 mm Hg with mean arterial pressure greater than 80 mm Hg if there was any manipulation of the optic nerves.[16]

Nasal restrictions include avoidance of nose blowing, use of straws, and positive pressure treatment at least 2 weeks after surgery and, if a patient requires a nasogastric tube, this should only be placed by an otolaryngologist under direct endoscopic visualization due to the presence of a skull base defect. Signage and communication to nursing and other care teams to avoid passing any tubes through the nasal cavity should be clear.

Postoperative medications include an oral corticosteroid taper over several days if the patient is believed to have adrenal insufficiency preoperatively and was treated with stress-dose hydrocortisone. A cortisol level can be checked on the first postoperative day in the absence of intraoperative steroids, which are generally only given in the setting of significant vision loss or 48 hours after any intraoperative steroid. Patients are given an appropriate bowel regimen and advised to avoid straining that may increase CSF pressure. Appropriate pain control and 0.65% saline nasal spray in both nostrils q8h is advised.

Patients with greater than 1 L of blood loss undergo coagulation panel checks every 6 hours and, in the morning, measurement of prolactin and serum cortisol as discussed earlier, as well as growth hormone if the patient has acromegaly. Prolactin is an excellent marker for overall pituitary gland function given its short half-life.

Patients with Cushing disease have serum cortisol levels checked every 6 hours.

Fluid status monitoring includes hourly intake and output evaluation followed by urine-specific gravity and serum sodium level checks.

If CSF leak is suspected, immediate otolaryngology evaluation with nasal endoscopy is performed and, if there is a leak, return to the operating theater for revision of the skull base reconstruction is performed.

Once discharged home, patients are advised to avoid lying flat but to sleep with the head elevated ("higher than the heart"). Activity restrictions include avoidance of lifting anything heavier than 5 pounds, bending at the waist, and to avoid driving if patients have severe visual deficits until cleared by ophthalmology. A bowel regimen to avoid straining is recommended.

Patients are seen in both the neurosurgery and otolaryngology clinics at 5 to 7 days postoperatively with packing removal at that time and discontinuation of prophylactic antibiotics. Splints, if present, are removed at 1 to 3 weeks depending on the septal reconstruction, and further follow-up is scheduled for evaluation and debridement. Patients generally undergo a postoperative MRI at 3 months in order to assess extent of resection and annually to assess for recurrence. Symptoms of recurrence that would prompt earlier imaging include return of or worsening headache, visual field deficits, or endocrinologic symptoms. Although long-term surveillance and radiologic, endocrine, and ophthalmologic follow-up is recommended, there is insufficient evidence regarding duration of time of surveillance and frequency. The first radiographic study is recommended at 3 months or longer after surgery for nonfunctioning pituitary adenomas.[31]

## SUMMARY

Postoperative care of patients undergoing TSS requires a team approach, capitalizing on the complementary knowledge and skills of surgical and medical disciplines. In the early postoperative period, endocrinologic problems and CSF leak are the major drivers of morbidity and need for readmission or revision surgery. With a team-based approach, most complications can be mitigated with a low risk of serious complications and excellent quality of life.

## DISCLOSURES

S.E. Lee: clinical trial funding and advisory boards for AstraZeneca, Genentech, GlaxoSmithKline, and Sanofi Regeneron. C.H. Snyderman: equity in SPIWay, LLC. P.A. Gardner: equity in SPIWay, LLC; Consultant Lazic.

## REFERENCES

1. Cote DJ, Alzarea A, Acosta MA, et al. Predictors and Rates of Delayed Symptomatic Hyponatremia after Transsphenoidal Surgery: A Systematic Review [corrected]. World Neurosurg 2016;88:1–6.
2. Cote DJ, Dasenbrock HH, Muskens IS, et al. Readmission and Other Adverse Events after Transsphenoidal Surgery: Prevalence, Timing, and Predictive Factors. J Am Coll Surg 2017;224(5):971–9.
3. Burke WT, Cote DJ, Iuliano SI, et al. A practical method for prevention of readmission for symptomatic hyponatremia following transsphenoidal surgery. Pituitary 2018;21(1):25–31.
4. Cote DJ, Iuliano SL, Catalino MP, et al. Optimizing pre-, intra-, and postoperative management of patients with sellar pathology undergoing transsphenoidal surgery. Neurosurg Focus 2020;48(6):E2.
5. Ausiello JC, Bruce JN, Freda PU. Postoperative assessment of the patient after transsphenoidal pituitary surgery. Pituitary 2008;11(4):391–401.
6. Voglis S, van Niftrik CHB, Staartjes VE, et al. Feasibility of machine learning based predictive modelling of postoperative hyponatremia after pituitary surgery. Pituitary 2020;23(5):543–51.
7. Burke WT, Cote DJ, Penn DL, et al. Diabetes Insipidus After Endoscopic Transsphenoidal Surgery. Neurosurgery 2020;87(5):949–55.
8. Paluzzi A, Fernandez-Miranda JC, Tonya Stefko S, et al. Endoscopic endonasal approach for pituitary adenomas: a series of 555 patients. Pituitary 2014;17(4): 307–19.
9. Wang F, Zhou T, Wei S, et al. Endoscopic endonasal transsphenoidal surgery of 1,166 pituitary adenomas. Surg Endosc 2015;29(6):1270–80.
10. Strickland BA, Lucas J, Harris B, et al. Identification and repair of intraoperative cerebrospinal fluid leaks in endonasal transsphenoidal pituitary surgery: surgical experience in a series of 1002 patients. J Neurosurg 2018;129(2):425–9.
11. Patel PN, Stafford AM, Patrinely JR, et al. Risk Factors for Intraoperative and Postoperative Cerebrospinal Fluid Leaks in Endoscopic Transsphenoidal Sellar Surgery. Otolaryngol Head Neck Surg 2018;158(5):952–60.
12. Zhou Q, Yang Z, Wang X, et al. Risk Factors and Management of Intraoperative Cerebrospinal Fluid Leaks in Endoscopic Treatment of Pituitary Adenoma: Analysis of 492 Patients. World Neurosurg 2017;101:390–5.
13. Parikh A, Adapa A, Sullivan SE, et al. Predictive Factors, 30-Day Clinical Outcomes, and Costs Associated with Cerebrospinal Fluid Leak in Pituitary Adenoma Resection. J Neurol Surg B Skull Base 2020;81(1):43–55.
14. Vimawala S, Chitguppi C, Reilly E, et al. Predicting prolonged length of stay after endoscopic transsphenoidal surgery for pituitary adenoma. Int Forum Allergy Rhinol 2020;10(6):785–90.
15. Chabot JD, Patel CR, Hughes MA, et al. Nasoseptal flap necrosis: a rare complication of endoscopic endonasal surgery. J Neurosurg 2018;128(5):1463–72.
16. Shutter LSCGP. Combined and Specialty surgery: otolaryngology and Plastics. Neurocritical Care Management of the Neurosurgical Patient. 2017:447-455. Available at: https://www.scopus.com/record/display.uri?eid=2-s2.0850405829 26&origin=inward&txGid=99726732aac1108609ca05c898769a3f.
17. Jandali D, Shearer S, Byrne R, et al. Assessment of post-operative healing following endoscopic, transnasal, transsphenoidal pituitary surgery without formal sellar grafting. Am J Otol 2020;41(2):102306.

18. Awad AJ, Mohyeldin A, El-Sayed IH, et al. Sinonasal morbidity following endoscopic endonasal skull base surgery. Clin Neurol Neurosurg 2015;130:162–7.
19. de Almeida JR, Snyderman CH, Gardner PA, et al. Nasal morbidity following endoscopic skull base surgery: a prospective cohort study. Head Neck 2011; 33(4):547–51.
20. Bhenswala PN, Schlosser RJ, Nguyen SA, et al. Sinonasal quality-of-life outcomes after endoscopic endonasal skull base surgery. Int Forum Allergy Rhinol 2019;9(10):1105–18.
21. Wu V, Cusimano MD, Lee JM. Extent of surgery in endoscopic transsphenoidal skull base approaches and the effects on sinonasal morbidity. Am J Rhinol Allergy 2018;32(1):52–6.
22. Zarino B, Verrua E, Ferrante E, et al. Cushing's disease: a prospective case-control study of health-related quality of life and cognitive status before and after surgery. J Neurosurg 2019;15:1–11.
23. Cusimano MD, Huang TQ, Marchie A, et al. Development and validation of the disease-specific QOL-CD quality of life questionnaire for patients with Cushing's disease. Neurosurg Focus 2020;48(6):E4.
24. Zeng L, Han S, Wu A. Long-term olfactory dysfunction after single-nostril endoscopic transnasal transsphenoidal pituitary adenoma surgery. J Clin Neurosci 2020;82(Pt A):166–72.
25. Chaaban MR, Chaudhry AL, Riley KO, et al. Objective assessment of olfaction after transsphenoidal pituitary surgery. Am J Rhinol Allergy 2015;29(5):365–8.
26. Upadhyay S, Buohliqah L, Dolci RLL, et al. Periodic olfactory assessment in patients undergoing skull base surgery with preservation of the olfactory strip. Laryngoscope 2017;127(9):1970–5.
27. Desai SV, Fang CH, Raikundalia MD, et al. Impact of postoperative pneumonia following pituitary surgery. Laryngoscope 2015;125(8):1792–7.
28. Manetti L, Bogazzi F, Giovannetti C, et al. Changes in coagulation indexes and occurrence of venous thromboembolism in patients with Cushing's syndrome: results from a prospective study before and after surgery. Eur J Endocrinol 2010; 163(5):783–91.
29. Suarez MG, Stack M, Hinojosa-Amaya JM, et al. Hypercoagulability in Cushing Syndrome, Prevalence of Thrombotic Events: A Large, Single-Center, Retrospective Study. J Endocr Soc 2020;4(2):bvz033.
30. van der Pas R, Leebeek FW, Hofland LJ, et al. Hypercoagulability in Cushing's syndrome: prevalence, pathogenesis and treatment. Clin Endocrinol (Oxf) 2013;78(4):481–8.
31. Ziu M, Dunn IF, Hess C, et al. Congress of Neurological Surgeons Systematic Review and Evidence-Based Guideline on Posttreatment Follow-up Evaluation of Patients With Nonfunctioning Pituitary Adenomas. Neurosurgery 2016;79(4): E541–3.

# Developing an Integrated Multidisciplinary Pituitary Management Team

Erin L. McKean, MD, MBA[a,b,]*, Stephen E. Sullivan, MD[a,b]

## KEYWORDS

• Teamwork • Pituitary • Team-based care • Multidisciplinary • Interdisciplinary

## KEY POINTS

• Team-based care allows for improved quality and value.
• Administrative and systemic support for multidisciplinary programs is essential for both short- and long-term success (through provision and alignment of resources, metrics, and incentives).
• Diverse qualities and values of team members can be leveraged for success in meeting metrics, providing high-touch patient care, innovating, and ensuring safety.
• Teams may find it useful to discuss and protocolize all aspects of patient care and follow-up.
• Coordination of time and space is important for team success and improved patient experience.

## INTRODUCTION

The treatment of pituitary disease is an excellent substrate on which to develop a multidisciplinary team approach in a large referral center. Pituitary disease is relatively uncommon, and few providers or institutions can care for a sufficient volume of these patients to justify a dedicated center. The Pituitary Society in 2017 put forth a statement defining the criteria for Pituitary Tumor Centers of Excellence, first and foremost acknowledging the consensus opinion that interdisciplinary team-based care provides improved outcomes and value.[1] One thousand four hundred pituitary operations are performed per year in the United States, and a center requires a referral base of greater than a 10 million in population to achieve the threshold of 50 pituitary operations performed annually to meet the criteria of a Pituitary Center of Excellence as defined by the Pituitary Society. Organizational logistics, attentive operations

[a] Department of Otolaryngology and Neurosurgery, 1904 Taubman Center, Reception Area A, 1500 East Medical Center Drive, Ann Arbor, MI 48109, USA; [b] University of Michigan, Ann Arbor, MI, USA
* Corresponding author. Department of Otolaryngology, 1904 Taubman Center, Reception Area A, 1500 East Medical Center Drive, Ann Arbor, MI 48109.
*E-mail address:* elmk@med.umich.edu
Twitter: @skullbasedoc (E.L.M.)

Otolaryngol Clin N Am 55 (2022) 469–476
https://doi.org/10.1016/j.otc.2021.12.013
0030-6665/22/© 2021 Elsevier Inc. All rights reserved.

management, facilitated collaboration, and clear communication are key teamwork tools in delivering requisite high-volume, team-based integrated care.

A pituitary program requires the commitment of a dedicated team of professionals and an institutional commitment to provide necessary substantial resources to support these professionals. If either of these conditions cannot be met, the program will not flourish, and patient care will suffer. A successful program is difficult to build but can be destroyed quite easily. There are many models for integration of these resources in excellent pituitary programs across the world. Here we describe general principles of teamwork, as well as the evolution and function of our program as a means of beginning the discussion.

## WHO IS ON THE TEAM?

Although defining our team seems simple at first glance, it is easy to overlook critically important team members. Although our "frontline" team for decision-making and intervention consists of faculty from divisions in Neurosurgery, Endocrinology, and Otolaryngology, we rely on colleagues in Neuroradiology, Anesthesiology, Neuroophthalmology, Neuropathology, Radiation oncology, and Neurooncology. Our direct patient-facing frontline also includes clinic nurses and advanced practice providers (APPs), perioperative nurses and APPs, medical assistants, intake coordinators, resident physicians, and social workers.

For us, the backbone of the program lies in our administrative and nursing support. This was a key first step in the institutional backing of our program. A single administrative assistant is the gateway to the program, providing an identifiable, friendly, and available point of contact for patients, as they face a stressful illness. This lynchpin of our program takes all the initial patient calls and schedules every clinical encounter. All our patients are seen by a pituitary neurosurgeon, neuroendocrinologist, and, as necessary, a dedicated otolaryngologist in the same clinic visit. In our opinion, no cost-optimizing call center can provide anywhere near the degree of patient care provided by this specialist administrative assistant who organizes efficient and effective team-based patient experiences. Lack of dedicated administrative support means that there is no institutional support for a dedicated pituitary center. Likewise, we have a specialized nurse practitioner who has worked directly with both neurosurgery and neuroendocrinology for patient concerns and needs, and we have an otolaryngology-based nurse coordinator for cranial base patients. In our medical system, nurse management is separate from department administration, and managerial alignment within and across departments and teams is crucial for aligning team resources.

## BENEFITS OF TEAMWORK

The benefits of teamwork include improved accessibility for patients, decreased medical errors, increased quality, decreased hospitalization duration and cost, decreased hospital readmission[2] or return to the emergency department, decreased burnout, and leveraging of competing values and skills. Retrospective and observational studies have shown that lack of teamwork and impaired communication are among the most frequent contributors to adverse events and malpractice claims.[3] The same review found that the team members' perceptions of teamwork and leadership style affect their well-being.

Another advantage of interdisciplinary teams that is less often discussed is the ability to leverage unique values, skills, knowledge, and behaviors. A business school mentor and collaborator of mine (ELM), Dr Jeff DeGraff, introduced me to the

Competing Values Framework (CVF) and its applications in teams and leadership (view introduction at https://www.youtube.com/watch?v=45veR-Se-rl).[4] This framework was based on early findings by Robert Quinn and John Rohrbaugh[5] and then by Robert Quinn and Kim Cameron at the University of Michigan's Ross School of Business in 1999,[6] finding that leaders create the culture, competencies, and practices that reflect themselves (rather than those that maximize value for an organization or team). Dr DeGraff and colleagues applied the model to innovation and teamwork generally,[7–9] as well as to health care teams, noting that as we build teams, we individually tend to create value for ourselves, and we have the potential to destroy value for another team member or unit. However, if we understand that our diverse values and skills allow us to enhance quality, we can leverage these to build robust, innovative, and high-value programs. The CVF highlights the tensions between short-term outcomes and long-term sustainability; innovation and scalability; collaboration and competition; and creativity and safety. In our team, we have *competitors* who focus on short-term outcomes, doing things first and doing things fast; *collaborators* who focus on relationships, sustainability, and long-term outcomes; *controllers* who focus on standardization, scalability, and safety; and *creators* who focus on innovation and have a vision for the future. Examples of how our diverse team members have added value in each domain is seen in **Fig. 1**.

**SETTING EXPECTATIONS AND PRINCIPLES FOR COMMUNICATION AND DECISION-MAKING**

Teams may find it useful to discuss and protocolize care. Our team found it useful to lay out expectations for new patient intake and evaluation, nonoperative care, preoperative assessment and management, intraoperative care (including complication and

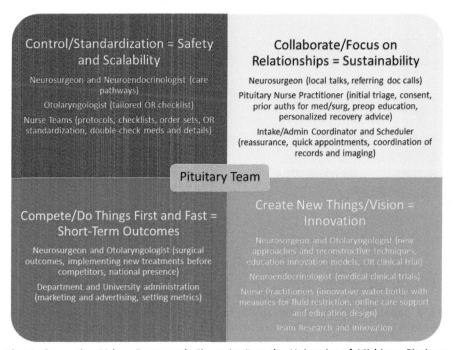

**Fig. 1.** Competing Values Framework "in action" at the University of Michigan Pituitary Program.

unexpected diagnosis management), inpatient postoperative care, early at-home postoperative care, and late postoperative management. Conversations about expectations and plans of care before enacting those plans allow for standardization where appropriate, input from all team members based on expertise and experience, and consensus formation in a stress-free environment. One example is our agreed-on preoperative and intraoperative management, with written expectations given to resident and operating room (OR) teams. **Fig. 2** shows our preoperative "timeout" in the OR for pituitary adenomectomy. The timeout is most often run by the otolaryngologist with the entire operative team engaged, with the details tailored for our specific cases, built on a hospital standard. Reconstruction has also been standardized with a decision-tree for cerebrospinal fluid leak repair based on size, location, and flow volume of the leak. Likewise, care pathways have been developed for outpatient management. This standardization does not take away the decision-making capacity of individual team members but rather allows the real-time decision-maker to have readily available knowledge of preferences and concerns of other team members.

Decisions may deviate from protocol as needed for a given situation, and we further agree on who is the ultimate decision-maker in specific instances. For example, for our team, the ultimate perioperative and surgical decision-maker for patients with pituitary adenomas is the neurosurgeon, and the ultimate decision-maker for patients with sinonasal malignancy is the otolaryngologist. Identification of the ultimate decision-maker for real-time decision-making (such as with intraoperative complications or

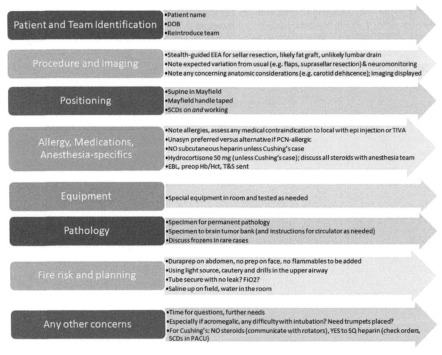

**Fig. 2.** Sample "time out" checklist specific to pituitary adenomectomy at the University of Michigan. DOB, date of birth; EEA, endoscopic endonasal approach; SCD, sequential compression device; TIVA, total intravenous anesthesia; PCN, penicillin; EBL, estimated blood loss; Hb, hemoglobin; Hct, hematocrit; T&S, type and screen; PACU, post-anesthesia care unit.

deciding on plans for a surprise intraoperative frozen section diagnosis) decreases acute stress and builds trust. Respectful discussions are a must, and open sharing and receiving of concerns and expertise is expected.

Finally, a pituitary team conference has been initiated weekly, allowing for validation of care pathways or reasoned deviation via team input; this is helpful also for education, research hypothesis generation, and onboarding of new team members.

## COORDINATION OF TIME AND SPACE

For our program, we were fortunate to build on the visions, hard work, and successes of our mentors, Dr Bill Chandler (neurosurgery—pituitary), Dr Ariel Barkan (neuroendocrinology—pituitary), and Dr Larry Marentette (otolaryngology—ventral cranial base). Clinical time and space ran concurrently for the pituitary surgeon and pituitary endocrinologist in the Neurosurgery Department space. Likewise, in the Otolaryngology Department space, the (ventral) Cranial Base Program had team clinic with the skull base otolaryngologist and neurosurgeon. As the programs evolved, we were able to align our clinical and operative time to assure all team members could be present and/or available to assure exceptional patient access and optimal team communication. Our system experienced changes over time, and there are increasing barriers to multidisciplinary clinics. Barriers include the following: determination of who pays for the APP and nurse support for the comprehensive program; payment to providers is not based on optimal patient experience but rather on distinct services; increased hospital metrics for space efficiency can lead to one team member being pushed out of clinic to increase throughput by other programs; not all space is outfitted with the tools necessary for all team members (eg, our neurosurgery clinic lacks endoscopes and a cleaning process, monitors, debridement equipment); and scheduling has to allow for time efficiency for all providers. Creative solutions can be found, but there is no substitute for strong administrative support and advocacy in the face of competing system metrics and demands.

Beyond clinic, concurrent OR block time and flexibility for urgent cases is critical. It is expected that we will have multiple pituitary cases each week. When the neurosurgeon books pituitary cases, he knows the otolaryngologist will be available (and likewise, the otolaryngologist can book sinonasal malignancy resections requiring craniotomy at parallel times, knowing that the neurosurgeon will be available). We are aware that this is not as smooth for some colleagues, and we do believe this is essential to our success.

## OTHER CONSIDERATIONS: DOCUMENTATION AND BILLING, RESEARCH, ONBOARDING
### Documentation and Billing

Setting expectations for billing multispecialty clinic visits and operative cases is also helpful in assuring team cohesion and shared expectations. It can be useful to engage institutional or other coding and billing experts in developing plans, and physicians should review current coding guidelines relevant to their cases. We have found it useful to give our coders the North American Skull Base Society white paper,[10] particularly when billing for challenging unlisted procedure codes, and we have established template letters to amend and append for each relevant case. We have discussed what to do for image-guidance codes and reconstruction codes that are not allowed to be shared. We alternate who codes for the image-guidance and any fat grafting (unless it is clear that one person or team has done the key work).

## Research

We have also found it helpful to reach agreement on research priorities and structure of projects, and this has improved patient experience and research success. Currently, we consent patients for our brain tumor bank tissue specimen collection, as well as for an olfactory preservation clinical trial. Particularly as our processes have changed during the Coronavirus-19 (COVID-19) pandemic and our preoperative in-person face time with patients has decreased (with the use of telemedicine), fully educating patients and consenting them for studies must be done via telehealth visits or in preoperative holding; this is performed along with other testing, such as smell testing. Consistent with what is well known in clinical research, we have found that patients cannot be consented for numerous studies without increasing their stress and risk of inadequate education. Although we have many ideas to consider, we agree on what is highest priority at the current moment and how to structure and resource (fund or provide human effort) the studies. Although we do not currently have a research coordinator dedicated to the Pituitary Program specifically, we continue to advocate for this resource. We aim to share time and funding between the Otolaryngology Cranial Base Program and the Neurosurgery Pituitary Program.

## Onboarding

When team members change, specific attention to team dynamics is important in reiterating and establishing expectations and processes. It can be very useful for new team members to spend additional time with Pituitary Program participants outside of the formal clinic or OR time. For example, our nurse practitioners and coordinators find it useful to gain experience in departments outside of their main "home" department or division, allowing for expansion of their knowledge base and a greater ability to answer patient questions and cross-cover when issues arise.

## SUSTAINABILITY

It is worth taking time to finally focus narrowly on sustainability. As noted previously, the foundation of our program lies in shared values and robust administrative and nursing support. Just before and then during the COVID-19 pandemic, our team changed dramatically, raising barriers to providing efficient, high-quality care. The single administrative assistant who provided frontline reassurance and expedited care moved to another unit; the Pituitary Clinic nurse practitioner retired; and the Otolaryngology Cranial Base nurse coordinator moved to another program while the role was being downsized and reorganized. There were also changes in providers: addition of a neurosurgeon, replacement of an otolaryngologist, and replacement of the specialized neuroendocrinologist. We are now revisiting our recruitment and onboarding processes, as well as our care pathways and consensus planning mechanisms. We are evaluating our time and space needs, figuring out how to best incorporate new team members in scarce OR and clinic resources. We are also assessing the cost to the system of losing experienced team members (eg, evaluating costs of emergency room return visits for what otherwise would previously be managed by phone consultation, number of calls to support staff, quality of education, and so forth). We will use this information to advocate for realignment and possible augmentation of resources, as well as for devising Lean models for efficiency and patient satisfaction.

Further threats to our program's sustainability occur when resources are allocated in ways that do not align for team members or when individual department–based incentives cause divergent values between team members. Alignment of resources and incentives across departments and team members is critical for team success.

Recently, our team was faced with several initiatives that seem good at face value, but competing values were destroyed when implementing those new initiatives. For example, each physician is now being measured on volume of outpatient new patient visits and wait times for new patient visits. During the COVID-19 pandemic, all of our Pituitary Program team physicians increased telemedicine volume, and the multidisciplinary clinic was no longer running concurrently, physically together. Individual physician wait times decreased, and new patient volumes increased. However, that did not necessarily provide an increase in communication and patient satisfaction with the visits themselves. In addition, OR access decreased for both the neurosurgeon and otolaryngologist, making it such that the new patients who were seen quickly in clinic could not get efficiently to the OR. Saturday OR times were offered by the health system and departments, but the otolaryngologist had a new administrative role that did not allow for a day off in lieu of the Saturday. Further, it is worth noting that our team coparents, and weekend childcare is more challenging. Our surgeons care deeply about spending time with their children when they are freely available. Although these personal factors may seem insignificant, autonomy and work-life balance are key to physician well-being, and patient care suffers when burnout occurs. Team members and administration should be sensitive to incorporating the wellness of others into resource and incentive planning, or there could be a risk to program sustainability.

When we speak of incentives, we must again acknowledge that incentives are not only financial. Other incentives include added human resources (eg, research coordinators and administrative or medical assistant support), autonomy and schedule flexibility, additional clinical and OR access, technical assistance, and electronic medical record support tools (**Fig. 3**). For our team, there is nothing more rewarding professionally than exceptional patient care. We do have competing priorities outside of the professional arena, and we recognize nonfinancial incentives for team success to be equally or more effective than financial incentives. When planning with team members, it is important to advocate for them in ways that are most meaningful to them.

Finally, in looking at the cost of incentives and program resources, the addition of human capital is generally costliest. Although adding team members can be expensive in the short term (and can increase fixed costs over the long term), program expansion and adequate resource allocation allows high volume care, which in turn provides an increase in quality of care and decrease in variable costs (through increase in efficiency and amortization over number of cases), thus increasing value over time. Costs

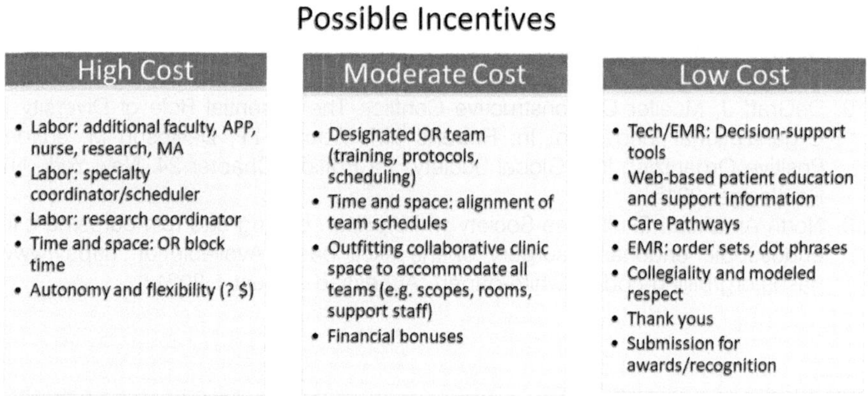

## Possible Incentives

| High Cost | Moderate Cost | Low Cost |
|---|---|---|
| • Labor: additional faculty, APP, nurse, research, MA<br>• Labor: specialty coordinator/scheduler<br>• Labor: research coordinator<br>• Time and space: OR block time<br>• Autonomy and flexibility (? $) | • Designated OR team (training, protocols, scheduling)<br>• Time and space: alignment of team schedules<br>• Outfitting collaborative clinic space to accommodate all teams (e.g. scopes, rooms, support staff)<br>• Financial bonuses | • Tech/EMR: Decision-support tools<br>• Web-based patient education and support information<br>• Care Pathways<br>• EMR: order sets, dot phrases<br>• Collegiality and modeled respect<br>• Thank yous<br>• Submission for awards/recognition |

**Fig. 3.** Possible pituitary team incentives (for individuals and teams). MA, medical assistant; EMR, electronic medical record.

must be balanced with return on investment. Alternatively, supplying additional shared nonhuman resources to streamline the care provided by the existing team is a very cost-effective way to build efficiency, collaboration, and trust.

## SUMMARY

Interdisciplinary teams have many potential and proven benefits, including decreased burnout, decreased medical errors, increased quality, and leveraging of competing values and skills. Pituitary Tumor Centers of Excellence must have adequate volumes and high-functioning teams to provide exceptional, high-value care. Organizational logistics, attentive operations management, facilitated collaboration, and clear communication are key teamwork tools in delivering that care.

## DISCLOSURE

The authors have nothing to disclose.

## REFERENCES

1. Casanueva FF, Barkan AL, Buchfelder M, et al. Expert Group on Pituitary Tumors. Criteria for the definition of Pituitary Tumor Centers of Excellence (PTCOE): A Pituitary Society Statement. Pituitary 2017;20(5):489–98. Erratum in: Pituitary. 2018 Sep 20.
2. Mickan Sharon M. Evaluating the effectiveness of health care teams. Aust Health Rev 2005;29(2):211–7.
3. Manser T. Teamwork and patient safety in dynamic domains of healthcare: a review of the literature. Acta Anaesthesiol Scand 2009;53(2):143–51.
4. DeGraff J. Competing Values Framework Introduction video. Available at: https://www.youtube.com/watch?v=45veR-Se-rl. Accessed August 1 2021.
5. Quinn RE, Rohrbaugh J. A spatial model of effectiveness criteria: Towards a competing values approach to organizational analysis. Management Sci 1983; 29(3):363–77.
6. Cameron KS, Quinn RE. Diagnosing and changing organizational culture. Reading: Addison-Wesley; 1999.
7. Cameron KS, Quinn RE, DeGraff J, et al. Competing values leadership. Cheltenham, United Kingdom: Edward Elgar Publishing Ltd; 2014.
8. DeGraff Jeff, Nathan-Roberts Dan. Innovativeness As Positive Deviance: Identifying and Operationalizing the Attributes, Functions, and Dynamics That Create Growth. In: Spreitzer Gretchen M, Cameron Kim S, editors. The Oxford Handbook of Positive organizational Scholarship. 2011.
9. DeGraff J, Mueller C. Constructive Conflict: The Essential Role of Diversity in Organizational Innovation. In: Roberts LM, Wooten LP, Davidson M, editors. Positive Organizing in a Global Society. 1st Edition. Chapter 24. New York, NY: Routledge; 2015.
10. North American Skull Base Society white paper: coding and reimbursement for endoscopic endonasal surgery of the skull base. Available at: https://www.nasbs.org/billing-coding-white-paper/. Accessed August 1 2021.

# Pediatric Pituitary Surgery

Peter J. Madsen, MD[a], Shih-Shan Lang, MD[a,b],
Nithin D. Adappa, MD[a,c], James N. Palmer, MD[a,c], Phillip B. Storm, MD[a,b],*

KEYWORDS

• Pediatric • Endonasal • Skull base • Craniopharyngioma • Rathke cleft cyst

KEY POINTS

- Common lesions that arise from the pituitary in children include craniopharyngioma, Rathke cleft cysts, pituitary adenomas, and inflammatory conditions.
- Other lesions of the sella, suprasellar, and parasellar region in children include germ cell tumors, optic pathway glioma, and hypothalamic hamartoma.
- Lack of sphenoid pneumatization in young children can present a challenge to endonasal skull base approaches but can be overcome by navigation-assisted drilling of the skull base.
- Preoperative tumor markers can be helpful in evaluating for germ cell tumors.
- Endonasal approaches to pediatric craniopharyngioma can improve extent of resection and lead to fewer vascular complications compared with open craniotomy.
- The use of nasoseptal flaps in patients with a high-flow cerebrospinal fluid leak can help decrease the rate of postoperative leak.
- A multidisciplinary approach to the evaluation and treatment of these patients is critical for optimal outcomes.

## INTRODUCTION

Tumors of the sella, suprasellar, and parasellar region are not infrequently encountered in children, as they account for approximately 10% of primary pediatric brain tumors.[1] Surgical approaches to these lesions have undergone major advances in the past decade. Once considered too challenging given the lack of sinus pneumatization often seen in children, advances in endonasal techniques and surgical navigation technology have made it possible to safely reach this region in children.[2] This has allowed surgeons to address a wide range of pathologic conditions, often achieving gross total resection with less morbidity than typically associated with traditional

[a] Division of Neurosurgery, Children's Hospital of Philadelphia, Wood Building, 3401 Civic Center Boulevard, Philadelphia, PA 19104, USA; [b] Department of Neurosurgery, Perelman School of Medicine at the University of Pennsylvania, Philadelphia, PA, USA; [c] Department of Otorhinolaryngology and Head and Neck Surgery, Perelman School of Medicine at the University of Pennsylvania, 3400 Spruce Street, Philadelphia, PA 19104, USA
* Corresponding author. Division of Neurosurgery, Children's Hospital of Philadelphia, Wood Building, 3401 Civic Center Boulevard, Philadelphia, PA 19104.
E-mail address: storm@chop.edu

Otolaryngol Clin N Am 55 (2022) 477–491
https://doi.org/10.1016/j.otc.2021.12.017
0030-6665/22/© 2022 Elsevier Inc. All rights reserved.

open craniotomy. In this review, the authors discuss the evaluation, perioperative management, surgical approaches, and considerations for typical lesions of the pituitary encountered in children. An understanding of anterior skull base reconstruction techniques is also essential for the successful management of these patients, and as such, is discussed. A highly specialized, multidisciplinary approach, involving neurosurgeons, rhinologists, endocrinologists, pediatric intensivist and anesthesiologists, oncologists, and ophthalmologists, is essential to optimize outcomes for pediatric patients with lesions of the pituitary region.

## BACKGROUND
### Anatomic Considerations

The use of endoscopic endonasal techniques in adults with lesions of the anterior skull base has become standardized and widely accepted. Adoption of such methodologies has been slower in the pediatric population, but this has undergone an evolution in the past decade. An often stated concern regarding endonasal skull base approaches in the pediatric population is the lack of pneumatization of the paranasal sinuses, particularly the sphenoid sinus.[3,4] Analysis of pneumatization patterns in children has shown that pneumatization of the sphenoid sinus typically begins at 3 years of age and is complete at approximately 10 to 14 years of age.[2] During this time, the extent of pneumatization can be quite variable, but typically begins in the presellar location and extends inferiorly and posterolaterally (**Fig. 1**).[3] For children with incomplete pneumatization, approaches to the sella and anterior skull base often require extensive drilling of the sphenoid bone, aided by the use of an intraoperative guidance system based on preoperative computed tomography (CT) imaging.[2] For conchal and presellar pneumatization patterns, image guidance is important given that normal sphenoidal landmarks, such as the opticocarotid recess, are obscured by bone.

Additional study of pediatric skull base anatomy has shown that intercarotid distance, once thought to be a limiting factor in accessing the skull base in children, is stable throughout much of childhood and into adulthood and does not seem to be a limiting factor.[3] This is especially true of the intercarotid distance at the level of the superior clivus, which seems to be fixed throughout life. Only in very young children,

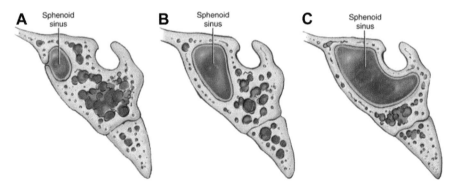

**Fig. 1.** Navigation-assisted endonasal surgery has enabled access to the anterior skull base in children at various stages of sphenoid sinus pneumatization. Pneumatization typically progresses from conchal pattern (not shown), where no pneumatization is present, to presellar (*A*), sellar (*B*), and eventually into a postsellar pattern (*C*). (*Adapted with permission from Joe, SA. Endoscopic Resection of Pituitary Tumors. Atlas of Endoscopic Sinus and Skull Base Surgery.* 2019.)

under 4 years of age, is there a decrease in intercarotid distance of the cavernous segment of the carotid artery when compared with adults.[2,5] Despite this narrower corridor, resection of lesions, even gross total resection, is still feasible for experienced surgeons.[3] Preoperative assessment of the course and location of the extracranial and petrous carotid arteries is important for planning the operative corridor and the amount of sphenoid bone drilling that will be possible. Intraoperative image guidance is again important when significant drilling is required between the carotid arteries.[2]

### Embryology and Development

As is the case with many pediatric pathologic conditions, an understanding of embryology and development is important for those treating lesions of the pituitary and parasellar region in children. Embryonic development of the pituitary occurs from the joining of the adenohypophysis (anterior pituitary) from Rathke pouch with an extension of the telencephalon that will become the infundibular stalk and neurohypophysis (posterior pituitary).[6] Remnants of Rathke pouch are the presumed origin for the development of Rathke cleft cysts (RCCs).[7] Childhood craniopharyngioma is thought to arise from the neoplastic transformation of a remnant of Rathke pouch.[8]

Unlike their adult counterparts, young children who have anterior skull base surgeries have not yet completed the growth and development of the midface and sinus regions. As such, some investigators have raised concerns that iatrogenic disruption of nasal growth zones with endonasal approaches may hinder this normal development process.[9] Fortunately, evaluations of midfacial growth following expanded endonasal surgery in children have suggested that there is no impact on facial growth.[9,10]

## PATHOLOGIC CONDITIONS
### Primary Pituitary Lesions in Children

Pathologic conditions of the pituitary in children maintain some overlap with those seen in adults, but significant differences in presentation and lesion type exist (**Table 1**).

Craniopharyngioma represents the most common tumor of the pituitary region in the pediatric age group. With a reported incidence of 0.5 to 2 cases per million in all age groups, 30% to 50% of cases occur in children.[11] Unlike the papillary-type craniopharyngioma typically seen in older adults, childhood-onset craniopharyngioma mostly comprises histologically of the adamantinomatous type.[11] This difference has significant implications for the treatment of craniopharyngioma with targeted therapies, as discussed later. Childhood craniopharyngioma is often quite cystic, and given its slow growth, can reach very large sizes. Common presentations of childhood craniopharyngioma include growth restriction or delayed puberty secondary to inadequate growth hormone production; symptomatic hydrocephalus with headaches, nausea, vomiting, lethargy, or more subtle cognitive changes; and visual changes from optic nerve compression or increased intracranial pressure.[8] On imaging (**Fig. 2**A, B), pediatric craniopharyngioma can be characterized by a mixed cystic-solid tumor arising from the sella with peripheral calcifications on CT imaging present in 93% of cases.[1,12] MRI shows enhancement of the solid component and cyst wall.[1] The lesion often extends into the suprasellar space and can occupy the third ventricle, where obstruction of cerebrospinal fluid (CSF) flow can occur, resulting in hydrocephalus.

Another primary pathologic condition of the pituitary encountered in children is RCC. This benign lesion arises from remnants of Rathke pouch, as discussed above.

**Table 1**
**Commonly encountered lesions of the pituitary and sellar region in children**

| | Common Presentation | Common Hormonal Changes | Imaging Features |
|---|---|---|---|
| Craniopharyngioma | Growth restriction Symptomatic hydrocephalus | Low growth hormone | Calcification Cystic |
| Rathke cleft cyst | Headache Hormonal disturbances | Variable | Cyst of variable protein density |
| Pituitary adenoma | Headache Bitemporal hemianopsia Galactorrhea (prolactinoma) | Elevated prolactin | Homogeneous enhancement, sellar expansion |
| Lymphocytic hypophysitis | DI | DI | Enhancing lesion of the infundibulum |
| Germ cell tumors | Headaches, hydrocephalus | DI (germinoma) | Infundibular involvement (germinoma) |
| Optic pathway/ hypothalamic glioma | Visual changes | Variable | Expansion of optic pathway, hypothalamic involvement |

They are a frequent incidental finding on imaging (with an incidence of 4%–33% in autopsy cases), but with growth can lead to symptoms secondary to mass effect on surrounding structures, causing headaches, visual changes, or pituitary hormone disruption.[13] Symptomatic RCCs account for 6% to 10% of symptomatic sellar and parasellar lesions.[14] Imaging demonstrates a cystic lesion centered on the pituitary stalk with variable intensity on MRI depending on protein concentrations within the cyst (**Fig. 2**C).[1] RCCs can be isolated to the sella, but the majority (87%) have suprasellar extension.[1]

Despite being the most common pathologic condition of the pituitary in adults, pituitary adenoma is relatively rare in children, making up only 4% of intracranial tumors in children.[1] Macroadenomas account for 60% of pituitary adenomas in children. Presenting signs and symptoms can be due to compression of adjacent structures, leading to visual changes (ie, bitemporal hemianopsia) and headaches. Hormonal disturbances owing to secreting adenomas can lead to the same array of pituitary syndromes seen in adults. Prolactinomas are the most common macroadenoma encountered in children, representing 50% of pediatric pituitary adenomas in the literature.[1,15] At the authors' institution, prolactinomas have made up an even larger proportion of adenomas, at close to 90%. The radiographic appearance of pediatric pituitary adenoma mimics their adult counterpart, demonstrating a solid enhancement pattern with expansion of the sella and extension into the suprasellar cistern in the case of macroadenomas (**Fig. 2**D).[12]

Several conditions in children can often lead to mass lesions of the pituitary and are important to differentiate from true tumors of the pituitary. Pituitary involvement in multicentric Langerhans cell histiocytosis (LCH) occurs in 20% to 25% of cases.[16] Patients with LCH of the pituitary often present with diabetes insipidus (DI), and imaging may show an enhancing mass of the infundibulum. Lymphocytic hypophysitis

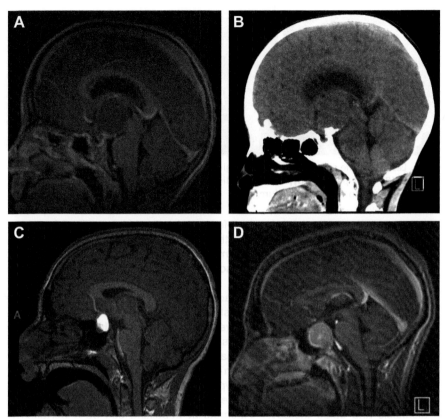

**Fig. 2.** Characteristic imaging of pediatric primary pituitary pathologic conditions. (*A*) Adamantinomatous-type pediatric craniopharyngioma showing cystic sellar mass with suprasellar extension on MRI, associated with calcifications of solitary sellar component and wall on CT imaging (*B*). (*C*) RCC. (*D*) Macroadenoma of the pituitary in a child.

(LH) typically refers to an autoimmune process affecting adolescent women more than men that leads to inflammation of the pituitary with thickening of the gland or infundibulum.[17] DI is also a common presenting sign of LH. Generalized hyperplasia of the anterior pituitary can be seen during puberty and is a normal finding but can mimic a mass lesion.[1]

### Pathologic Conditions of the Sellar and Parasellar Region in Children

There are several unique lesions of the sella and parasellar region that arise in children (see **Table 1**), whose treatment can be quite varied depending on pathologic condition, and are important to consider when evaluating a child with a lesion in this region.

Intracranial germ cell tumors (GCTs) account for 3% to 11% of pediatric brain tumors, of which approximately 30% occur in the sellar region.[18,19] Female patients with GCTs tend to present with lesions of the sella, whereas male patients tend to present with pineal region tumors. Simultaneous GCTs of the sellar and pineal regions occur in 5% to 10% of patients.[18] Sellar GCTs can be isolated to the pituitary gland or stalk or fill the sella and extend into the suprasellar space (**Fig. 3**A). DI is a common presentation for patients with sellar GCTs, especially germinoma. Tumor marker levels

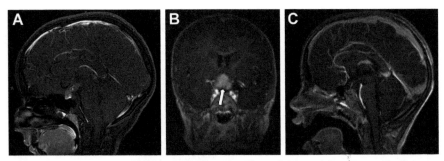

**Fig. 3.** Lesions of the sella and parasellar region seen in children. (*A*) GCT, specifically a germinoma. (*B*) Optic pathway/hypothalamic glioma; note expansion of optic chiasm (*arrow*). (*C*) HH posterior to the infundibulum.

(β-human chorionic gonadotropin and α-fetoprotein) should be obtained from blood and CSF when possible to determine if the lesion is a nongerminomatous GCT, as this has major implications on treatment strategies. Lack of or equivocal tumor markers should prompt biopsy, and an endonasal approach can be considered for lesions in the sella.

Optic pathway/hypothalamic gliomas account for 7% of glioma diagnoses and are low-grade lesions, typically pilocytic astrocytoma.[20] They can fill the sellar and suprasellar space and lead to obstructive hydrocephalus. Involvement of the optic apparatus can lead to visual disturbances, and baseline visual assessments are critical. Imaging often demonstrates an enhancing lesion of the suprasellar region that expands the optic nerves and/or chiasm (**Fig. 3**B). Optic pathway glioma is a very frequent feature of neurofibromatosis type 1, and biopsy is typically not required for diagnosis in this population. In other settings, biopsy is often required to establish a diagnosis and guide therapy.[20] Attempts at debulking can be undertaken for lesions causing significant mass effect or obstructive hydrocephalus, but care should be taken to avoid disruption of the optic apparatus, pituitary stalk, and hypothalamus.

Although considered dysplastic rather than neoplastic lesions, hypothalamic hamartomas (HH) represent another mass lesion of the suprasellar region. Children with HH often present with precocious puberty and gelastic seizures. The lesions can enter the suprasellar space but have a clear hypothalamic origin and have imaging characteristics similar to adjacent brain tissue (**Fig. 3**C). They can be classified as either sessile or pedunculated. Open craniotomy has been the more traditional approach and is aimed at disconnecting the lesion from the hypothalamus. The pedunculated type is more amenable to disconnection than the sessile type. Because of the morbidity associated with open craniotomy and the poor long-term results, MR-guided laser ablation of these lesions is becoming the preferred treatment of choice. Recent series of laser ablation for HH have shown improvements in seizure freedom rates with rates as high as 93%.[21]

Other lesions of the sellar and suprasellar region encountered in children include arachnoid cysts, lipomas, epidermoids, and atypical teratoid/rhabdoid tumors.[1,22]

## PREOPERATIVE EVALUATION AND PERIOPERATIVE MANAGEMENT

The preoperative evaluation of children with lesions of the pituitary and parasellar region requires a multidisciplinary approach, involving endocrinologists, ophthalmologists, and anesthesiologists in addition to the surgical team. With few exceptions, evaluation of endocrinologic function is important to help distinguish between possible pathologic conditions, identify and correct any hormonal deficiencies before surgery, and establish a preoperative baseline function of the hypothalamic pituitary axis. A full endocrinologic panel should be obtained in the workup. Common hormonal changes seen with the various pathologic conditions discussed can be found in **Table 1**. Life-threatening hormonal disturbances can occur, especially in the case of children presenting with DI. Prompt diagnosis and treatment with hormone replacement is critical to avoid complications of severe hypernatremia, hypothyroidism, or hypocortisolism.

Preoperative laboratory evaluation of pediatric sellar masses with GCT marker levels is very important. Elevation of these markers in the blood and/or CSF can lead to a diagnosis, particularly in the case of nongerminomatous GCTs, and allow for transition to chemotherapy or radiation therapy without the need for surgical biopsy.[18] Many of the above lesions can appear similar on imaging, so these simple tests can be crucial in quickly making a diagnosis and avoiding unnecessary surgery.

Ophthalmologic evaluation is also important to establish baseline function before surgical or other interventions.[23] Many lesions of this region, especially optic pathway/hypothalamic gliomas, can progressively affect the optic apparatus over time, so serial ophthalmologic evaluations are therefore important to monitor for deterioration in vision. Fundoscopic examination can also be used to evaluate for the presence of papilledema as a sign of raised intracranial pressure.

Decisions about the need for CSF diversion should also be made promptly for any child presenting with signs and symptoms of hydrocephalus. Emergent CSF diversion can be achieved with the placement of an external ventricular drain. This may often happen before undergoing endocrine laboratory tests, but they are still imperative and should be obtained as quickly as possible. Frequently, lesions in this location can grow to a size that fills the third ventricle and occlude both foramen of Monro. When this occurs, it is necessary to either place bilateral ventricular drains or communicate between the 2 lateral ventricles via a septotomy. These temporizing measures can be undertaken until definitive diagnosis is made with either biopsy or tumor marker analysis. Patients with tumors that can be completely resected or debulked enough to allow for reestablishment of normal CSF pathways may be able to avoid permanent CSF diversion, but patients with surgically challenging lesions that may take time to respond to chemotherapy or radiotherapy may require ventriculoperitoneal shunt placement to manage their hydrocephalus.

Children who undergo biopsy or resection of pituitary and sellar tumors can have complicated postoperative courses that require the input from multiple surgical and medical providers. Depending on the extent of resection and location of the tumor, permanent or transient DI is commonly encountered and can be particularly challenging to manage in this population. Input from critical care medicine and endocrinology is important, but surgeons should also be comfortable managing this often expected complication.

## TREATMENT PARADIGMS AND TECHNIQUES

When managing a child with a lesion of the pituitary or sellar region, it is important to establish the goal of intervention, as many entities are better suited for biopsy or upfront chemotherapy or radiotherapy. Tumor markers play an important first step in this process, as discussed above with regards to GCTs. Inconclusive markers or a profile that points toward a germinoma should prompt plans for biopsy. Other lesions of this region for which biopsy should be considered include optic pathway/hypothalamic gliomas and inflammatory pathologic conditions, such as LCH. The endoscopic endonasal approach should be considered as a means of obtaining tissue, as it allows excellent access to the sellar and suprasellar region without the morbidities associated with open craniotomy.

When planning an endonasal biopsy, it is important to define the relationship of the tumor to the critical structures of the region, such as the optic chiasm and pituitary stalk. With regard to the optic chiasm, lesions can be accessed via either an infrachiasmatic or A suprachiasmatic approach. Either approach will require entry into the subarachnoid space and therefore will result in a CSF leak that will require management, as described later. In cases whereby pituitary function is still grossly intact, especially neurohypophysis function, care should be taken to avoid excessive manipulation or injury to the pituitary stalk. Trajectories to the lesion should be planned to avoid the infundibulum.

Lesions that are amenable to resection or more definitive management can be approached from an endonasal corridor, and techniques for the successful removal are discussed later.

### Surgical Techniques

Resective approaches to the sella and sellar region in children require many of the same techniques as those used in the adult population, but with an added emphasis on the safe but extensive drilling of the skull base as well as a "two-nostril-four-hand" approach to tumor resection.[24] Pediatric pituitary and skull base tumors can often reach large sizes given their slow growth characteristics and delayed symptom development (**Fig. 4**). Attempts at gross total resection of such lesions require an adequate working corridor and are typically performed with a binostril technique. To allow for binostril work, a posterior septectomy should be performed (**Fig. 5**).[25] Once a wide nasal corridor has been established, the sphenoid sinus should be opened widely or the sphenoid bone drilled extensively depending on the lack of pneumatization as previously discussed. Navigated drilling is crucial for these situations as well as identification of the midline to stay between the critical neurovascular structures of the skull base. Once the face of the sella has been drilled away, the dura should be exposed along the intercarotid distance as much as possible (**Fig. 6**A). Children often have a significant intercavernous or circular sinus located within the dura along the anterior sella turcica.[26] This will often require hemostatic control, typically achieved with cautery (**Fig. 6**B), before incising the dura and extending the dural opening ventrally across the sinus (**Fig. 6**C).

Tumor resection can be aided by the fact that lesions of this region, especially craniopharyngioma, often develop in the subarachnoid plane. As such, they tend to preserve an arachnoid barrier between tumor, blood vessels, and brain parenchyma. This allows a tumor to be delivered, hand over hand, through the dural opening using slow, gentle traction without the need to completely visualize and dissect the deep and lateral borders of the lesion. Of course, care must be taken to maintain separation between the tumor and normal structures during delivery, which is often made more difficult in the setting of recurrent tumor surgery or after radiation.[27]

### Cyst Drainage Techniques

When addressing symptomatic RCCs, a main goal of intervention is to drain the cyst and prevent reaccumulation of cyst contents.[13] Some have advocated for resection of the cyst wall as a means of preventing recurrence, but this has come at the cost of increasing postoperative DI rates.[13,28] An alternative to cyst wall resection, marsupialization, involves the use of pedicled nasoseptal flaps (NSF) to create a path into the sphenoid sinus for continued drainage of cyst contents and prevention of cyst recurrence. Results of this technique have shown excellent cyst control rates with

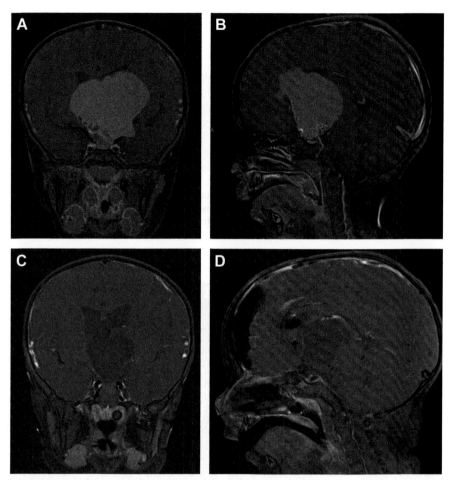

**Fig. 4.** Pediatric pituitary lesions, especially craniopharyngioma, can reach large sizes with extension lateral to the carotid arteries but are still amenable to endonasal resection. Pre-operative coronal (*A*) and sagittal (*B*) T1-weighted, postcontrast MRI showing a large cystic, solid craniopharyngioma in a 2-year-old girl with significant suprasellar and lateral extension. Immediate postoperative imaging (*C, D*) shows complete resection of the lesion using an endoscopic endonasal approach.

lower risk of hypopituitarism encountered with cyst wall resection.[29,30] This technique can be augmented by the use of a silastic stent that can hold open the drainage tract while the NSFs heal (**Fig. 7**), after which the stent can be removed, leaving behind an open and mucosalized drainage pathway from the cyst.

### Skull Base Repair

A common concern regarding endonasal surgeries, especially extended approaches and those in children, is the feasibility and durability of repair techniques to prevent CSF leak. Resection of pituitary and sellar lesions in children often results in the creation of a high-flow CSF leak, as entry into the subarachnoid space is often required.[31] This is especially true for pediatric craniopharyngioma in the supradiaphragmatic region. The use of a pedicled NSF has dramatically improved the postoperative CSF leak rate in

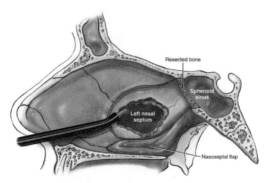

**Fig. 5.** Resection of large pituitary or sellar tumors in children often requires a significant working corridor and removal of the posterior nasal septum to allow for binostril resection. (*Used with permission from* Joe, SA. Endoscopic Resection of Pituitary Tumors. *Atlas of Endoscopic Sinus and Skull Base Surgery.* 2019.).

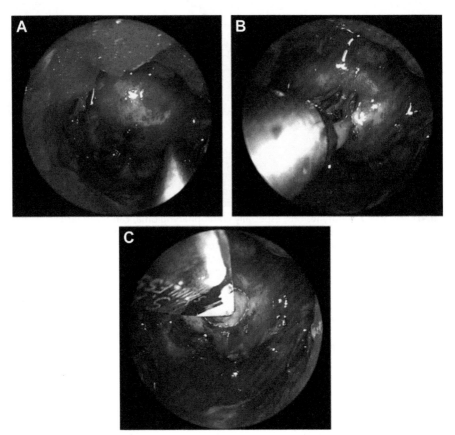

**Fig. 6.** (*A*) Exposed dura of the sella after drilling of the sphenoid bone. (*B*) Bipolar cautery is often required to prevent significant bleeding from the intercavernous sinus before opening with a retractable knife (*C*). (*Used with permission from* Joe, SA. Endoscopic Resection of Pituitary Tumors. *Atlas of Endoscopic Sinus and Skull Base Surgery.* 2019.)

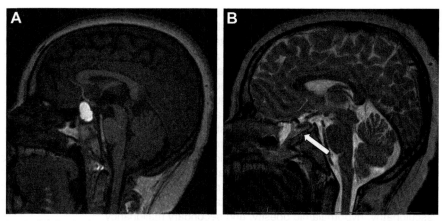

**Fig. 7.** (*A*) Sagittal T1-weighted MRI showing a hyperintense cystic lesion of the pituitary stalk consistent with a RCC. (*B*). Postoperative T2-weighted MRI after cyst drainage and marsupialization with NSF as well as placement of a silastic stent (*arrow*) into the cyst to keep the drainage pathway open while the flaps heal in place.

both adult and pediatric patients.[31–34] NSFs should be harvested and placed using well-established techniques (**Fig. 8**).[35] Repair of large defects can also be augmented with the use of fascia lata and fat graft. This combined approach to anterior skull defect repair has proven quite successful even with large defects, large resection cavities, and the presence of preoperative hydrocephalus. As the technique for repair has evolved, the average rate of postoperative CSF leak has been reported at under 7% even in cases of high-flow intraoperative CSF leak.[36] The use of lumbar drain at the time of resection and repair remains controversial, with some investigators advocating its use in all high-flow CSF leak settings, whereas others find its use to be largely unnecessary.[32,33,36–40] In the authors' practice, they do not routinely place lumbar drains upfront or when a repair requires revision, but consider ventriculostomies and lumbar drains for recalcitrant leaks. Their institutional CSF leak rate is approximately 5%.

## CONTROVERSIES: PEDIATRIC CRANIOPHARYNGIOMA

One of the major points of contention regarding pediatric skull base tumor resection lies in the optimal treatment of pediatric craniopharyngioma. Historically, open

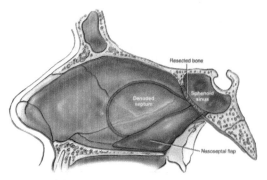

**Fig. 8.** The NSF often required for anterior skull base repair following lesion resection or biopsy. (*Adapted with permission from* Joe, SA. Endoscopic Resection of Pituitary Tumors. *Atlas of Endoscopic Sinus and Skull Base Surgery.* 2019.).

surgical resection via craniotomy was standard, but with this approach came significant morbidity and mortality associated with neurovascular injuries. As an alternative, many investigators have proposed subtotal resection or targeted cyst drainage followed by radiotherapy as a less morbid alternative to attempted open gross total resection.[41,42] The adoption of endonasal techniques in the pediatric age group, though, opened the door to a method of achieving gross total resection that theoretically carries less risk for neurovascular injury given that the tumor has a tendency to push critical neurovascular structures up and away from the surgical entry corridor. This concept was borne out from studies showing a lower rate of neurovascular complications in endonasal versus open approaches to pediatric craniopharyngioma.[33] This lower rate of neurovascular complication, as measured by the volume of ischemia associated with resection, was also correlated with a lower incidence of hypothalamic obesity. The ability to achieve a gross total resection with fewer surgical complications also spares the patient from the detrimental delayed effects of radiotherapy, such as vasculopathy, hypothalamic obesity, and secondary malignancy.[43]

## FUTURE DIRECTIONS

The establishment of multi-institutional collaborative research initiatives has led to the creation of large-scale genomic, transcriptomic, and proteomic data sets to cohort data from rare pediatric tumors, such as craniopharyngioma. This has allowed for the identification of new therapeutic targets that may obviate surgical interventions and avoid their associated risks. Adult craniopharyngioma, which is typically the papillary subtype, has been found to harbor recurrent point mutations in the BRAF gene and has been susceptible to small molecule inhibitors targeting BRAF and other members of the MAP kinase pathway.[44,45] Childhood craniopharyngioma, though, did not show similar or other recurrent targetable mutations, but more recent work has demonstrated a proteomic signature that suggests these tumors may also be susceptible to drugs targeting the MAP kinase pathway.[46] Further collaborative work is needed to better define childhood craniopharyngioma, as well as the other tumors of this region, to further advance the care of children with pituitary and sellar region tumors.

## SUMMARY

Pediatric pituitary surgery has evolved to address a wide range of pathologic conditions, and the techniques developed over the past decade have allowed for access to these lesions, enabling surgical results once thought impossible. Concerns regarding the lack of sphenoid pneumatization and risks of CSF leak have been overcome with advances in technology and technique. A complex understanding of the pathologic conditions that occur in this region is important for an appropriate workup and determination of initial surgical intervention. Although controversies still exist, especially with regards to the management of pediatric craniopharyngioma, endoscopic endonasal approaches to pediatric pituitary and sellar lesions have become well-established tools that will continue to undergo further advancement and refinement.

## CLINICS CARE POINTS

- Evaluation of a pediatric patient with a pituitary or sellar region tumor should begin with an ophthalmologic examination, complete endocrinologic evaluation, and possibly tumor markers.

- Elevation in tumor markers may indicate a nongerminomatous germ cell tumor and obviate surgical intervention.
- Extensive navigation-assisted drilling of the sphenoid bone is often required for children without pneumatization of the sphenoid sinus.
- A large working corridor and binostril technique is often required to allow for four-handed resection of large tumors.
- Marsupialization of Rathke cleft cysts with a nasoseptal flap and silastic stenting is a viable alternative to cyst wall resection as a means of minimizing cyst recurrence.
- Skull base repair often requires the use of a nasoseptal flap, especially in the setting of high-flow cerebrospinal fluid leak.
- Close postoperative management of endocrinologic changes, especially diabetes insipidus, is essential given the high rate of postoperative hypopituitarism in these patients.
- Endonasal resection of pediatric craniopharyngioma is associated with lower incidence of neurovascular injury compared with open surgery.

## DISCLOSURE

The authors have no relevant financial or other conflict of interest to disclose.

## REFERENCES

1. Schroeder JW, Vezina LG. Pediatric sellar and suprasellar lesions. Pediatr Radiol 2011;41(3):287–98.
2. Kuan EC, Kaufman AC, Lerner D, et al. Lack of sphenoid pneumatization does not affect endoscopic endonasal pediatric skull base surgery outcomes. Laryngoscope 2019;129(4):832–6.
3. Tatreau JR, Patel MR, Shah RN, et al. Anatomical considerations for endoscopic endonasal skull base surgery in pediatric patients. The Laryngoscope 2010; 120(9):1730–7.
4. Hamid O, El Fiky L, Hassan O, et al. Anatomic variations of the sphenoid sinus and their impact on trans-sphenoid pituitary surgery. Skull Base 2008;18(1):9–15.
5. Banu MA, Guerrero-Maldonado A, McCrea HJ, et al. Impact of skull base development on endonasal endoscopic surgical corridors. J Neurosurg Pediatr 2014; 13(2):155–69.
6. Amar AP, Weiss MH. Pituitary anatomy and physiology. Neurosurg Clin N Am 2003;14(1):11–23, v.
7. Trifanescu R, Ansorge O, Wass JAH, et al. Rathke's cleft cysts. Clin Endocrinol (Oxf) 2012;76(2):151–60.
8. Drapeau A, Walz PC, Eide JG, et al. Pediatric craniopharyngioma. Childs Nerv Syst 2019;35(11):2133–45.
9. Parasher AK, Lerner DK, Glicksman JT, et al. The impact of expanded endonasal skull base surgery on midfacial growth in pediatric patients. Laryngoscope 2020; 130(2):338–42.
10. Chen W, Gardner PA, Branstetter BF, et al. Long-term impact of pediatric endoscopic endonasal skull base surgery on midface growth. J Neurosurg Pediatr 2019;23(4):523–30.
11. Bogusz A, Müller HL. Childhood-onset craniopharyngioma: latest insights into pathology, diagnostics, treatment, and follow-up. Expert Rev Neurother 2018; 18(10):793–806.

12.. Evanson J. Radiology of the pituitary. In: Feingold KR, Anawalt B, Boyce A, et al, editors. Endotext. South Dartmouth, MA: MDText.com, Inc; 2000. Available at: http://www.ncbi.nlm.nih.gov/books/NBK279161/. Accessed August 9, 2021.

13. Han SJ, Rolston JD, Jahangiri A, et al. Rathke's cleft cysts: review of natural history and surgical outcomes. J Neurooncol 2014;117(2):197–203.

14. Ross DA, Norman D, Wilson CB. Radiologic characteristics and results of surgical management of Rathke's cysts in 43 patients. Neurosurgery 1992;30(2): 173–8.

15. Hoffmann A, Adelmann S, Lohle K, et al. Pediatric prolactinoma: initial presentation, treatment, and long-term prognosis. Eur J Pediatr 2018;177(1):125–32.

16. Leung AKC, Lam JM, Leong KF. Childhood Langerhans cell histiocytosis: a disease with many faces. World J Pediatr 2019;15(6):536–45.

17. Gellner V, Kurschel S, Scarpatetti M, et al. Lymphocytic hypophysitis in the pediatric population. Child's Nervous Syst 2008;24(7):785–92.

18. Echevarría ME, Fangusaro J, Goldman S. Pediatric central nervous system germ cell tumors: a review. Oncologist 2008;13(6):690–9.

19. Mesquita Filho PM, Santos FP, Köhler LR, et al. Suprasellar germinomas: 2 case reports and literature review. World Neurosurg 2018;117:165–71.

20. Rasool N, Odel JG, Kazim M. Optic pathway glioma of childhood. Curr Opin Ophthalmol 2017;28(3):289–95.

21. Curry DJ, Raskin J, Ali I, et al. MR-guided laser ablation for the treatment of hypothalamic hamartomas. Epilepsy Res 2018;142:131–4.

22. McCrea HJ, George E, Settler A, et al. Pediatric suprasellar tumors. J Child Neurol 2016;31(12):1367–76.

23. Nuijts MA, Veldhuis N, Stegeman I, et al. Visual functions in children with craniopharyngioma at diagnosis: a systematic review. PLoS One 2020;15(10): e0240016.

24. Ali ZS, Lang S-S, Kamat AR, et al. Suprasellar pediatric craniopharyngioma resection via endonasal endoscopic approach. Childs Nerv Syst 2013;29(11): 2065–70.

25.. Joe SA. Endoscopic resection of pituitary tumors. In: Atlas of endoscopic sinus and skull base surgery. Philadelphia, PA: Elsevier; 2019. p. 245–54.

26. Tubbs RS, Griessenauer C, Loukas M, et al. The circular sinus: an anatomic study with neurosurgical and neurointerventional applications. World Neurosurg 2014; 82(3–4):e475–8.

27. Dhandapani S, Singh H, Negm HM, et al. Endonasal endoscopic reoperation for residual or recurrent craniopharyngiomas. J Neurosurg 2017;126(2):418–30.

28. Lu VM, Ravindran K, Perry A, et al. Recurrence of Rathke's cleft cysts based on gross total resection of cyst wall: a meta-analysis. Neurosurg Rev 2020;43(3): 957–66.

29. Kuan EC, Trent MS, Luu NN, et al. Preventing restenosis of marsupialized Rathke cleft cysts using a nasoseptal flap lining. Laryngoscope 2019;129(10):2258–61.

30. Kuan EC, Palmer JN, Adappa ND. The rhinologist's role in the management of Rathke's cleft cysts. Curr Opin Otolaryngol Head Neck Surg 2019;27(1):67–71.

31. Rastatter JC, Snyderman CH, Gardner PA, et al. Endoscopic endonasal surgery for sinonasal and skull base lesions in the pediatric population. Otolaryngol Clin North Am 2015;48(1):79–99.

32. Nation J, Schupper AJ, Deconde A, et al. CSF leak after endoscopic skull base surgery in children: a single institution experience. Int J Pediatr Otorhinolaryngol 2019;119:22–6.

33. Madsen PJ, Buch VP, Douglas JE, et al. Endoscopic endonasal resection versus open surgery for pediatric craniopharyngioma: comparison of outcomes and complications. J Neurosurg Pediatr 2019;1–10. https://doi.org/10.3171/2019.4.PEDS18612.
34. Ghosh A, Hatten K, Learned KO, et al. Pediatric nasoseptal flap reconstruction for suprasellar approaches. Laryngoscope 2015;125(11):2451–6.
35. Sansoni ER, Harvey RJ. Large skull base defect reconstruction with and without pedicled flaps. In: Endoscopic sinus and skull base surgery. Elsevier; 2019. p. 285–98.
36. London NR, Rangel GG, Walz PC. The expanded endonasal approach in pediatric skull base surgery: a review. Laryngoscope Investig Otolaryngol 2020;5(2):313–25.
37. Yamada S, Fukuhara N, Yamaguchi-Okada M, et al. Therapeutic outcomes of transsphenoidal surgery in pediatric patients with craniopharyngiomas: a single-center study. J Neurosurg Pediatr 2018;1–14. https://doi.org/10.3171/2017.10.PEDS17254.
38. Stapleton AL, Tyler-Kabara EC, Gardner PA, et al. Risk factors for cerebrospinal fluid leak in pediatric patients undergoing endoscopic endonasal skull base surgery. Int J Pediatr Otorhinolaryngol 2017;93:163–6.
39. Chivukula S, Koutourousiou M, Snyderman C, et al. Endoscopic endonasal skull base surgery in the pediatric population. J Neurol Surg B 2012;73(S 01). s-0032-1312130.
40. Zwagerman NT, Wang EW, Shin SS, et al. Does lumbar drainage reduce postoperative cerebrospinal fluid leak after endoscopic endonasal skull base surgery? A prospective, randomized controlled trial. J Neurosurg 2018;1–7. https://doi.org/10.3171/2018.4.JNS172447.
41. Clark AJ, Cage TA, Aranda D, et al. A systematic review of the results of surgery and radiotherapy on tumor control for pediatric craniopharyngioma. Childs Nerv Syst 2013;29(2):231–8.
42. Kanesaka N, Mikami R, Nakayama H, et al. Preliminary results of fractionated stereotactic radiotherapy after cyst drainage for craniopharyngioma in adults. Int J Radiat Oncol Biol Phys 2012;82(4):1356–60.
43. Kiehna EN, Merchant TE. Radiation therapy for pediatric craniopharyngioma. Neurosurg Focus 2010;28(4):E10.
44. Brastianos PK, Santagata S. ENDOCRINE TUMORS: BRAF V600E mutations in papillary craniopharyngioma. Eur J Endocrinol 2016;174(4):R139–44.
45. Brastianos PK, Taylor-Weiner A, Manley PE, et al. Exome sequencing identifies BRAF mutations in papillary craniopharyngiomas. Nat Genet 2014;46(2):161–5.
46. Petralia F, Tignor N, Reva B, et al. Integrated proteogenomic characterization across major histological types of pediatric brain cancer. Cell 2020;183(7):1962–85.e31.